FOOD AND HEALTH IN EARLY
MODERN EUROPE

FOOD AND HEALTH IN EARLY MODERN EUROPE

DIET, MEDICINE AND SOCIETY, 1450–1800

David Gentilcore

Bloomsbury Academic
An imprint of Bloomsbury Publishing Plc

B L O O M S B U R Y
LONDON · NEW DELHI · NEW YORK · SYDNEY

Bloomsbury Academic

An imprint of Bloomsbury Publishing Plc

50 Bedford Square
London
WC1B 3DP
UK

1385 Broadway
New York
NY 10018
USA

www.bloomsbury.com

BLOOMSBURY and the Diana logo are trademarks of Bloomsbury Publishing Plc

First published 2016

British Library Cataloguing-in-Publication Data
A catalogue record for this book is available from the British Library.

ISBN: HB: 978-1-4725-2889-6
PB: 978-1-4725-3497-2
ePDF: 978-1-4725-3319-7
ePub: 978-1-4725-2842-1

Library of Congress Cataloging-in-Publication Data
Gentilcore, David.
Food and health in early modern Europe / David Gentilcore.
pages cm
Includes bibliographical references and index.
ISBN 978-1-4725-2889-6 (HB) – ISBN 978-1-4725-3497-2 (PB) – ISBN 978-1-4725-3319-7
(ePDF) – ISBN 978-1-4725-2842-1 (ePUB) 1. Health promotion–Europe. 2. Nutrition–Europe.
3. Food supply–Europe. 4. Food consumption–Europe. I. Title.
RA427.8.G42 2015
613.094–dc23
2015004354

Typeset by Integra Software Services Pvt. Ltd.
Printed and bound in India

For Fabiana, of course

CONTENTS

LIST OF FIGURES

INTRODUCTION

In 1786 the French surgeon Jean Baptiste Pressavin wrote, 'there is only one way to be in perfect health, but a thousand ways to be ill'. His was a plea for preventive medicine, which, Pressavin argued, was 'the surest and least conjectural part of medicine'.[1] In addition to being effective, it was also safe. Preventive medicine, or hygiene, had none of the risks and dangers of curative medicine, where disease treatments were frequently as harmful as the illness itself.

Food was at the heart of staying healthy. In the words of the Spanish doctor and theologian Álvarez de Miraval, 'almost all of the maintenance of our health consists in the good ordering and administration of food and drink'.[2] There was nothing new in this; from the time of Hippocrates, medical authors had counselled their readers on what, how and when to eat. You might think: *plus ça change...* After all, we seem to be concerned with the link between food, diet and health as never before. Our own obsession with 'nutritionism' – the focus on the nutrition different foodstuffs provide (or not), as opposed to the pleasure they might give or the social aspects related to their consumption – derives from the medicalization of diet and food intake. More or less authoritative medical and dietary advice competes with a plethora of self-help books, media coverage, internet bloggers and food packaging information for our attention, resulting in today's 'food anxiety'. The questions asked of French physician Laurent Joubert in the sixteenth century remain our own: 'is this [food] good, is this bad or unhealthy? What does this do?'[3]

And yet, if human concern with food and health is a constant, it also has a history. Long before the discovery of nutrition by laboratory science in the nineteenth century, medical authorities offered detailed advice to an eager and anxious public. What 'experts' considered 'good to eat', and why, changed over time.[4] Advice on eating for health was also subject to a range of conditioning factors, such as rank and occupation, nation and region, religion and morality, and the reaction to novelty. In the early modern period, as now, information on healthy eating was both abundant and much in demand, just as it was often contradictory. Doctors agreed: there was no perfect dietary regime. Early modern Europeans may not have had to contend with the tussle between government agencies and health organizations (on the one hand) and food industry lobbies and marketing (on the other), as we do.[5] They were not faced with today's corporate obfuscation strategies and the confusing array of roles and positions taken up by medical professionals and the media, where the constructive generation of information meets the 'cultural production of ignorance'.[6] But early modern Europeans did have to contend with the vagaries of knowledge production, beginning with differing medical opinions. On a broader scale, they had to make sense of some quite radical shifts in the medical understanding of foods and how they worked in the human body, to say nothing of how these ideas engaged with changing food availability, habits and preferences. Just as now, healthy eating was socially constructed.[7] Of course, it was a very different construct from our own: and understanding that construct is what this book is about.

Food and Health in Early Modern Europe is the first in-depth study of printed dietary advice over the entire early modern period, here taking us from the late fifteenth century to the early nineteenth. It is also the first to trace the history of European foodways as seen through the prism of this advice. It offers a doctor's eye view of changing food and diet. Jean Céard's suggestion, made at a conference back in 1979, that 'a methodical study of health regimens would doubtless provide many elements for a history of food', is still a work in progress.[8] In addition to studying European regimens spanning the early modern period, I have considered works of materia medica, botany, agronomy and horticulture, which likewise abound in dietary advice. This is enriched with comments from a range of other printed sources, such as travel accounts, cookery books and literary works.

The relationship between food and medicine has often been obscured, for the two tend to be seen as separate arenas. Approaching them instead as part of a continuum, as anthropologist Nancy Chen has suggested, offers insights into both food consumption and the process of health maintenance.[9] Following their advice, this book is thus both a history of food practices and history of the medical discourse about that food. As a result, it is also an exploration of the interaction between the two: the relationship between evolving foodways and shifting medical advice on what to eat in order to stay healthy. I have structured this book so that the first two chapters examine the changing nature of the regimen genre in the context of wider medical trends. These are followed by a series of thematic chapters in which the dietary advice is related to changes in food perceptions, practices and preferences. The themes were chosen to reflect the main concerns of the regimens themselves: the differences between rich and poor, elites and labourers; the role of origin and nationality in diet; the benefits (or not) of a religiously inspired asceticism and fasting; the reversal in attitudes to fruit and vegetable consumption; the response to the new foods from the Americas; and the place of beverages in a healthy diet. The medical advice, opinions and preoccupations are all discussed against a backdrop of wider changes in food practices over the early modern period.

Food and Health in Early Modern Europe would not have been possible without recent work by historians in a range of fields, two of which are relatively new. 'Although historians study change, a survey of historiographical literature shows that we usually find it hard to accept something new in our own backyard', Kyri Claflin has observed.[10] This book emerges out of two separate, occasionally intersecting, sub-disciplines and historiographical traditions that were both once the focus of attempts at marginalization by mainstream historians: the social history of medicine and food history.

The history of medicine has flourished like few other branches of history in the last thirty years, generating a wealth of new approaches, influenced by wider historiographical trends while also contributing to them. These include the study of learned medical discourse and the social history of medicine. The former has taken more the traditional history of ideas approach in ever new directions, where medical knowledge encounters the 'social',[11] such as in biographical studies and the reconstruction of scholarly networks. The social history of medicine, for its part, was first proclaimed to have 'come of age' some twenty years ago.[12] Since then both directions have developed their own corpuses of primary sources, a varied secondary literature and lively debates among specialists. As these have both thrived, and despite the vaguely social orientation of both, a gap between the two – between the study of change in the theory and practice of medicine – has developed and widened, to the point that it now seems unbridgeable. One of the aims of this book is a modest, tentative contribution at bringing these two fundamental but now distinct branches of the history of medicine back into contact with one another, by exploring how the medical discourse of regimen shaped and was shaped by changing food perceptions and practices in the wider society of early modern Europe.

The history of food and diet in early modern Europe, as a field of exploration, only became of interest in the 1960s, when it was the subject of study by French *Annales* scholars.[13] Their interest lay mainly in reconstructing food production and consumption rates. The emphasis was on demographic and epidemiological crises, such as famine and dearth, and on prices and wages. Similar work was being done by British social and economic historians. The approach was largely quantitative. The 'cultural turn' of the 1980s brought with it a move to a more qualitative approach and a study of food practices and beliefs, at different ranks and among different elements of society.[14] This came together with an older history of high cuisine and gastronomy, sometimes the preserve of 'foodies' and local historians, to produce today's thriving discipline.[15]

The earliest historical investigations into the genre of dietetics and regimen (in English) were actually carried out by a sociologist, Bryan Turner. His focus was on food discourses and social practices, in particular as suggested by the work of the physician George Cheyne (who will feature much in this book).[16] One of the first historians to devote serious attention to the genre has been Andrew Wear, in a chapter of his book *Knowledge and Practice in English Medicine*.[17] Wear wanted to redress the balance of the dominant social approach to the history of medicine by focusing on 'knowledge', on what people 'knew', without forgetting its links to practice. The study of preventive medicine was an ideal way of doing this, not least because so much history of medicine had been on the therapeutic side of things, on changing healing activities and therapies, consistent with the focus of twentieth-century medicine itself.

Most of twentieth-century medicine had been a story of 'magic bullets' and miracle cures conquering diseases, that it must have been natural for historians studying earlier periods to see medicine in that therapeutic way. Medicine focused on curing of sick, and so the history of medicine did likewise. Just as preventive medicine took a sideline to therapeutics in the twentieth-century present, so it lay forgotten in studies of the earlier past. But with declining confidence in medicine's all-conquering march of progress, first evident in the 1970s, we can pinpoint a corresponding resurgence in the notion and practice of preventive medicine. Journals, associations and university departments of preventive medicine were all founded in the 1970s, devoted to the prevention of disease and the promotion of health.

With the exception of an important survey of 'vernacular medicine' by Paul Slack, it took somewhat longer for historians of medicine to shift their gaze from therapeutics to prevention, however.[18] Thus Erwin Ackerknecht's important but unashamedly presentist study of therapeutics completely missed the revival of diet and regimen in the eighteenth century.[19] And this brings us back to Wear. Wear's chapter on preventive medicine is important because it identifies the key themes: (1) the fact that this literature was addressed to the middling and upper sections of society: it provided for choices in diet and lifestyle for those who were able to make such choices; (2) that, while there may have been great interest in the literature, few people took up the advice it contained (a debateable point, it turns out); (3) that it provided a vehicle for the circulation of canonical medical ideas while allowing people to make choices for themselves, thus bringing together learned and popular, university and domestic, medicine.

The contents of this dietary advice are increasingly well known to early modern historians, thanks to a variety of studies over the past decade or so. Scholars as diverse as Fin Heikki Mikkeli, the American food historian Ken Albala, the German historian of medicine Klaus Bergdolt, the French medievalist Marilyn Nicoud and the American historian and sociologist of science Steven Shapin have explored different aspects of the genre and the advice it provided.[20] They have brought to the fore the importance people in the past placed on the complexities of the *ars vivendi*, and the role of moderation, balance and regularity in structuring one's daily life in order to stay healthy, as well as the social and cultural constraints affecting the responses to and implementation of these ideas.

The early modern period has proved a particularly fertile ground for exploration – both in the history of medicine and the history of food – given the many changes and shifts which occurred in this time of transition and tension. In terms of its print culture the early modern period saw changes in society throughout Europe (albeit with regional variations), such as vernacularization, print dissemination and reading patterns. Vernacular languages gradually replaced Latin. Latin retained its function as a language of institutionalized learning, as a lingua franca in the European context and in the use of specialized terminology, but the vernaculars were increasingly used for the communication of knowledge. Print technology made texts more widely available in multiple copies and accessible to an ever more heterogeneous public, especially of non-professional readers. This went hand in hand with increasing literacy rates, as well as the participation of the semi-literate in knowledge exchange. Useful texts like regimens were frequently read aloud. Publishers sought to meet the demands of a growing middle class of merchants, lawyers and other middling groups, even (occasionally) women, in particular during the second half of our period.

The academic outlook changed significantly, from the recovery of classical civilization that characterized the humanist movement to the ideology of natural knowledge, based on direct observation, investigation and experimentation. This was also a time of changing world views: on a global scale, brought on by contacts with non-Europeans and new worlds, and the challenges these brought about, and on a miniscule scale, due to new technical instruments like the microscope.

There were also changes in medicine, in terms of knowledge and practice. Humours and complexions, differing from person to person, gave way to a universal physiology. Not only did the place of preventive medicine shift vis à vis curative medicine, but the content and stress of preventive medicine changed. The Renaissance 'hot regimen' of abundant warm meals, exercise and hot baths was replaced by a 'cool regimen' of light meals, fresh air and cold baths in the eighteenth century.[21]

Notions surrounding the preservation of health went back to the ancient idea of 'hygiene'. Rather than being reduced to simple cleanliness, hygiene – from the Greek *hygeia*, or health – was the belief that staying healthy had a lot to do with one's way of life. Of all different facets of medical education, preventive hygiene was the one most open to the non-medical public. As John Sinclair put it in the introduction to his massive survey of the genre, the 'preservation of health and the prevention of disease, is a kind of neutral ground, between the several branches of medicine, and the common sense and daily observation of well informed men, and of course is open to everyone'.[22]

Before health became a goal for concerted social action, in the nineteenth century, it was a concern of individuals. What typifies the relationship between people and health during the early modern period was a concern for their own individual health. It was literally axiomatic: 'Every man is a fool or a physician, to himself at least'. This saying had its origins in the *Annals* of Tacitus, who said that by the age thirty every man ought to know what was best and worst for his own constitution.[23] It was reiterated throughout the early modern period whenever a medical author wanted to stress the importance of self-regulation. The forms that this personal interest in health took varied widely from person to person and over time, of course, but a commitment to the maintenance of one's own health and the treatment of disease remained.

There is ample historical evidence of both the desire to learn about and follow such advice, just as there is evidence of a resistance to the detailed minutiae of it. On the one hand, we have growing evidence of a 'culture of prevention', as Sandra Cavallo and Tessa Storey have recently put it.[24] Although their focus is on late Renaissance Italy, the notion can be applied to the entire early modern period, even considering the vagaries in shifting medical fashions and preferences. Not that we should expect early modern patients to be the willing and passive recipients of medical advice. As Alisha Rankin has recently shown, individually tailored dietary advice could be the subject of intense negotiation and, indeed, rejection.[25] There is also evidence of increasing dissatisfaction in learned circles with the fundamental nature of dietary advice: 'an exact ordering of our life and diet … such progidy, tediousness, and inconvenience', in the words of Francis Bacon, writing in the early seventeenth century.[26] But as if to answer Bacon's concerns, when there was a renewal of the regimen genre in the mid-eighteenth century, it had shed its Renaissance exactness and tedium, replaced by more generalized and simplified rules of life, as we shall see.

The demand for information and guidance was certainly there and medical authors rushed in to satisfy it. Sinclair listed 1,878 titles, overwhelmingly for the period from the sixteenth to the eighteenth centuries.[27] Admittedly, it is an eccentric and selective list, including numerous titles which are not regimens at all – but it provides a good indication of the sheer scale of the genre at a Europe-wide level. What Nancy Siraisi has said with respect to a fairly early title, Girolamo Cardano's *De sanitate tuenda* (On the maintenance of health), is pertinent to the genre as a whole: '[Cardano's] writings on nourishment and the body cross and re-cross – in both genre and content – the boundaries between academic medicine and the culture of cities and courts, between natural history and medicine, between medicine and moral or political philosophy, between the care of others and the examination of the self'.[28]

From the sixteenth century medical authors increasingly made their regimens and health guides accessible by writing in the vernacular. They developed enticing titles like 'haven of health', 'medicinal anchor', 'health's improvement' and 'portrait of health' – even if the bulk had more prosaic titles along the lines of 'preservation of health'. Publishers contributed to their success by printing them in inexpensive octavo (or smaller) formats. Thomas Moulton's *Mirror or Glass of Health*, which went through at least seventeen editions between 1530 and 1580, was as cheap as any book on the English market, at 2d or 3d.[29] Not only were there multiple editions of the more successful regimens, but these could long outlast the time of their printing. Castore Durante's *Il tesoro della sanità*, first published in Rome in 1586, went through an extraordinary thirty-four editions in Italy over the next ninety-three years (the last being in 1679).[30] A copy of the English translation, printed in 1686, was inscribed by a William Davis in 1798.[31]

This longevity was possible because the notion of regimen and the literary genre associated with it held sway throughout the early modern period, whether 'as a holistic metaphysical paradigm or a practical set of rules'.[32] However, the most successful and long-lived of all, still regularly reprinted, was not written by a physician at all and for the simple nature of its advice constitutes almost a sort of non-regimen: Alvise Cornaro's *Della vita sobria* (1558). In English alone, 'on the sober life' went through twenty-five editions between 1634 and 1777 and a further thirty over the next 55 years – not to mention a 'ten cent pocket series' edition published in Girard, Kansas, in 1918, which brings us back to the popularizing spirit of many of these titles.[33]

But was the pursuit of health and physical well-being truly open to everyone, as Sinclair claimed? It was certainly far from being 'neutral' and 'common sense', Sinclair's other descriptors. An interest in the intricacies of such advice, to say nothing of the wherewithal to put it into practice, presumed a degree of wealth, leisure and education. Before health became an essential human right, at least as an ideal, it was recognized as a preserve of the elites: a luxury for those spared the necessity of long hours of toil, poor living conditions and little choice in matters of food consumption. Only the well-off and the educated had the luxury of worrying about what they ate and drank; the poor simply worried about staving off hunger. As a result, our authors addressed a limited readership (unlike today's nutritionists and health educationalists who aim to reach a much broader public). The beneficiaries, to judge from the book titles and dedications, were variously, princes, magistrates and scholars. They were the elites, leisured and urban. During the eighteenth century this category swelled to include the expanding bourgeoisie. That said, access to the information contained in these regimens was not just the preserve of those who could read and afford books. Just as one book could pass through many hands, so its contents could also be transmitted orally. In a world where books were frequently read aloud, and where literacy and illiteracy overlapped, information circulated widely.

The extent to which these supposedly popular medical books were targeted at the 'popular classes' remains a matter for speculation. The rural population is mentioned often, but only as a foil for the urban elites (such as 'this foodstuff is suitable only for peasants'). The first, and perhaps only, regimen directed at 'country-dwellers' was published late in the eighteenth century, in the context of an Enlightenment concern with the health of the lower orders.[34] By this time, the poor were becoming the targets of well-intended efforts by the elites, the objects of medical reforms, but still did not feature as subjects in health regimens.

I have made especial effort in this book to cover the full chronology of the early modern period, charting the many significant changes, as well as the continuities. I have also tried to do justice to the 'Europe' of the title, ranging from Portugal to Poland and Scotland to Sicily. But if French, Italian and English material tends to predominate, this is only in part the result of the limits of my linguistic abilities; it also reflects both the culinary importance of, first, Italy and then France during the period, as well as the emerging historiography of the field of food history. Finally, a word on what *Food and Health in Early Modern Europe* is not. This is not a book on the role of dietary recommendations as a part of medical therapeutics, which would (and should) require a book of its own. Thus I have not done justice to manuscript regimens penned for specific people; in fact, I have had to ignore manuscript altogether in favour of print. Nor does this book explore works recommended for special categories of people, such as children or the elderly.[35] For our medical authors writing on how to preserve health only male adults corresponded to the healthy ideal – and the regimens were written to help them stay that way. This also explains why there is no thematic chapter on food and gender, as one might have expected, given the importance of the subject. Dietary advice was not written with women in mind; indeed, the first regimen directed at women was only written at the end of our period, as we shall see. That said, there is (of course) a gendering of many of the topics explored in the book, and this has been discussed where pertinent.

Acknowledgements

The writing of this book was made possible by a semester's teaching buy-out courtesy of the Centre for Medical Humanities at the University of Leicester, in 2012, for which I would like to thank the Centre's director, Professor Steve King, and a semester of university study leave, in 2014, for which I would like to thank the University of Leicester.

Colleagues across Europe and North America have generously shared their work and provided valuable advice and suggestions: Ken Albala (University of the Pacific, CA), Melissa Calaresu (University of Cambridge), Brian Cowan (McGill University), Trudy Eden (University of Northern Iowa), Violaine Giacomotto-Charra (Université Michel de Montaigne, Bordeaux), Elizabeth Hurren (University of Leicester), Michael LaCombe (Adelphi University, NY), Paul Lloyd (University of Leicester), Philippe

Meyzie (Université Michel de Montaigne, Bordeaux), Heikki Mikkeli (Finnish Academy of Science and Letters), William O'Reilly (University of Cambridge), Steven Shapin (Harvard University), Peter Scholliers (Vrije Universiteit Brussel), Emma Spary (University of Cambridge) and Irma Taavitsainen (University of Helsinki). I am also grateful to the staff at Bloomsbury, in particular Rhodri Mogford and Emma Goode, for expertly guiding this book through the editorial process.

In this strange new e-world in which we live (for better or for worse), the primary resources for this book are almost all available electronically, many as a result of excellent digitalizations done in the last few years. Thankfully, for my purposes, the David Wilson Library at the University of Leicester has subscriptions to both Early English Books online (EEBO) and Eighteenth Century Collections Online (ECCO), which together provide access to all works published in English for the course of the early modern period; all the rest are freely available courtesy of sites such as 'Gallica' (Bibliothèque Nationale de France), the Münchener DigitalisierungsZentrum of the Bayerische Staatsbibliothek (BSB), 'Medic@' (BIU Santé, Paris), the Biblioteca Virtual Miguel Cervantes and, of course, Google.

David Gentilcore, Leicester, September 2014

CHAPTER 1
HEALTHY FOOD: RENAISSANCE DIETETICS, c.1450–c.1650

Introduction

> There is nothing more useful in medicine than knowing the qualities of the things that we use in life, whether to avoid those which are harmful or to take those which are beneficial. This is what has obliged wise men to express their sentiments on all that which is eaten, always making use of their knowledge and experience.[1]

So proclaimed the French doctor Nicolas Venette from his chair of regius professor of anatomy and surgery. Fine sentiments indeed, but, as is the way with these things, the devil was in the detail. The nature of this detail and lay reactions to it are illustrated in the following two examples.

It is usually a good idea to begin with Michel de Montaigne, one of the most influential writers of the French Renaissance, sometimes referred to as the father of modern scepticism. In 1580 he published his *Essais* (literally, 'attempts'), which dealt with a wide range of topics. The final one is on the subject of 'experience'.[2] In it Montaigne deals with his lifelong search for knowledge via experience. He uses disease and health, medicine and doctors as a means of demonstrating what he himself has learned from living. Montaigne reveals his own failure to follow dietary rules, trusting his own personal experience over the strictures of the learned physicians. Experience was the best guide to what habits and foods were best for one, and which ones should be avoided, whereas the usefulness of medical advice was limited. 'The art of medicine', Montaigne wrote, 'is not so rigid that we cannot find an authority for anything that we may do.... If your doctor does not think it good for you to sleep, to take wine or some particular meat, do not worry; I will find you another who will disagree with him'.

Our second example comes from *Don Quixote*, by Miguel de Cervantes, one of the classics of not just Spanish, but world literature, written between 1605 and 1615. This mock-heroic knightly chronicle has the knight's squire, Sancho Panza (*panza* meaning 'belly'), being promised an island to rule over, as a reward for his service. The portly and dull-witted Sancho is a kind of 'everyman', a realistic and practical side-kick to the knight's idealism and naïveté. When Sancho finally gets his island, of which he is governor, he also gets his very own court physician. The physician torments Sancho by keeping him from eating a variety of delightful foods. To a frustrated Sancho, the physician explains the nature of his duties:

I, señor, am a physician, and I am paid a salary in this island to serve its governors as such, and I have a much greater regard for their health than for my own, studying day and night and making myself acquainted with the governor's constitution, in order to be able to cure him when he falls sick. The chief thing I have to do is to attend at his dinners and suppers and allow him to eat what appears to me to be fit for him, and keep from him what I think will do him harm and be injurious to his stomach; and therefore I ordered that plate of fruit to be removed as being too moist, and that other dish I ordered to be removed as being too hot and containing many spices that stimulate thirst; for he who drinks much kills and consumes the radical moisture wherein life consists.[3]

Supporting his prohibitions with axioms quoted from Hippocrates, the doctor first has Sancho's fruit taken away, then the meats – the partridge, the rabbit, the veal, the *olla podrida* (stew) – then everything else, until the doctor finally has himself removed (Figure 1.1).

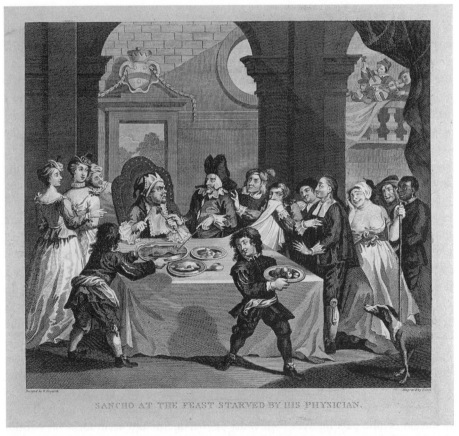

SANCHO AT THE FEAST STARVED BY HIS PHYSICIAN.

Figure 1.1 'Sancho at the feast starved by his physician'. Engraving by T. Cook after W. Hogarth, late eighteenth century (Wellcome Library, London).

These two examples – the first a sceptical criticism, the second a parody – attest to the widespread nature of medical advice on diet during the Renaissance. They suggest that physicians pronouncing on dietary matters, as well as the content of the advice itself, would have been well known to the reading public of the time. In addition to its familiarity to readers, the dietary literature of the Renaissance reveals much more than what the physicians thought was good to eat. They also give us a glimpse of the most basic fears, prejudices and preoccupations of the culture of the time. As Ken Albala has observed, modern nutritionists might promise a slimmer waistline, increased stamina or freedom from heart disease; Renaissance physicians, by contrast, spoke of clear and rational thought, the avoidance of putrefaction and fevers, and the maintenance of a balance of humours in the body. The framework differed, as did the goals.[4] In the Renaissance a certain food might be condemned because of an association with the lower ranks society, or because of a foreign or exotic origin, or because it had been denounced by some ancient authority. These dietary criteria reflect the social, national, scholarly, even aesthetic concerns of their authors as clearly as any artwork or poem.

It is common to see the field of hygiene – preventive medicine – as static during the early modern period, with only minor changes to the framework based on the writings of Hippocrates and Galen of Pergamum (died 200 AD). Surviving throughout the Middle Ages, it was revived during the Renaissance, only to be challenged during the seventeenth century. Even if many other features of Galenism were rejected, however, the code of hygiene retained its hold. Erwin Ackerknecht simply referred to it as 'the so-called Greek diet, which lasted into the eighteenth century'.[5] Superficially, this is true; but, as Heikki Mikkeli has argued, the framework's malleability and adaptability hide some substantial developments and shifts. Moreover, the whole area of preventive medicine was called into question from the mid-seventeenth century. The result, almost as a backlash, was that a whole new science of hygiene was developed during the eighteenth century, which fulfilled the scientific requirements of that time.[6] This chapter and the next will outline and make sense of these changes, in particular with regard to shifting ideas about food and diet. To understand the nature of Renaissance dietary advice this chapter will consider the theory, its application and the genre and its reception.

The theory: The Galenic revival and the six non-naturals

In medieval Western Europe most medical texts were based on translations or interpretations of Arabic authors, further codified and developed, themselves based on the surviving writings of ancient Greece and Rome. These medieval texts included over one hundred regimens written between the twelfth and fifteenth centuries, in Latin and the vernacular, by both famous doctors and anonymous authors.[7] An interest in such texts was part of the medicalization of urban society towards the end of the Middle Ages, and in particular a developing courtly tradition.

Emblematic of the different traditions which came together during the Middle Ages in this tradition is the most successful of these works, which came out of the medical school of Salerno: the *Regimen sanitatis salernitatem*.[8] For many centuries portions of this Latin medical poem were as common in the mouths of physicians all over Europe as the aphorisms of Hippocrates or the sayings of Galen. Editions continued to be printed throughout the early modern period, such as the 1608 translation by John Harrington, which includes Harrington's rendering of advice regarding leeks:

Green leeks are good, as some physicians say,
Yet I would choose howe'er I them believe,
To wear leeks rather on St. David's Day,
Than eat the leek upon St. David's Eve.[9]

By Harrington's day another intellectual and cultural force had been adding to this regimen tradition for well over a century: humanism. Humanists sought to restore the body of classical learning and place it at the centre of their own educational curriculum. This was accompanied by a search for as many of the original texts of antiquity as possible, and in the original Greek, unsullied by medieval translations and commentaries. In medicine, learned physicians began to study Greek, abandoning the translations and interpretations for the original Greek texts, which they believed closer to the original source of knowledge. 'Knowledge' meant looking back to the ancient past, in contrast to our own view of knowledge, which is based on progression and the future.

In 1525 the Venetian librarian and printer Aldo Manuzio published the complete works of Galen. And by the middle of the century all the major classical sources on dietetics had been edited and translated into Latin, as well as into some of the European vernacular languages. This included individual editions of what would prove to be the two most influential works on early modern regimen: Galen's *Hygiene*, known in Latin as *De sanitate tuenda* (On the preservation of health) and his *De alimentorum facultatibus* (On the faculties or powers of aliments).[10] Galen in particular was a prolific author and his writings overshadowed those of his predecessors. As a result of the Galenic revival, sometimes referred to as neo-Galenism, Renaissance medical ideas about health and diet adhered more strictly to the theories of Galen than ever before (or since).

Galenic writings formed the basis of elaborate theories about how foods affect the human body and what combinations of food would foster optimal health. The effects of the Galenic revival are apparent not only in the success of regimens as a literary genre but also in changes in their approach and content. What is the subject of a few words in Michele Savonarola's courtly regimen of the mid-fifteenth century, commenting on the values of particular foodstuffs, becomes the subject and raison d'être for an entire, detailed treatise by Baldassare Pisanelli, writing in the late sixteenth century (Figure 1.2).[11]

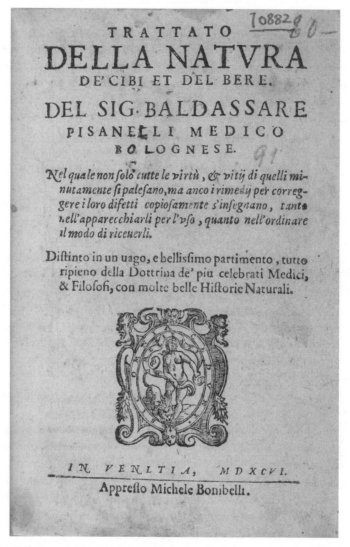

Figure 1.2 Title page of Baldassare Pisanelli's *Trattato della natura de' cibi et del bere*, 1586 (Wellcome Library, London).

In his study of the genre, Albala divides Renaissance regimens into three periods.[12] It is possible to question the overly schematic nature of the division, as Mikkeli has done, but as a broad guide to the main phases, Albala's periodization works.[13] Dietaries of period one (1470–1530s), prior to the Galenic revival, were similar to the medieval predecessors. They were often written in a courtly context, like Savonarola's, with the exception of being printed and circulating more widely. Those of period two (1530–1570s) coincided with the Galenic revival and were more philologically orientated, first establishing and then defending a Galenic orthodoxy. The regimens of this period are the most uniform, across Europe. Pisanelli's is an example of this, both in its Galenic influence and the fact that it, in turn, influenced other published regimens.

Period three regimens (1570–1650s) demonstrate the gradual breakdown of this Galenic hegemony. Reverence for classical authorities was tempered by a realization that they had sometimes erred, as new discoveries came to light. The Oxford doctor Walter Baley pointed to how 'the navigations in these later yeeres made by the Portingales into the east Indians, and by the Spaniards into the west Indians, hath made manifest to us how greatly the old authors, I meane Dioscorides, Galen, Plinie, Avicenna, Serapio, and the other writers of the former time were deceived'.[14] There was more open criticism of the ancients and the expression of opinion based on personal experience, experiment and the circulation of knowledge. Pietro Andrea Mattioli's commentaries on materia medica increasingly dwarf the original text of Dioscorides.[15] Renaissance regimens come to an end with the new models of digestion and nutrition, ushered in by Santorio Santorio and Jan Baptist van Helmont, as we shall see in the following chapter.

But let us return to the regimens themselves and their rationale. According to medical teaching, the body was constituted by: (i) 'natural things': that is, things which make up the individual body, namely, the elements, humours, faculties and spirits; (ii) 'non-natural things': things which affect bodily health; and (iii) 'things against nature': illnesses and their causes and sequels. The field of hygiene or dietetics was concerned with the second of these, the so-called 'non-naturals' (the *res non naturales*). I say so-called, because the expression may need explaining. In this case, 'non-natural' did not mean 'unnatural', but referred to a special category of things separate from one's own bodily make-up. These things external to the body were responsible for either health or illness and there were six of them: air, food and drink, motion and rest, sleep and waking, repletion and evacuation, and strong emotions or passions. The preservation of the individual was tied to the intrinsic nature, daily activities and particular circumstances surrounding that person.[16] Galen referred to the sorts of external factors that might determine a healthy life, but it was his followers who coined the expression 'the six non-natural things'.[17]

Humanist medicine of the Renaissance inherited this outlook, with two defining characteristics. First of all, nourishment tended to take up most space within this framework due to its sheer complexity. Secondly, as revived during the Renaissance, the Galenic system was intensely individualistic. Foods like cheese and wine might be converted into nourishing foods in some bodies but could be poisons in others, as an anonymous French treatise reminded its readers.[18] Accurate diagnosis of the individual and a tailor-made regimen for each person were therefore regarded as crucial. Unlike our own nutritional theory, in Galenic medicine there could be no universal set of prescribed nutritional guidelines, or even an idea of good or bad foods that would apply to all people.[19]

The idea of the six non-naturals remained in place throughout the early modern period, forming the bedrock upon which preventive medicine was based. As a doctrine, it 'provided a concise, flexible, and widely accepted framework for articulating the primary demands imposed by the conditions of existence upon men and women who sought seriously to preserve their physical well-being'.[20] That said, its importance waxed and waned throughout the period, in line with the fortunes of preventive medicine. The Protestant and Catholic Reformations Christianized them. The Tyrolean doctor Ippolito Guarinoni put God at the top of the list, so that the six became seven. In order to remember them, Guarinoni pointed out to his readers that the first letters of each spelt out the Old German word for 'healthy', *gesondt*, beginning with *Gott* (God), *essen* (eating) and so on.[21] During the mid-seventeenth century the Cartesian influence of the 'body as machine' notion undermined their relevance. Then they resurface with the Hippocratic revival and the importance of the environment in medicine which characterizes the eighteenth century.

To understand why the six non-naturals affected each body differently we need to understand Galenic medicine, based on four physiological principles that remained more or less intact throughout the Renaissance. The first of these was that the body was understood to be regulated by four basic fluids or humours: blood, phlegm, yellow bile (choler) and black bile (melancholy). Health was defined as the proportional balance of these four fluids. Secondly, each person was born with a predominance of one particular humour, or at least a tendency for that humour to be produced in excess. People with a predominance of the blood humour were characterized as 'sanguine', for example; people could also be phlegmatic, choleric or melancholic. An individual's humoural make-up – called complexion, constitution or temperament – determined the diseases to which they would be subject, their character and emotional state. It also determined what sort of diet they should follow to stay healthy. These humoural labels have survived long past the medical system of which they were a part. We still use them to describe mood and character types: a sanguine person is cheery and optimistic, phlegmatics are lazy and slothful, cholerics are prone to outbursts of anger and melancholics are, of course, sad.[22]

This was because – and this is the third point – each humour had qualitative properties. Blood was hot and moist, phlegm was cold and moist, choler was hot and dry, and melancholy was cold and dry. These properties were not so much actual tactile measurements of temperature and humidity as the effect each humour was perceived to have on the body. An individual's humoural make-up, their 'complexion', would affect their appearance. Thus sanguine people would logically appear ruddy, whereas phlegmatics would be pale, with a watery, washed-out colour. Tobias Venner described cider- and perry-drinkers in exactly these terms. Because both cider and perry were 'cold in operation', Venner explained, 'the much and often use of them is very hurtfull to the liver, which by over-cooling, it doth so enfeeble and dispoliate of its sanguifying [i.e. blood making] facultie, that the colour of the face becommeth pale and riveled [wrinkled].'[23]

The final aspect of Galenic physiology we need to understand is that the humoural system had its parallels throughout the natural world. Just as human bodies were regulated by the four humours, so all organic matter, including animals and plants – and thus foods – were composed of elements that gave them their own humoural properties. These were called 'qualities'. In the same way that a person could be described as 'phlegmatic', so a cucumber would be described as cold and moist in its quality. These qualities shaped the nature and content of dietary advice.

The application: Galenism and dietary advice

Matching the proper foods to the individual was the key to this entire system. And this was precisely where things began to get difficult – the 'detail' mentioned in the introductory section of this chapter. It raised two fundamental questions. The first was that of 'maintenance' versus 'correction'.[24] This question hinged on whether one believed the body's natural state to be one of health or, rather, a tendency towards illness, if not illness itself. Galen's *De sanitate tuenda* was a regimen intended for the perfect constitution: the well-balanced, healthy body with no congenital tendency towards disease. But how many people were really like that? As a result, was it better to feed one's complexion, ingesting foods consistent with it, thus presuming a state of health, or attempt to temper it by eating foods of a different nature, thus presuming a tendency to certain illnesses or conditions? For example, should the elderly, who were considered dry and cold by nature, eat dry and cold foods, which were most in keeping with their own bodily make-up; or, if old age was to be considered a kind of disease, should they eat warm and moist foods to counter its deleterious effects? The Anglo-Welsh historian and political writer James Howell put it this way: 'For as the physitians hold there is no perfection of corporall health in this life, but a convalessence at best, which is a medium 'twixt health and sicknesse'.[25]

Given that most bodies were considered unhealthy and thus to some extent unbalanced, correction tended to occupy pride of place in Renaissance regimens. This system is known as allopathic: ailments and symptoms are corrected by applying remedies opposite to the sufferer's imbalance. Eating opposites was essential in order to maintain balance, part of a 'praiseworthy regimen of living', to use the words of *Le thresor de santé* (1607). For people of a melancholic humour, naturally cold and dry, foods of a 'moist and warm quality' were recommended; for cholerics, naturally hot and dry, cold and moist foods were best; while for phlegmatics, naturally cold and moist, hot and dry foods should be consumed; and the sanguine, naturally hot and moist, should eat dry and light foods.[26]

The second question for the regimens brings us back to the nature of individuality. If each person was different how could one write a health guide for more than a single reader? While the personal physician to a prince or well-off individual would tailor their handwritten medical advice to fit one person, the authors of printed regimens could not afford this luxury – at least not if they wanted to sell their books. Renaissance authors approached the problem in different ways. First of all, they limited the variables by writing for particular social groups or professions (scholars, magistrates),[27] geographical settings (the inhabitants of particular cities, like Rome or Lisbon),[28] or age groups (the elderly, or to be more exact, those who aspired to become so).[29] They also aimed to have it both ways: one of their selling points was to write for large groups while also giving the impression of tailoring advice to the individual. Readers could always find advice that was specific enough to their own bodies to make the regimen relevant to them.

Occupation and social status were major factors in dietary recommendations and conditioned the target readership of regimens. In addition to the qualities of the foods they ate, people were advised to consider the texture and consistency of foods. How quickly something passed through the body and how easily it could be digested were just as important as its humoural qualities. People who toiled or took exercise, such as labourers, were advised to eat solid and sustaining foods: beans or root vegetables or beef, for example. These kinds of foods were generally known as 'gross' or 'crass' in the literature, without today's connotations of disgusting (but you can see the link). More sedentary people, like students and aristocrats, were advised to eat lighter foods that were more easily digested and offered less nourishment: eggs or chicken, for example.

Students and scholars were one especially at-risk group, and several regimens were devoted especially to them. Their mental exertion posed a serious threat to health, combined with a sedentary lifestyle and a predisposition to melancholy. Thinking itself was believed to disturb the digestive process, which is why studying right after a meal was absolutely forbidden. Excessive study also exhausted the body, leaving no energy left for processing food. In the words of Guglielmo Grataroli, 'Orderlie diet quickeneth the spirits and reviveth the minde, making it more active and coragious to know and practize vertuous operations'.[30] In addition to favouring 'light' foods, the scholar was advised to beware of foods harmful to the brain, like onions and garlic, whose fumes smothered the intellect and understanding. Poorly prepared food could also spoil one's thoughts and gluttony was obviously lethal to the intellect.

Renaissance authors also considered a person's age and gender as having an influence on their humoural make-up. Young people tended to be hotter and more sanguine; as people aged, the body's vital fluid and heat were consumed, and so they became increasingly colder and drier. As a result, younger people were allowed to eat colder foods, while the elderly were given warmer and more easily digested foods as their capacity to digest and assimilate foods gradually diminished, as we have seen. Numerous regimens promised to help their readers live to a ripe old age.

Women were regarded as being generally colder and moister than men in complexion. This was used to explain why women were considered softer, weaker and less intelligent than men. Medical theory may have been an evident tool of subjugation, with its roots in Aristotelian philosophy, but it also meant that a woman's diet should be different from a man's. That said, most of the dietary literature was written by men, with other men in mind, and rarely dealt with women's needs. As a result, no Renaissance regimen was published with women specifically in mind. Savonarola came close, writing a regimen for pregnant women, in Italian (c.1460), but it was not published until our own times.[31] Given this, the historian needs to look elsewhere for references to the kinds of food women should eat. As Laura Prosperi has shown, medical writers only considered the topic worthy of elaboration when discussing women's procreative functions. Thus in treatises on 'women's diseases' or midwifery we find recommendations on what to eat during pregnancy or when trying to conceive.[32] Somewhat paradoxically, the suggested diet tends to consist of the sorts of nourishing 'peasant' foods that the elites were normally advised to avoid. One of the most successful of these, eventually translated into eight European languages, was the evocatively titled *Der Swangern Frauwen und*

Hebammen Rosegarten (Rose garden for pregnant women and midwives), first printed in Strasbourg and Hagenau in 1513.[33]

Finally, regimens enforced the idea that diet should vary by season. Weather conditions would naturally affect a person's internal temperature and humidity. Foods that heated the body were more appropriate during winter, and cooling foods during summer. People were also advised to eat more food in the colder months of the year and, conversely, eat both less as well as lighter foods during the hotter months. People in the colder regions of Europe could eat much more food than inhabitants of the south, without suffering the consequences (a theme we shall return to in Chapter 4). The Spaniard Juan Valverda noted how fierce Scots and Britons could consume vast quantities of semi-raw flesh, so that a single Scotsman's portion of meat would stuff four Spaniards.[34]

Physic and cookery: The Renaissance medical understanding of foods

In practical terms, it seems unlikely that in any given household an entire family could be served different foods to suit each individual's unique complexion or make-up. But for those people with the wealth to serve many different foods in each course, or for those people who could freely choose what they ate, these medical theories offered a powerful system for categorizing foods and deciding what to eat, and when, and what to avoid. It is why Jesuit colleges offered a range of dishes at each course, so individuals could choose according to their own bodies, needs and tastes.[35]

During the Renaissance cookery and physic were perceived as closely connected. 'A good coke is halfe a physycyon', wrote Andrew Boorde, while Thomas Cogan affirmed that 'the learned physitian ... is or ought to be a perfect cooke in many points'.[36] There were limitations to this cosy relationship. These are evident in the increasing tensions between a refined and variegated courtly cookery, one the one hand, and the moderation and temperance advocated by medicine, on the other.

Moreover, Renaissance medical advice was not easy or even consistent. Just as today, during the Renaissance there were a variety of different food ideologies that made eating a potentially confusing (and even hazardous) enterprise. Even for the dietary writers themselves, their own native customs and habits often coloured their recommendations. Galen might have thought beef too difficult to digest for the average person, as we shall see in Chapter 4, but why then could Englishmen eat it without harm (asked English authors)? Fish might be dangerously cold and moist, but it had its defenders, as we shall see in Chapter 5.

Furthermore, ideas about certain foodstuffs could change over time. In the early sixteenth century sugar was considered an ideal aliment, but by the seventeenth-century physicians claimed it made teeth black and burned in the digestive system, causing blockages to form. Ideas could vary according to confessional beliefs. For instance, wine was considered among the substances most analogous to human blood and so an ideal foodstuff, since it was evidently transformed easily into blood. And yet, as we shall see in Chapter 8, for the pen of puritanically orientated authors wine could be seen as a debilitating vice, best avoided. Differences like these suggest that physicians were anything but united in their opinions about food. Like today, readers had a variety of opinions to choose from. These disagreements also make generalization about the dietary literature difficult; and yet, beyond these variations, certain basic nutritional ideas about food were held by all Renaissance authors, from the late 1400s up until the mid-1600s.[37]

The first of these was that bread was absolutely essential for proper nourishment. Bread was not just the 'staff of life'; it was considered a kind of glue that kept all the other foods in place. Writing in the 1590s, the English physician Thomas Moffett believed bread to be absolutely indispensable to good 'concoction': this refers to the cooking of the foods in the stomach, before our modern theory of digestion. Without bread, 'all other meats [foods] would either quickly putrifie in our stomachs, or sooner pass thorough them then they should'. And the result of this would be 'crudities, belly-worms and fluxes', as we see in those people who 'eat none or too little bread'.[38]

Meat was equally important. Since nourishment was defined as the ability for a food to be converted into the substance and fabric of the human body, those substances most similar to the body were also considered the most nourishing, and so the most healthy. To quote Moffett again, because animal flesh is 'in substance and essence most like our own', it can, 'with le[a]st loss and labour of natural heat be converted and transubstantiated into our flesh'.[39] Providing the body of the right complexion to digest the meat, it was the perfect foodstuff. That said, not all meats were equal, and a weaker, more sedentary individual would require lighter meats than a well-exercised labourer. There was absolutely no question that the human body needed some form of meat to stay healthy; a vegetable-based diet, the subject of Chapter 6, was practically unthinkable.

If meat was good, fish was problematic. Fish qualified as a nutritious form of flesh, but their cold and moist qualities, like the element in which they lived, and their excessively gluey texture meant that they could provoke an overabundance of phlegm. Worse still, fish might get stuck at some stage during the digestive process, forming a clog or blockage, considered one of the major causes of disease, from gout to fevers. To counteract these harmful effects, proper seasonings or condiments should always accompany fish: lemons, heating spices and sugar. These were seasonings that would cut through the gluey substance of the fish and balance its coldness, and were thought of as medicinal ingredients rather than just flavour enhancers.

As this use of condiments to temper the potentially harmful effects of fish suggests, another widely held notion was that any potentially unhealthy food could be 'corrected' or adjusted. Renaissance nutritional theory incorporated a culinary system as well. Indeed it is quite possible that medicine lay at the root of European cookery practices. Thus the abundant use of spices, particularly on foods classified as cold or difficult to digest, quite probably has a medical origin. Even the very idea that moist foods like fresh pork or lamb should be roasted to dry them out, or that dry foods should be boiled, acquires a certain logic according to the Galenic system. Each procedure made the dish a more humourally balanced whole, more easily assimilated and more fit to nourish the body. Thus condiments and seasonings were defined not only as spices and sauces, but as any food that was served with, or used to correct, another one. As a result something like lettuce was often considered a condiment, used to correct something else, rather than a foodstuff in its own right.

This approach is most evident in the attitude to vegetables and fruit, a topic of which dietary authors were generally quite wary. In addition to being too far down the Aristotelian 'chain of being' for comfort, as Allen Grieco has suggested, vegetables and fruit were far too cold and watery for frequent consumption, offering little nourishment and producing only a watery, thin blood.[40] Renaissance medical authors were not opposed to fruits and vegetables per se, however. For hot-complexioned people, or in summer, or to counterbalance 'hot' foods, vegetables were considered fine as a condiment. Fruits were best eaten cooked and corrected with spices. And for choleric people, or for hardy labourers, fruits were believed not to pose a threat. They could also be corrected by drying, which is why raisins were preferred to grapes, as raisins had less noxious moisture than grapes and their sweetness was more concentrated, making them hotter in quality.

As this suggests, very few foods were condemned outright by Renaissance physicians. Some of the foods considered positively harmful were those it was hard to place as either flesh, fish or fruit. Mushrooms, for example, were thought to be excrements of the earth, and the fact that so many mushrooms were poisonous was taken as a clear sign that all varieties were dangerous. Frogs were another almost universally condemned food, again partly because they were so difficult to categorize. Any food that lived or was raised in an unwholesome environment was suspect, like eels, thought to reproduce asexually from rotting organic matter, or waterfowl that feed on muck in stagnant pools. The defects of the environment, fodder and even mood would eventually be passed on to the person who ate such foods.

How did the dietary authors assign foods to their respective categories? First and foremost, they relied on the ancients, such as Galen and the writer on materia medica Dioscorides. To this, they added their own observations and experience. The most important criterion for assigning foods their respective 'qualities' (*facultates*) was taste. Sweet and savoury (or meaty) flavours usually led to those foods being classified as hot and moist. Because heat and moisture were the two fundamental requisites for life, they were also considered the most nourishing. Milder flavours, like chicken or light-fleshed fish, were considered more temperate, possessing moderate heating and warming qualities. Foods that had a bite or that one could feel heating the body were considered hot and dry: most spices, hot herbs (like garlic) and salt. Foods that constrict the body's passages and make the tongue pucker, with sour and bitter flavours, were categorized as cold and dry. Finally, insipid flavours and watery foods were placed in the cold and moist category, which included most leafy vegetables and fruits. If you are 'as cool as a cucumber' or use the term 'hot' to describe black pepper or chilli or refer to some wines as 'dry', you are employing remnants of humoural theory.

With qualities determined by taste, disagreement and questioning often resulted. New plants and foodstuffs from the Americas occasioned a range of different responses as medical writers sought to classify them in comparison to those they already knew (something we shall return to in Chapter 7). As a result, towards the end of the Renaissance, the means of determining qualities was called into question. For instance, in 1558 Giambattista Della Porta proposed adopting distillation as a means of more accurately determining the qualities of plants. 'There are no surer searchers out of the virtues of the plants than our hands and eyes', Della Porta wrote. 'The taste is more fallible: for, if in distillation, the hottest parts evaporate first, we may conclude that it consisteth of hot and thin parts'.[41]

We have been considering single foodstuffs thus far, but physicians' recommendations went beyond considerations of individual ingredients. A 'balanced' dish meant combining hot and moist staples with cold and dry condiments, such as vinegar; correcting cold and moist foods with hot and dry spices; improving foods that were thick and crass with cutting and sharp flavours that would help them pass through the body (such as mustard on pork); and giving body and substance to very light foods like small birds by serving them with a thickened sauce made with breadcrumbs or ground almonds. The same applied to the meal as a whole. Renaissance physicians believed that a strict order of foods was crucial. Thus raw fruit was not to be eaten at the end of a meal, for it would float on top of the contents of the stomach and eventually putrefy, sending noxious vapours into the brain and disrupt the entire bodily system.

Although there was a close fit between elite cookery and medical advice, not every dish or menu was based on some kind of medicinal logic. Savonarola would not be the last court doctor to have to reconcile advice on how to stay healthy with the pleasures of courtly life, somehow producing a regimen which promised its reader to be able 'to live longer and more joyfully'.[42] Physicians made frequent tirades against dining practices at Renaissance courts, enough to show that not all cooking practices qualified as acceptable. Doctors were especially frustrated by the courtly practice of eating too many different kinds of foods in one sitting, mixing meat and fish in one meal and heaping on all sorts of sweet confections (as we shall see in Chapter 3). The result was disruption in the stomach, since medical theory argued that each food required a different amount of time to be properly 'concocted'.

Court physicians and medical authors were aware that that many of their recommendations went unheeded. Worse still was the ridicule they received. As the French physician Laurent Joubert complained in 1587, 'Many [courtiers] never cease interrogating physicians when at table: is this [food] good, is this bad or unhealthy? What does this do? Most of those who ask have no desire to follow what the physician says, but they take pleasure in doing it, for entertainment'. The result of all these interruptions and distractions, according to Joubert, was that physicians got up from the table only half fed.[43]

Indeed it was a commonplace of physicians that people did not take enough heed of dietary advice, or of their own health in general. This was a mixture of the truth, as medical authors saw it, and a rhetorical strategy to claim the reader's attention and boost sales. The royal physician John Archer, never one to undersell his own abilities, was well aware that 'people of all qualities do commonly feed upon what comes to table, be what it will, without considering the nature or qualities of any thing, or agreements or disagreements to their constitutions, so it do but please their pallat'. But in so doing,

Archer warned, they 'do dig their graves with their teeth'.[44] In other words, buy my book if you do not want to suffer the same fate. In a similar vein, the author of what would be the most successful health guide of all, Alvise Cornaro, bemoaned afterwards that 'although it is praised by all, it was nonetheless avoided by all'.[45] While recognizing the difficulty in following his recommendations for sobriety, Cornaro was also pleading for greater recognition of it.

Renaissance regimens and their readership

Dietary advice was at once something you might receive from your physician (for the elite who had one) and a successful literary genre. Several hundred regimens were published during the Renaissance, both in Latin and in most of the vernacular languages of Europe. To give an idea, regimens and health guides represent 10 per cent of the entire corpus of medical texts published in England during the sixteenth and seventeenth centuries. They were published evenly over the two centuries, although slightly more published in the sixteenth century.[46] Most were written by doctors, although there are a scattering of clerics, lawyers and schoolmasters.

Various characterizing features of this genre suggest that a substantial portion of the literate population of Europe took an avid interest in regimen and diet. To make their books easy to follow and consult, medical authors wrote their regimens in didactic prose, sometimes adopting a dialogue form or verse. Readers were not assumed to have specialized medical knowledge: the theoretical underpinnings of knowledge were explained and references to authorities and use of Latin terms were usually interpreted or translated. Authors divided their books into chapters according to the different non-naturals, foodstuffs (grouped according to category) and complexions. Some medical authors made a virtue of brevity. The Spanish doctor Gregorio Méndez boasted that his versified regimen might have been 'small in quantity' but it was 'great in its benefits'.[47] And those authors who wrote at great length and went into considerable detail provided tables of contents or indexes, even on occasion using a flowchart to structure the text. Another Spaniard, Blas Álvarez de Miraval, went further than most, producing a 'table of notable things' (*tabla de las cosas dignas de notar*) that was over ninety pages long – but, then, it was a long regimen![48] The books themselves tended to be printed in a small format, octavo or less, without illustrations or embellishment, in order to keep costs down. And their authors wrote in the vernacular. If the earliest vernacular regimens were simply medieval texts translated from Latin, the first original regimen written in English was Thomas Elyot's *Castel of Helth* of 1539. From then on English predominated, including a few translations from contemporary works in Latin and French.[49] The same trend is evident elsewhere in Europe (Figure 1.3).

Renaissance doctors claimed to write in the vernacular in order to be read by all people, regardless of their medical learning and training. That said, the books did not usually aim at supplanting the role of the physician, but rather contributing to it. Elyot hoped that his regimen would enable the layperson 'to instructe his

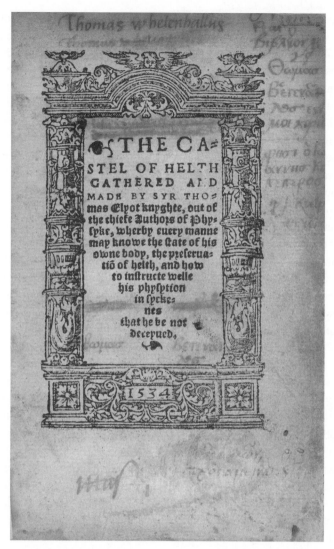

Figure 1.3 Title page of Thomas Elyot's *Castel of Helth*, 1539 (Wellcome Library, London).

phisition, wherunto he maye adapt his counsayle and remedies'.[50] The influence of the Reformations meant that this was combined with a sense of Christian charity and a concern for the public good. From the end of the sixteenth century nationalism also became a motive, particularly in France and England, as the public good became the good of the nation-state.

When it came to readership, the nature of the genre imposed its own limitations. The Veronese physician Bartolomeo Paschetti argued that paying attention to one's health was a sign of nobility and virtue. Patricians, like those of his adopted city of Genoa, had a particular obligation to stay healthy, in their role as public officials.[51] In his regimen, Tommaso Rangoni had humanist scholars like himself in mind, for he regarded good health as necessary to creative thought and a humanist way of life.[52] Medical authors aimed their works at literate people with the leisure and financial means to think about their health: the middling and upper ranks of society. Joseph Du Chesne (Quercetanus), who had practised medicine widely before being appointed physician to the French king Henri IV, was quite explicit about his readership: 'seeking to address myself particularly to the rich, not too the poor and labourers for whom such regimens are not suited since they do not have the means to put them into practice, obliged to live as they can and not as they want, and that is to say quite badly and unthinkingly, instead of well and medically.'[53]

Even when authors made claims to write for 'the poor' or 'the unlearned' in their prefaces, these were mainly rhetorical. The poor were considered incapable of making choices about their health; as a result, there was either no point in writing for them. Luckily, there was no need, for they were healthy enough already! So wrote the Coimbra professor Fernando Rodriguez Cardoso in his study of the six non-naturals.[54] Urban artisans and the rural poor ate cheap food, did not see physicians and still lived a healthy life, Cardoso argued. Noblemen, by contrast, ate a regulated diet, saw their doctors periodically and yet still had many illnesses. Cardoso explained that the regular habits of labourers and the exercise they got at their jobs was enough to keep them well.

Not everyone had such a rosy-eyed view of the poor, however. Girolamo Cardano believed that while the labouring poor might be healthier in theory, in reality they were more prone to disease and early death. 'Poverty is a great evil', Cardano wrote, 'which itself brings diseases, and death, and mourning.'[55] And a handful of authors did write with the poor in mind, with an imagined readership of those who were responsible for, or in contact with, the poor. The Parisian doctor Jacques Dubois (Jacobus Sylvius) was driven to write a short 'health regimen for the poor' by the 'calamity and wretchedness of the poor, both in this city of Paris, as in other towns and villages.'[56] For 'poor', Dubois had labourers in mind – 'gentz de peine et travail' – as opposed to the indigent. The role of the doctor was not to advise the avoidance of excess and all the other niceties of the usual regimens, but to assist them in finding sufficient nourishment. Dubois recommended very simple foods, like soups and stews, which had water as a base, to which were added root vegetables and herbs, bits of offal and stale bread or cereals. Such foods had the advantage that they 'are of great nourishment and last a long time in the body.'[57]

While the intended objects of his study would certainly have known all this, by dint of hard experience and necessity, Dubois's treatise did manage to turn standard regimens on their head. Where they dismissed certain foodstuffs as suitable only for the poor, Dubois made a virtue of this negative characterization and built a treatise around it. At the same time, his book only served to reinforce the notion that the labouring poor had a different constitution from the leisured rich, which necessitated the consumption of quite different foodstuffs, as we shall see in Chapter 3.

When it comes to readership, in a Europe characterized by semi-literacy, where different levels of literacy mixed with none, and where reading was a collective and collaborative activity, accessibility to these books and the information they contained was broader than might at first seem. In aristocratic households, for example, the servants may also have benefited from this widespread 'culture of prevention', as Sandra

Cavallo and Tessa Storey argue.[58] The letters of the Spada-Veralli family in Rome reveal how food intake in this aristocratic household 'was constantly being monitored, advised upon, and reported within the family'.[59] But they go further. An analysis of the letters together with household inventories, as well as the rationale behind the contents and arrangement of domestic interiors, allows them to analyse the extent to which preventive medical advice was variously ignored, followed or appropriated. People worried about the quality of the air around them, about getting a good night's sleep, about the kind of exercise suitable to their rank and about the hygiene of the body. They sought some kind of control over these facets of their lives in the pursuit of health: determining where to site their houses, whether to sleep during the day, what games to play and how best to cleanse the body. Paying attention to one's health empowered both laypeople, giving them a degree of control over the maintenance of their own health, and doctors, who alone had the learning and expertise necessary to dispense and interpret the often complex advice.

It is certainly easier for the historian to demonstrate the importance regimen played in people's lives than to show a clear link to specific texts. We shall have to content ourselves with the former. An understanding of regimen enabled lay people 'to correlate two crucial aspects of their lives: their everyday bodily habits and their anxieties about health'.[60] This medical advice was followed, and at least engaged with, by those sections of society who had the means to make food choices. Those who made use of preventive medicine were also those most likely to buy medicines – from apothecaries, grocers, charlatans and pedlars alike – and hire medical practitioners. This practice was not confined to the elites, but extended down to the level of tradesman. Clearly, the more disposable income people had, the greater the possibility to exercise choice.

As first-person documents reveal, early modern Europeans had assimilated this understanding of the body and disease, even if they shaped it according to their own needs and interpretations. Diaries reveal how this might work in practice. A retired Sussex barrister, Timothy Burrell, confided the following in his diary: 'Yesterday having wetted my feet by walking out in the dew and having eaten a small piece of new cheese, I have been today been tortured with flatulent spasms'.[61] The exact cause and effect of Burrell's suffering is largely lost on us (we are left wondering if, had the cheese been aged, he might have been spared). Similarly, Gilles de Gouberville, a well-fed country squire in Normandy, diagnosed and treated himself – both the cause and the cure being food. On eating a piece of cold beef after dinner, and in a draughty kitchen, Gouberville found himself with a cold which gripped him in the head, kidneys, heart and limbs. His remedy consisted of sugar-plums, raisins and old wine. When his stomach bothered him, Gouberville ate large amounts of calf-foot jelly; and when he vomited, he prescribed shoulder of mutton, liberally doused with wine, for himself.[62] Joubert's *Erreurs populaires* is full of such esoteric causal connections, some with learned origins, others the fruit of popular lore.[63]

These first-person sources prompt the larger question of how preventive and curative forms of medicine, regimen and remedy might interact with one another in daily life. The records of the duchess of Saxony, Elisabeth of Rochlitz (1502–57), provide one possible answer. As reconstructed and analysed by Alisha Rankin,

Elisabeth kept a detailed account of her illnesses and medical treatments.[64] Elisabeth was an 'active' patient: she compiled a collection of medical recipes, from a wide range of sources, for her own personal use, and kept a substantial supply of medicines and medicinal ingredients, bought from at least six different apothecaries. She was treated by a wide variety of healers, including physicians, surgeons and barbers, most notably the doctor Sebastian Roth von Auerbach and a 'Jewish doctor' named Hirsch. In addition, as a devout Lutheran, Elisabeth frequently sought recourse to divine help.

Auerbach wrote to Elisabeth that 'medicament without regimen cannot bring true health'.[65] To treat her 'flux in the breast', Auerbach recommended that she avoid, as unhealthy, onions, garlic, mustard and horseradish, foods seasoned with pepper, cinnamon, cardamom and other fragrant spices, smoked meat, fish and game, all stuffed dishes, all foods fried in butter, as well as beans, lentils and sauerkraut. That did not leave much, given the culinary options available in sixteenth-century Germany; and indeed Elisabeth may not have followed Auerbach's recommendations. We know that the duchess was a lover of food and drink who disliked any form of strict dietary regulation. She rarely kept to a regimen for more than a few days. Thus Elisabeth argued with Hirsch, who briefly treated her in 1556, complaining to her brother Philip that Hirsch had forbidden her from drinking wine and asking Philip to send her beer instead. Elisabeth expressed initial optimism about her ability to keep to the diet, but was glad when Hirsch left and she could return to her normal eating habits. 'Food and drink still taste good to us', she wrote, 'whether the Jew likes it or not, and as proof of this we ate five [game] birds for lunch today'.[66]

One has the impression that for the duchess of Saxony her collection of medical recipes was more important to her health than the regimens she was recommended by her doctors. This may be typical of lay attitudes to preventive medicine. It helps us keep the historical importance of the genre in perspective. Regimens were undoubtedly a best-selling literary form but we should not exaggerate the importance of books on preventive medicine to the public, as compared to curative medicine (the treatment of illness or therapeutics). In England, regimens and health guides made up one out of ten medical books printed, as we have seen, which is certainly a substantial proportion. However, books of curative medicine – such as recipe collections, treatises on materia medica and pamphlets for proprietary medicines – together made up 23 per cent of the entire corpus of medical titles, or over twice that of the regimens.[67]

By the 1650s, according to Albala, 'enough had been written on diet', which serves to explain the decline of the printed regimen as a genre.[68] To market saturation, Cavallo and Storey add a declining interest in preventive medicine as a possible explanation.[69] Both are true, even if the decline was only relative and short-lived, as we shall see in the following chapter. The seventeenth century did see an increasing shift towards curative medicine at the expense of preventive medicine, both in terms of medical practice and in patients' own expectations. But if there was a slowdown in the publication of regimens, it was only a temporary one. The eighteenth century experienced a renewed demand for titles on the subject, though much changed in content and style, as part of a renascence of preventive medicine.

CHAPTER 2
HEALTHY FOOD: THE FALL AND RISE
OF DIETETICS, c.1650–c.1800

Introduction

In 1763 a 44-year-old miller in the Essex town of Billericay decided he had had enough of his obesity. The sense of suffocation Thomas Wood felt after eating only added to his head and stomach aches, disturbed sleep, vertigo, constant thirst, rheumatism, gout and epileptic fits. A local clergyman recommended an 'exact regimen', advising Wood to read 'Cornaro's book', which would 'suggest to him a salutary course of living'. The simple advice of Alvise Cornaro – to embrace sobriety and avoid excess – evidently retained its appeal, despite being written two hundred years earlier. Wood became so enthused by the book's contents that he immediately gave up his fatty meats, which 'he ate voraciously three times a day', his butter, cheese and large amounts of strong ale, in favour of a strict diet. Within a few years Wood was restored to perfect health, in body and spirit: enough to feature in an article of the London College of Physicians' *Medical Transactions*, signed by reliable witnesses. To achieve this, Wood did not give up on physicians – indeed one of the signatories of the article was his doctor, Benjamin Pugh – but the go-it-alone philosophy struck a chord with eighteenth-century eaters, determined to reduce and regulate their intake of food and drink (Figure 2.1).[1]

One of the reasons for Conaro's continued appeal to British readers was due to the work of a Scottish doctor earlier in the eighteenth century, George Cheyne. Waging an ongoing war with his own obesity, and having become a Bath-based society doctor, Cheyne asserted that health was the individual's responsibility. He stressed the old idea that ''tis easier to *preserve* health than to *recover* it'.[2] Like Cornaro, Cheyne stressed that temperance was the key to staying healthy, the quantity of the food consumed being just as important as the 'quality' (nature) of the foods consumed. For the healthy, the point was to avoid excess and choose foods that would maintain bodily 'juices' in the right consistency. Cheyne was convinced that most people above the class of labourer ate too much food, and he calculated the ideal daily ration of food and drink. Particularly once illness took over, rigorous measures were necessary. At the outset, Cheyne would advise a patient to cut back on meats and alcohol, and increase intake of vegetables, cereals, dairy products and mineral water. In more extreme cases, he would recommend a 'lowering diet', which might consist only of milk and 'seeds' (meaning oatmeal or rice).

Cheyne was one of a cluster of physicians interested in diet as the key to health during the middle decades of the eighteenth century. The regimen as espoused in these works

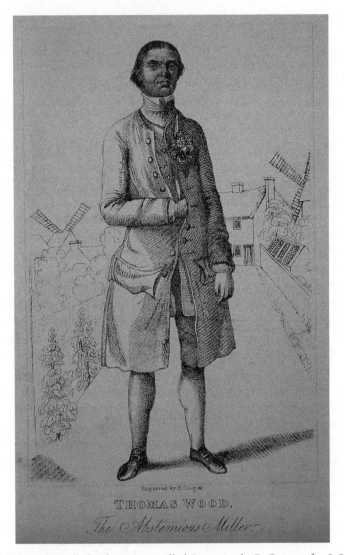

Figure 2.1 'Thomas Wood, the abstemious miller'. Engraving by R. Cooper after J. Ogborne, 1773 (Wellcome Library, London).

was just the sort of thing to appeal to the rising Enlightenment bourgeoisie in England and France. The good life resulted in increasing rates of corpulence.[3] Well-off and well-fed they may have been, but on both sides of the Channel the growing middle classes were also self-aware and cultured, in tune with a message of prevention, regulation and moderation.[4] They had a spate of new dietary manuals at their disposal – significantly slimmer than those of old, as if in line with their reducing intentions. They also had additional sources of information to satisfy their medical curiosity, such as new periodicals like the *Journal de Trévoux* in Paris and the *Gentlemen's Magazine* in London (and of course numerous others elsewhere in Europe).[5]

The message that they should trust in the power of nature, as represented by philosophers like Jean-Jacques Rousseau, struck a chord with this audience. Doctors ensured they had a role in this back-to-nature trend, both as authors advocating it and as practitioners putting it into practice for their patients. Just as our miller Wood did not intend to do without the services of a physician, so Rousseau had his own doctor, the Parisian Achille Le Bègue de Presle. Le Bègue stressed the importance of preventive medicine. But while his regimen offered detailed advice on the regulation of the six non-naturals, Le Bègue also warned of the 'dangers' of tampering with them, through 'imprudence, temerity or ignorance'.[6] His book aimed to provide the necessary expert advice, while suggesting that it was no replacement for the physician's role. Why not seek a doctor's advice 'on the means of maintaining health' and 'the rules of life relative to one's temperament' while one was still healthy, Le Bègue asked, rather than wait until one was well and truly sick before consulting the doctor?[7] His treatise devotes ample space – over one hundred pages – to a discussion of food and drink, all couched in terms of the 'dangers' to health different foodstuffs might pose. Le Bègue surveyed the dangers of eating too much or too little, of too many different foods or too much of the same food, too many acid foods and too many alkaline and so on.

If Cheyne's very specific and often bizarre advice predates the faddish diets of our own times, and if Le Bègue predates some of our own food anxieties, together they give the impression that books on regimen had remained influential in Europe since Renaissance times. The language of both Cheyne and Le Bègue may be different, in line with the latest understanding of digestion and the nature of foods; but their approaches to regimen would have been recognizable to a Renaissance doctor. And yet this impression of continuity is a false one.

As this chapter will show, no sooner had Galenism been revived in the early sixteenth century, producing the Renaissance notion of dietetics we explored in Chapter 1, then there were challenges to it. Renaissance investigators often found themselves disagreeing with the ancient authorities, taking them in new directions, leading to a break with tradition. New theories resulted in new ways of explaining the natural world. In a range of fields, from anatomy to astrology, new findings would lead to what historians often refer to as the 'scientific revolution', even if it was not so much as a revolution, as an evolution. Radical, new ideas and theories co-existed with accepted, traditional ones. Nowhere is this more evident than in the understanding of diet and physiology. Here there was no revolution, no sudden abandonment of Galenic and Hippocratic ideas; indeed older humoural notions persisted right into the nineteenth century, even if shorn of explicit references to the underlying system of the humours. However, these references were accompanied by new theories and ideas, which sought to explain the effects of food on the human body in very different terms.

The challenges to Galenism were so effective that, during the seventeenth century, preventive medicine gave way to an emphasis on therapeutics. Medicine became increasingly associated with *medicines*. Regimen was sidelined, as the focus shifted away from how to take care of healthy bodies to how to cure particular diseases. Anatomy and chemistry were seen as the most important, innovative and scientific parts of medicine, with dietetics relegated to crafts like cookery.[8] This faith in medicines, which seems so modern, was itself eventually challenged, as these often harsh remedies failed to keep pace with the rising expectations of society. Beginning in the early decades of the eighteenth century, a backlash ensued, with doctors and patients alike advocating a greater place for the curative powers of nature and the body itself. With the turn to a more natural and environmental medicine from the middle decades of the eighteenth century, preventive medicine underwent a resurgence and hygiene became an important part of the medical curriculum. A return to regimen – albeit one quite different from that of the Galenic orthodoxy – was the result. The revival lasted for the rest of the eighteenth and well into the nineteenth century, until the arrival of a new concept of disease in the form of germ theory.

In order to understand these changes, this chapter will survey the main medical developments characterizing the latter century and a half of the early modern period. It will ask how this affected the nature of medical advice on food and diet and its impact on food habits themselves.

Paracelsus and iatrochemistry

The first significant challenge to the nascent Galenic orthodoxy really belongs to the previous chapter, at least in terms of its chronology. Its proponent, Paracelsus, was a creature of the early sixteenth century, with its multiplicity of radical religious movements; but its main impact was felt during the seventeenth century. The new theory Paracelsus advocated is very difficult to assess fairly. On the one hand, it represents without doubt the first major leap towards modern pharmaceutical chemistry (i.e., chemical drugs); but, on the other hand, its founder was a religious mystic and showman, who wrote in an all but impenetrable language, with more than the odd contradiction.

Out of this bizarre combination of spiritualism, alchemy, folk medicine and observation of the natural world came an entirely new vision of health, disease and the process of healing. The Swiss German Theophrastus Bombastus von Hohenheim, calling himself Paracelsus, was a pioneer in suggesting that physicians abandon the ancient authorities like Galen and instead rely on direct observation, trial and error. He was the first physician to reject humoural physiology outright, replacing it with a chemical, or better alchemical, system. In this system three elements were considered the basic constituents of life: sulphur, mercury and salt. All food could thus be assessed in terms of its chemical components. Paracelsus believed that disease was caused by an invasion from outside, instead of an interior imbalance. He proclaimed that every disease had its own remedy, one that would work in every human body; he also targeted specific organs of the body as sites of disease, rather than the bodily constitution as a whole (which Galenists looked at). In terms of the remedies, he believed in treating diseases with concentrated doses of a plant or mineral's chemical essence, rather than the herbal remedies of Galenism.

Paracelsus advocated local remedies for local diseases. There was no need to rely on expensive and rare imported remedies, since German drugs were as good, if not better, as those imported from Italy or France. As he wrote, probably in the late 1520s, to think otherwise:

> is the fault of Italy, the mother of ignorance and inexperience. For the Italians saw to it that the Germans thought of nothing of their own plants, but rather took everything from Italy itself or from beyond the sea. This, they realized, was to their own advantage and thus they pursued it, not out of brotherly love to be sure, which in them has wholly or almost entirely grown cold'.[9]

At the same time, on a more traditional note, Paracelsus was a firm supporter of regimen. It was everyone's responsibility to follow regimen in order to 'conserve' the body. In his two short treatises 'On the long life', written in 1526–1527 but only published some forty years later, Paracelsus wrote that everyone should know what they ate and drank. The reasoning behind it, however, is more radical: through regimen, the individual became his own doctor, assisting nature to stay healthy and live longer. There was also a spiritual side to regimen, since how one lived one's mortal life was intimately connected with the hereafter, which he argued was something the ancients ignored. Paracelsus also posited a connection of the physical body to the cosmos, the microcosm to the macrocosm, an astrological medicine shared by few writers of regimens.[10]

Paracelsus' theories only acquired some degree of influence a generation or two after his death in 1541. It was only towards the end of the sixteenth century, and then during the seventeenth century that a school of followers came into being. The Paracelsians were also known as iatrochemsists (healing chemists), presenting a rival, chemical, system to that of Galenic humouralism. The iatrochemical school refined Paracelsus' ideas and jettisoned some of the mystical context. Sulphur, mercury and salt were seen not so much as elements but as transformative processes. Sulphur was regarded as the key to all combustion, flammability and change within the human body; mercury was the volatile principle, explaining how things move through the body; salt provided structure and solidity within the body. In this system, digestion was considered a threefold process which transformed food, transported it through our body and became our solid 'parts'. The iatrochemists developed a whole new system of medicines and therapies, while beginning to think about the human body in very different terms.

One follower of Paracelsus was the Flemish physician Jan Baptist van Helmont, who studied processes of fermentation and the effects of what he termed 'acids' and 'alkalis'. Van Helmont theorized that digestion was a breaking down of food particles by means of acid in the stomach – rather than by heat, as Galen believed. This was the first chemical account of the process of digestion. So important was the process that, as van Helmont argued, 'digestions do prescribe the rules of diet', rather than physicians or books.[11] In addition to positing the centrality of digestion, van Helmont was dismissive of preventive medicine, seeing it as ineffective and a mask for physicians' lack of worthwhile medicines.

Van Helmont's philosophy ought to have spelt the end for the need for dietary advice, but the diet–health–illness link was too strong for the Helmontians to do away with it completely.[12] One English Helmontian, George Thomson, wrote at considerable length about diet and regimen. While Thomson's categories and structure remained essentially Galenic, his advice was radically different. With appetite and digestion as a guide, one could eat just about anything: no foods were completely harmful as and of themselves. Gone were the 'rule of contraries' and the 'contrived cookeries' of Galenic regimens. Thomson may have demonstrated a preference for 'simple home-bred food' and 'moderation … in all things', but he wrote that personal pleasure and appetite should be our guide as to what foods are best for us. 'To be rigidly kept from what is lawful and useful', Thomson affirmed, 'is little better than Turkish slavery'.[13]

The long-term impact of Paracelsus and his followers was nothing less than the 'invention' of modern chemistry, at least in the sense that they were interested in exploring things from a chemical dimension. They originated new chemical therapies and investigated chemical reactions taking place in the human body. It would lead to seeing food in chemical terms, investigating and analysing the chemical constituents of food. And yet, despite all of this, the Paracelsians did not construct a new dietary system. They did not even suggest a radically new way of assessing and understanding foods. The French Paracelsian Joseph Du Chesne is illustrative of this.

Du Chesne may have replaced the humours of Galen with the three chemical elements of Paracelsus (salt, sulphur and mercury), but he kept the Galenic 'qualities' (hot, cold, dry and moist) and their varying degrees. The old concept of heating or cooling foods remained firmly in place, even if the explanatory model and language changed. Consider the example of black pepper:

> The great piquant or piercing quality of pepper, which one perceives in the taste and burning sensation it leaves on the tongue, stems from what chemical physicians call an aronic salt, which is subtle and penetrating and therefore cuts into, attenuates, and dissolves the tartars and viscidities of the stomach and other parts, and this is why the ancients found it to be good for the treatment of quartain fevers and various other maladies.[14]

In other words, Du Chesne thought that the ancients might have been wrong about the reasons, but he agreed with pepper's beneficial effects. In this process, traditional characterizations and uses were re-tooled and reconciled with new Paracelsian theories. Elsewhere, the difference is in style. When it came to describing bread, Du Chesne agreed with Galen on its importance for health. However, he eschewed a comparative discussion of the merits of different grains, cereal-by-cereal, as a Galenic physician would have done, for a geographical survey of France's many different breads.[15]

The iatromechanists

Just as significant to a shift in ideas about diet, and indeed preventive medicine in general, was mechanical medicine. It had its beginnings with Santorio Santorio (Sanctorius), professor of theoretical medicine in Padua. For thirty years or so, he tells us, Santorio regularly sat on his 'weighing chair', weighing himself several times every single day. Santorio would compare the weight of the food he ate each day with what he expelled. He noted a discrepancy in the latter and so surmised that the body must also excrete waste in other ways. Santorio called this extra excretion 'insensible perspiration': waste that evaporated off the surface of the body and by exhalation during the course of the day. Because some foods caused a greater weight of insensible perspiration, he concluded that less of that particular food's nutrients were actually absorbed by the body. As a result, foods that caused less perspiration were actually more nourishing, sometimes too much so, since more of them was absorbed; foods that were lighter in texture were generally processed more efficiently than denser foods.

Santorio's *Ars de statica medica* (1614) represents both the culmination of the commentary tradition on classical texts, which we associate with Renaissance humanism, and an attempt to establish a new doctrine, in his case a 'statistical medicine' founded on measureable principles. Like Paracelsus, Santorio eschewed ancient authority for direct experience and reasoning. 'It does not follow, Galen said nothing of it, therefore it is vain', Santorio argued, noting that 'we have found out many instruments, and those not contemptible, which were not known before our times'.[16] Instruments like Santorio's weighing chair provide evidence of how methods of investigation took a decidedly novel turn (Figure 2.2).

Santorio's own dietary recommendations, his notion of 'concoction', as well as his view of the place evacuation had in the structure of the non-naturals, remained firmly in the Hippocratic-Galenic tradition. But Santorio was the first person to believe that the quantification of physiological functions was the best way to understand them. Rather than the traditional elements and qualities, what underpinned Santorio's ideas was a vision of the body and its functions in terms of mathematical functions. Even more important than what he discovered or his ideas on insensible perspiration was thus the methodology and approach he introduced. This stressed the mechanical nature of the body and its functions.

Iatromechanics, or mechanical medicine, saw the body as a machine and sought to explain human life in terms of physics and mathematics. From this point of view, the point of medicine was to restore the proper functioning of the human machine by tightening or loosening or otherwise tinkering with the mechanism. Drawing on the ideas of natural philosophers like Isaac Newton, René Descartes and Giovanni Alfonso Borelli, iatromechanics was used to explain all physiological and pathological processes. Unlocking the secrets of the functioning of the human body was a matter of determining how the machine worked, such as the mechanical breaking down of food to explain digestion. It also took medical investigations to a whole new level: less concerned with the time-worn business of prescribing individual regimens and theorizing about the nature of foods, and more concerned with therapeutics. Medicine became more interested in investigating the physical causes of particular diseases, and curing them via drug therapies. It became more interested in curing than in regulating health, as evident in the medical textbooks which devoted more and more space to therapeutics and less

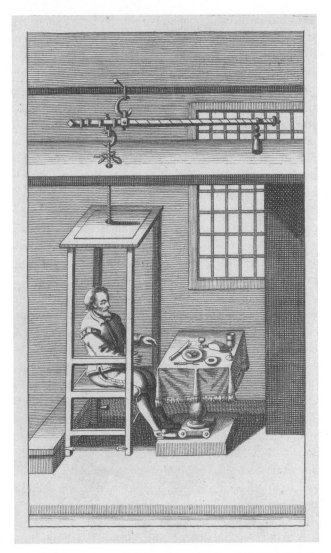

Figure 2.2 Santorio Santorio (Sanctorius) on his weighing chair, 1718 (Wellcome Library, London).

to regimen. The Parisian physician Philippe Hecquet concluded that the prophylactic potential of diet was being completely ignored by contemporary doctors.[17]

This relegation of regimen to a minor role is evident in the mechanistic approach that focused on the fabric of the body itself. From the end of the seventeenth century, and the work of the Halle-based doctor Friedrich Hoffmann, the operative words relative to the body and health were nerves, vessels, tubes and fibres. The body was healthy when blood and 'nerve fluids' circulated freely in the body and when excreta were expelled freely from it. As Hoffmann put it in his influential treatise of 1695, 'whoever eats well, digests well and excretes well, is healthy'.[18]

Transition: Reconciling old and new

Both chemical medicine and mechanical medicine, in their different ways, stressed the curative power of medicine over the preventive. This meant a decline in the number of published regimens across Europe, but certainly not their disappearance as a literary genre. Authors adapted to the new medical philosophies in two quite different ways: on the one hand changing the medical language and interpretative model, but leaving the dietary structure and framework relatively untouched and, on the other hand, altering the format and approach to produce a new kind of regimen.

In terms of the first strategy, what is intriguing about many regimens is how they tried to incorporate the latest scientific theories into what was still an ancient humoural framework. The best attempted to harmonize the older and newer theories into a convincing whole. Such was a work by the Parisian physician Louis Lémery, first published in French in 1702, and widely translated thereafter. Lémery's *Traité des aliments* not only sought to combine iatrochemical and iatromechanical ideas, but it did so on a Galenic framework. Lémery admits in the preface that the structure and method of his work entirely follow that of Baldassare Pisanelli's. If comparing himself to such a Galenist as Pisanelli, published over one hundred years earlier, seems a step too far, Lémery is quick to distance himself from him. 'In short, [the method] is the only thing that I have taken out of that author, and any one may easily see, how little like we are to one another, in any thing else, and especially in the way of our explaining the nature and properties of foods' (Figure 2.3).[19]

Lémery makes extensive use of new chemical theories, incorporating 'fermentation' into his discussion of digestion. He also mentions the role of respiration and circulation of the blood in distributing nutrients throughout the body, something absent in earlier dietary writings. When it comes to foods, Lémery discusses them in series, as in any Renaissance regimen, but gone are food 'qualities', with their relative 'degrees', replaced by four 'chemical constituents': the terrestrial, aqueous, oily and saline 'parts'. These are certainly a step beyond humouralism, though no laboratory-based chemical analysis was as yet involved. Indeed the constituents of foods are still determined mainly by taste, which Lémery divides into bitter, acid, sharp, salt, acerbic, harsh, sweet and oily.[20] He offers chemical or sometimes mechanical characterizations and explanations of how individual foods work in the body. And yet, what Lémery actually says about the foods, and the advice he gives about their consumption, is little changed. In his entry on 'cucumbers', for instance, Lémery mentions how they were made up of 'a little oyl, much phlegm, and an indifferent measure of essential salt' and contained 'a viscous and thick juice'.[21] What this means, however, is entirely Galenic: that their moistness makes them difficult to digest and they are best eaten during summer and seasoned with onions, salt and pepper.

We are evidently in a typical intermediary phase of change and continuity. What changes most in seventeenth-century regimens is language, with the vocabulary of chemical constituents and mechanical processes taking the place of fluids and elements. New medical terms find their way in, such as 'symptom'.[22] At the same

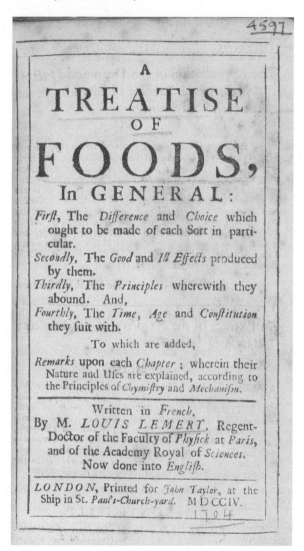

A

TREATISE

OF

FOODS,

In GENERAL:

Firſt, The *Difference* and *Choice* which ought to be made of each Sort in particular.

Secondly, The *Good* and *Ill Effects* produced by them.

Thirdly, The *Principles* wherewith they abound. And,

Fourthly, The *Time*, *Age* and *Conſtitution* they ſuit with.

To which are added,

Remarks upon each *Chapter* ; wherein their Nature and Uſes are explained, according to the Principles of *Chymiſtry* and *Mechaniſm*.

Written in *French*,

By M. *LOUIS LEMERT*, Regent-Doctor of the Faculty of *Phyſick* at *Paris*, and of the Academy Royal of *Sciences*. Now done into *Engliſh*.

LONDON, Printed for *John Taylor*, at the Ship in St. *Paul's-Church-yard*. MDCCIV.

Figure 2.3 Title page of the 1704 English translation of Louis Lémery's *Traité des aliments* (Wellcome Library, London).

time, Lémery's treatise illustrates how, despite the twin onslaughts of chemical and mechanical medicine, the basic foundations of humoural physiology remained more or less intact into the eighteenth century. Despite the rise and fall of new theories throughout the course of the previous century, no one had yet devised a completely new way of thinking about food and its role in health.

The second strategy medical authors pursued was to revisit the regimen format itself. The books became less concerned with the intricacies of food and drink, resulting in a more even exploration of the role of all six non-naturals as a whole. The specifically dietary advice given was much more generalized, often summed up in a few pithy rules.

As a result, late seventeenth-century regimens are much shorter than their Renaissance predecessors, more like extended pamphlets than treatises. For instance, François Pinsonnat prohibits nothing: 'I am not of the sentiment of those who say that fish, pastry, ham, sauces, butter, salt and pepper are like as many poisons in the body... All these foods are good or bad according to the good or bad use made of them'.[23] Rather, Pinsonnat's message is about moderation; when in doubt, err on the side of frugality over excess. All of this is to be determined by the reader himself, within the context of an intimate understanding of what is good and what is bad for our own individual bodies, built up over the experience of years.

Pinsonnat's approach and content have more in common with the bare-bones simplicity of Alvise Cornaro than the rich complexity of neo-Galenic texts:

> Examine yourself, observe yourself, deny yourself that which harms you, eat those foods which do you good: that is the best that medicine has been able to come up with for those people who are in good health, in order to maintain their health. Everything I have said hitherto and everything I shall say below will be a continual repetition of this incomparable maxim.[24]

Since, for Pinsonnat, there had been no better advice since the time of Hippocrates, a healthy man should rightly strive to be his own doctor, calling on medical aid only when he falls ill. The issue of whether one could be one's own doctor was much debated in the period, by physicians and with wider public.[25] One could argue that the whole point of a book on regimen was always to be one's own physician; but Renaissance dietaries were so complex, not to mention contradictory, that one might need a doctor to apply them in practice. The simplicity beginning in the late seventeenth century made this a real possibility.

The eighteenth century

Among the educated classes, knowledge of dietary principles remained widespread, as letters to doctors all over Europe demonstrate.[26] A series of consultation letters written between 1680 and 1720 to the Spanish doctor Juan Muñoz y Peralta, a native of Seville and based in Madrid, reveal the continuing dominance of hygiene in both lay and professional understanding of disease and the body. A recent study of the collection notes how 'references to habits of eating and drinking and to irregular patterns of sleep, exercise and rest are incessant in nearly all of the letters'.[27]

In addition to shedding light on the continuing attention to regimen, the letters reveal how traditional the nature of that regimen continued to be – certainly at the lay level, and perhaps among many practitioners, too. An unnamed friar from Bilbao wrote to Muñoz y Peralta, introducing his complaint in these terms:

> Taking my bilious, sanguine constitution, the fact I am forty-eight years old and that for thirty years of my life I have lived on crass, salty and spicy food, which is

common in the Order, despite all that, I have remained robust, with just a nasty sty in the right eye and some very occasional pains.[28]

Both the language and conceptions would have been familiar to a Renaissance physician of a hundred or even two hundred years earlier.

Diaries provide a similar impression of enduring Galenism. Those kept by a native of the American colony of Virginia for thirty-five years, between 1709 and his death in 1744, remind one of Samuel Pepys: as political observer, office-holder – and womaniser. But they also reveal the diarist's constant attempt to order his diet and the careful planning behind his meals.[29] William Byrd Jr., the diarist in question, was born in Virginia and educated in England, where he was elected a fellow of the Royal Society. He returned to the colony to manage his estate in 1705, at the age of thirty-one. Despite possessing a copy of Cheyne's 1724 dietary in his well-stocked library, Byrd's approach to regimen remained entirely traditional throughout, consistent with the theory of the non-naturals. In addition to recording the foods he eats, Byrd detailed the amount of sleep he received, his emotional states, his physical and sexual activities and the weather. It has to be said that the earlier diaries are more detailed than the later ones, not to mention a large gap in what survives from the late 1720s, so it may be too early to expect Cheyne's iatromechanical views to creep into Byrd's entries. One thing his clear: by his own reckoning, Byrd had greater success in managing his culinary appetites than his sexual ones.

Later on in the century, the 'culture of prevention' was still central but its contours were increasingly shaped by the new medical hygiene. This is evident in the letters of those who wrote to Samuel-Auguste Tissot in Lausanne in the second half of the eighteenth century.[30] Writing to this 'epitome of the enlightened, philanthropic medical man with a genuine understanding of nature',[31] these sufferers knew their own bodies and knew what Tissot expected of them. The correspondents provided ample detail of their food habits and preferences in their letters, related sudden changes in diet and lifestyle which brought on disease, and even referred to the notions and recommendations of Tissot himself, with their stress on simplicity, frugality and moderation.

The letters reveal a real concern with diet as a cause – as well as a cure – for illness. This contrasts strongly with Erwin Ackerknecht's conclusion that 'during the eighteenth century the prescribing of a diet in disease continued to become rarer and rarer'.[32] Never mind that Ackerknecht then follows this assertion with a long list of important exceptions, which includes Cheyne, Hoffmann and Tissot; because quite the opposite is true, as Robert Weston has suggested more recently. Based on a study of some 2,500 letters to and from doctors during the period 1655–1789, Weston finds that 'patients were almost always advised to adopt dietary restrictions in order to regain their health'.[33] What is less clear is what role regimen, in general, and food and drink, in particular, played when these people were *healthy*. Michael Stollberg has suggested that these things only became important when they sickened and sought treatment.[34] Mind you, we cannot expect people to write to important doctors when they are healthy. As a result, I would say that it is a question of degree. The letter-writers frequently point to sudden changes in diet as the cause of illness. They were certainly aware of the regimen they followed when they were healthy, even if they admitted to not always following the learned advice on such matters as they should have.

What is clear is how the regimens themselves became the site for two areas of tension. The first concerns the differing approaches of chemical and mechanical medicine, which occurred during the late seventeenth and early eighteenth century. The second regards the relative importance of curative over preventive medicine, a tussle which dominated the second half of the eighteenth century.

The eighteenth century began with an attempt to reconcile the two main schools, chemical and mechanical medicine. At the University of Leiden, Hermann Boerhaave, along the lines proposed by Hoffmann, suggested that bodily functions were controlled by a system of hydraulics, with vascular channels sucking up fluids or gases which are themselves subject to chemical change. In terms of the physiology of digestion, this inspired the thinking of the French physician Jacques-Jean Bruhier. In Galenic physiology the stomach was considered a sort of pot, forever bubbling away, and digestion was seen as a form of cooking ('concoction'). It followed that cooking foods in the kitchen, even overcooking them, was regarded as a good thing, because it meant less work for the stomach. By 1755, however, a physician such as Bruhier could confidently remark that certain foods could be eaten raw – such as fruits or oysters – and that for those which needed to be cooked, it was preferable 'for reasons of health as well as taste' not to overcook them.[35] In that year Bruhier produced a third edition of Lémery's *Traité des aliments*, with commentary, in which he did not shy from criticizing specific points of Lémery's work. This change in opinion was made possible by an accompanying shift in the understanding of the digestive process.[36] The action of the stomach was no longer seen in terms of concoction, but as the dissolving of food by the gastric juices.

In the end, the iatromechanical school would have the upper hand, even if it was a iatromechanism influenced by chemical ideas. We see this in the increased emphasis placed on the flux of fluids and substances throughout the body, with humoural language giving way to a discourse on hydraulics. But the dominance of mechanical processes did not override chemical interpretations. Indeed, the rise of modern chemistry influenced medical notions of foods. In a process begun by Lémery, foods were re-classified along chemical lines. Later in the century, the London physician William Forster similarly postulated a division of foods into eight chemically based categories: acidic, alkaline, salty, acrid and aromatic, spirituous, viscous and glutinous, oily, and acqueous.[37] Not everyone followed Forster's system, but most physicians adopted something like it. Thus for William Smith, another London doctor, the key to health was achieving a balance between in the consumption of acid foods (vegetables) and alkaline foods (meats).[38]

This chemical interpretation of foods, along with a mechanical concern for bodily processes, and in particular the flow of fluids through the body, affected ideas regarding diet and health. For instance, the eighteenth century saw a new attention on diseases like scurvy and gout, which were put down to an excessive of tartar deposits, caused in turn by an overly rich and abundant diet. This could be corrected, it was thought, by eating a diet which promoted the passage of fluids. This became a source of concern, and profit, for regimen-minded physicians, who recommended diets stressing the importance of fluid transport for their sick and corpulent patients. The most colourful of these diet practitioners, cited by Bruhier, was Cheyne. If other physicians embracing a mechanistic view of the body also affirmed the general notion that a proper diet was the key to maintaining good health, they did not give a systematic explanation of why and how dietary therapies worked. If they lost interest in the daily intricacies of diet, in their pursuit of medicines and therapies targeted at curing specific diseases, Cheyne was different. Over a period of twenty years Cheyne published a number of works in which he recast the study of dietetics. His most famous and influential work was the *Essay of Health and Long Life* (1724), written early in his career. In addition to giving an iatromechanical explanation of the relationship between diet and health, the book also set forth some simple rules of thumb for deciding what and, in particular, how much to eat.

For Cheyne, the human body was composed of solids and juices. Disease occurred when the juices became blocked or gluey (viscous) or encrusted to the body's tubes. This caused chronic ailments like gout, constipation, kidney stones, joint pain and nervous complaints. Cheyne prescribed drugs and bloodletting for his patients with such diseases; but changes in diet, aimed at restoring free flow of fluids through the tubes, were necessary to bring about long-term improvements. Fatty or oily foods, composed of large, gluey particles, were to be avoided in favour of lean or starchy ones. For example, the flesh of smaller, younger animals was preferable to that of larger, older animals. Beef was out: it was far too full of large particles and salts. Similarly, spring-ripening vegetables and fruits had less corrosive salt than those which ripened later in the year, for the sun concentrated the latter.[39] Foods that were lighter in colour were healthier than darker ones, because they were composed of finer particles and contained fewer salts. Hence Cheyne's preference for milk and eggs. Spices and strong flavours were to be avoided, a sign they were bad for one. 'Plain roasting and boiling' were to be preferred to 'made dishes, rich soop, high sauces, baking, smoking, salting, and pickling', which were 'the inventions of luxury', encouraging one to eat more, and harmful, foods.[40]

For all its innovations, however, Cheyne's treatise was a traditional regimen in structure. The focus was on the maintenance of health and the prevention of disease, by regulation of the six non-naturals. It was directed at a specific class of people, 'the studious' and 'gentlemen of the learned professions', like Guglielmo Grataroli's treatise of two centuries earlier. There are some similarities in the actual advice, too: not in the language and rationale, but in the foods recommended or best avoided.

Cheyne himself conducted a lifelong battle with his own obesity, which may help explain the interest in food quantities. Far from discrediting him in the eyes of potential patients and readers of his books, Cheyne's own obesity and gout seemed to bolster his success, as Anita Guerrini has noted.[41] People believed he understood their plight. Cheyne also understood his market. The more practical in nature the advice, the more receptive the public seemed to have been. Cheyne complained that his eminently practical *Natural Method*, which went into three editions in its first year (1742), 'was a more popular and consequently better bookseller's book' than his *Essay on Regimen* (1740), more theoretical in nature[42] (Figure 2.4).

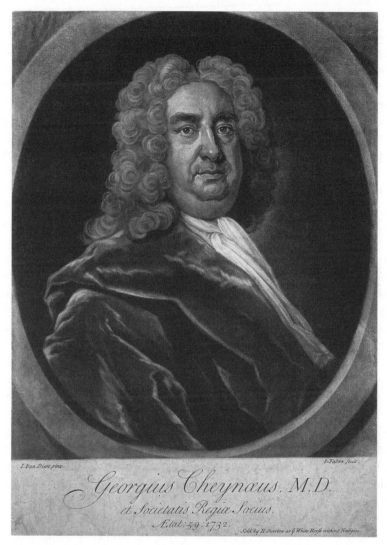

I. Von Diest pinx.   *I. Faber fecit*

Georgius Cheynæus. M.D.
et Societatis Regiæ Socius.
Ætat: 59 : 1732.

Sold by H. Overton at ye White Horse without Newgate.

Figure 2.4 George Cheyne. Mezzotint by J. Faber after Johan van Diest, 1732 (Wellcome Library, London).

There are numerous examples of people attempting to follow Cheyne's advice, from the founder of Methodism John Wesley to the writer and printer Samuel Richardson. Cheyne's influence on Wesley was twofold. Wesley attempted to follow Cheyne's dietary advice himself – his generally abstemious habits interrupted only during his stay in America in the 1730s, when Wesley admitted to eating 'animal food' and drinking wine.[43] He also wrote about it. Wesley encouraged the readers of his *Primitive Physic* (1747) to 'observe all the time the greatest exactness in your regimen or manner of living'. He even provided them with a list of 'plain easy rules, briefly transcribed from Dr Cheyne'.[44] Later in his life, at the age of sixty-eight, Wesley attributed his lasting health to the moderate eating advocated by Cheyne.[45]

When it came to Richardson, Cheyne was less effective. Richardson admitted to being 'a staunch epicure' and to disliking exercise, and was notably less successful than Wesley in following Cheyne's advice to relax, eat and drink less, and to exercise.[46] Although Cheyne tailored his advice to suit Richardson's tastes, and although 'exercise' meant being moved about rather than our more strenuous modern usage of the term, Richardson managed to follow Cheyne's advice only intermittently.

It was all too easy to satirize this. From the start of our period dietary advice and the doctor–patient relationship among the privileged remained a ready target, as we saw in the previous chapter, now increasingly represented in popular prints. The French printmaker Louis-François Charon paired a corpulent, hungry doctor (perhaps inspired by Cheyne) with an emaciated, dieting patient, setting the scene over dinner in England. As he greedily eats and drinks, the doctor says to the patient, 'Do as I prescribe, not as I do'. And in fact, the patient holds a sheet of paper advising a diet of only dandelion tisane to drink (a noted diuretic) and *bouillon pointu* to eat (not broth as this might suggest but slang for a rectal injection used as a laxative). The patient thinks, 'To see someone eat so much and not be allowed to eat. Damn! I would rather be in the Thames' (Figure 2.5).

Satire or not, Cheyne's continuing influence is evident in a concern for spelling out the exact quantities of food to be eaten in order to stay healthy. Referring back to Cornaro and Santorio, measuring quantities turned into something of an obsession for mechanical medicine. An anonymous French author even criticized Cornaro for not providing more precise information about quantities. What was the good of advocating frugality and self-control as the key to health maintenance if the amounts were not clearly itemized? What was the use of telling us he reduced his food intake to twelve ounces if we were not told what sorts of food it was and how it was prepared?[47]

Cheyne was partly responsible for the continuing attention paid to dietetics and preventive medicine as we near the end of the eighteenth century. This saw a backlash against the reliance on harsh medicines, the use of which had dominated medical practice from the mid-seventeenth century. Therapeutics was perceived – not without some reason – as the site of most advances in medicine. As William Falconer put it, 'It must be obvious to every person conversant in the science of medicine, that the dietetic part of it, or that which respects our regimen and way of life, has not been improved in equal proportion with that which regards the administration of medicines'.[48] But powerful medicines did not always live up to their promises. The semi-mystic James Graham, advocate of a vegetable regimen and cooling baths, considered 'your general manner of living and conducting yourselves to be of far greater consequence ... than loads of harsh, nauseous, and unnatural medicines from doctors and apothecaries'.[49] And, towards the end of his life, in his 'dietetic maxims', the poet and professor of medicine at Wittenburg University Daniel Wilhem Triller warned people against taking 'medicaments' when healthy; they merely destroyed 'the order of nature for nothing'. Moderation was all that was needed to keep what he called the bodily clock in correct working order.[50]

Better than harsh medicines was to trust in the spontaneous healing power of nature: Herman Boerhaave's 'vis mediatrix naturae'.[51] The phrase itself was attributed to Hippocrates and its use signals the Hippocratic revival of the eighteenth century.

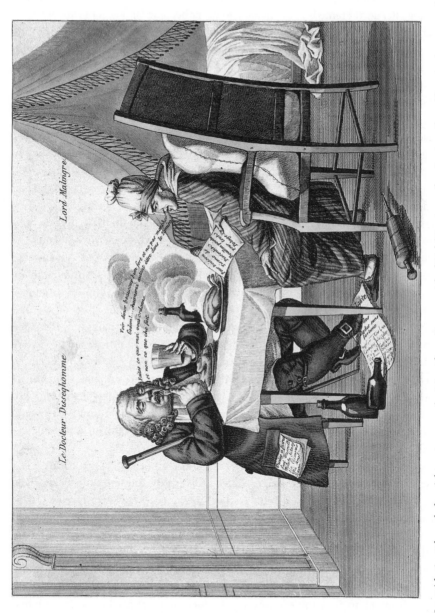

Figure 2.5 'Le médecin et le malade, où le gastronome égoïste et le gastronome à la diète' (Doctor and patient, or the self-centred gourmand and the dieting gastronome). Engraving by L.-F. Charon, late eighteenth century (Wellcome Library, London).

Chemical and mechanical processes were fused into a divinely regulated natural system, in which preventive medicine had pride of place. Relying on the health-giving powers of nature, William Buchan argued in 1769, was 'in every way consistent with reason and common sense'; indeed, 'had men been more attentive to [regimen], and less solicitous in hunting after secret remedies, medicine had never become an object of ridicule.'[52]

Buchan is indicative of both a renewed and a new attitude to regimen. While putting dietetics centre stage, Buchan did so in a context of a reform of medical provision and advice for all ranks of society. Diet presupposed the material possibility of making choices, an inescapable aspect of writing on dietetics that had plagued the genre since its Renaissance revival. 'To read over some specious systems of diet', the London physician William Black wrote in 1782, 'one could only conclude that they were written for those who had a coach and six at their doors, and a French cook at their kitchens'. While the privileged in society had the luxury of being able to take the dietary advice, if they so chose, and shape their habits accordingly, every one else 'must rest satisfied with the food which is cheapest and easiest procured'.[53] In chasing after the privileged, medicine had shirked its social duties.

The sign of a new trend, inspired by the reforming ideals of the Enlightenment, is evident in Buchan's *Domestic Medicine*, first published in Edinburgh in 1769 and the most successful general guide to health of the late eighteenth century, widely translated and frequently reprinted. Buchan advocated a kind of holistic environmentalism, in which the well-balanced body interacted with the surrounding environment, suggesting prudence and moderation. Food suggestions abound. Buchan poured scorn on the idle and luxury-loving rich for adopting a way of living that damaged their own health and was sympathetic towards the poor conditions of the urban and rural poor. Indeed, Buchan added a chapter to the 1797 edition, describing the diet of the poor, particularly in England, and offering recommendations for its improvement.[54] If England's poor ate 'badly', it was because they knew no better – not because eating such foods was somehow in keeping with their constitutions, as would have been argued earlier in our period. Enlightenment medical reformers like Buchan claimed to offer the poor a dietary choice.

This is not completely new: the seventeenth and eighteenth centuries saw a few regimens purporting to supplant the physician's role in advising about diet, especially among Paracelsians. The aims of John Archer's *Every Man His Own Doctor* (1671) are evident from the title. Or was it just a rhetorical strategy, a snappy title designed to sell more copies? If Archer had really intended to do away with the need to consult practitioners like him, there would surely have been no reason to inscribe a copy with this sales pitch: 'The author is to be spoke with at his chamber in a sadlers house overagainst the mewes gate next the Black Horse nigh Charing Cross [;] his howers there are from 11 to 5 in the evening [,] at other times at his howse in Knights-bridge'.[55]

Generally speaking, doctors were not comfortable with putting individuals in charge. According to Andrew Harper, writing in 1785, 'regimen…can produce the most salutary effects, but it needs particular skill to direct it'.[56] And, in case, if the claim to be one's own doctor was sometimes stated in eighteenth-century regimens, it was limited to prophylaxis; treatment remained the purview of doctors. Buchan's Swiss counterpart is evidence of this more cautious approach, both towards diet and in his intended readership. In his widely translated *Avis au peuple sur sa santé* (1761), Tissot provided very little information about either food or locale, much less on the link between the two. What limited dietary advice there is in Tissot is very much targeted at responding to particular diseases, such as what to eat and what not to in case of fever.[57] Indeed Tissot openly criticizes 'the great dangers of the regimen, or diet, and of the principal medicines' too often used in cases of illness.[58]

This sort of instruction was entirely consistent with a book which, as its extended title proclaimed, was 'particularly calculated for those, who, by their distance from regular physicians, or other very experienced practitioners, are the most unlikely to be seasonably provided with the best advice and assistance, in acute diseases, or upon any sudden inward or outward accident'. It is typical of the well-intentioned efforts of Enlightenment-inspired medical reformers: who wrote for the benefit of the poor, if not for the poor themselves. The hope was that cultural intermediaries, medical and otherwise, would apply these guidelines on preventive medicine in their care of the poor – not that the poor would take health and medicine into their own hands.[59]

Tissot's concern for diet found expression in a more focused work directed at thinkers, scholars and writers, or *gens de lettres*.[60] They too often took their meals in haste, without due attention to what was being eaten, resulting in stomach aches, Tissot argued. Worse still was the fashion for hot drinks like coffee and tea, with Tissot pointing to the political boycott of tea in the Thirteen Colonies as a wise health measure worth copying.[61] Providing health advice for this group of 'literary and sedentary' people had a long tradition in regimen treatises, going back to Grataroli, which Tissot however updated with a discussion of the importance of environment. He urged them to live as close as possible to nature, eschewing the artificiality and luxury of urban living.

The Hippocratic emphasis on the role of the environment in determining individual health, evident in Buchan and Tissot, also applied to entire societies. Our survey of the regimen ends with the 1790s, when the approach to hygiene shifted away from the individual and towards society. Hygiene was increasingly construed as a matter for public health. In virtually all European countries a diverse group of authors – including medical practitioners, government officials and statisticians – devoted their attention to a range of topics relating to the health of populations, as opposed to that of individuals. If private hygiene involved regimen, according to the French physician Jean Noël Hallé, public hygiene included the analysis of general environmental factors and those features of social structure deemed to determine health.[62]

In the meantime, the medical popularizing literature spread throughout Europe, leading to a resurgence in preventive medicine, but also increasing concern about its application.[63] In addition to a new concern for the poor, attention is also paid another group hitherto little addressed in regimens: women. The beneficiaries of the literature had always been largely male. Women had played a very small part: rarely discussed, aside from occasional advice relevant to female physiology, and even more rarely addressed. It was only in 1771 that the first regimen dedicated entirely to women appeared, *Le médecin des dames* (the women's doctor).[64] However, starting with the title, this volume addresses women as 'them', not as 'you', which brings us back to the role of the authoritative intermediary (men, in this case). In terms of content, the book's concern is just as much with the armoury of the female *toilette* as with the maintenance of health.[65] The Enlightenment produced various works directed at women of the 'science for ladies' type and it became something of a sub-genre within the field of popularizing literature; so the paucity of regimens written specifically for women to read is rather surprising.[66] It is even more so when we consider the rising role of the salon in the dining culture of eighteenth-century France, as we shall see in Chapter 3, to say nothing of the contribution made by actual women to the collaborative scientific endeavour, as reconstructed by Patricia Fara.[67]

What of the eighteenth-century regimens themselves? Francisco da Fonseca Henriques' charmingly titled *Âncora medicinal* (medicinal anchor) has all the appearance, structure and content of a Renaissance dietary, where food occupies pride of place over the other non-naturals.[68] The two-volume *Diaetetica* by the Transylvanian town physician István Mátyus is more up to date, citing the works of many other European writers and offering a more balanced approach to all of the non naturals.[69] Generally speaking, the revival in regimen was much less concerned than its Renaissance predecessor with spelling out the dangers and benefits of individual foodstuffs than earlier dietaries. Instead they stressed the importance of regulating the quantity of food ingested, emphasizing moderation and lightness. In his thirty-three densely written pages of dietary advice, Giuseppe Pujati mentions hardly a single food by name (with the exception of a warning against the dangers of mushrooms).[70] A concern with the broader theme of hunger and thirst dwarfed advice on which foods to eat and which to avoid. In his treatise of 1776, William Smith paid more attention to the health-related characteristics of different foodstuffs than most eighteenth-century physicians, yet he managed to survey them all in just eight pages.[71] In our final example, the French doctor and botanist Pierre Buc'hoz exemplifies the tendency for medical authors to be less concerned about the minutiae of diet even while they are purporting to write dietaries. In the preface to his *L'art alimentaire* of 1783, Buc'hoz modestly proclaims that 'this work is of the utmost interest to men, in that it treats of foods which are the healthiest for his life and shows the methods of preparing them'.[72] In fact, his treatise is little more than a ramshackle collection of recipes, with little explanation of why the dishes described are healthy. Perhaps Buc'hoz assumes his readers will know why.

Medical change and cookery

Although his title promises much more than it delivers, Buc'hoz leads us to the important theme of the relationship between the culinary arts and medicine. As a way of concluding these first two introductory chapters and opening out towards the rest of the book, this final section explores the effects of the changing medical philosophies on cookery.

The 'decline' of Renaissance dietetics helps explain the turn away from the spicy and sweet cooking and that dominated hitherto. This shift began in the middle of the seventeenth century, when cookery books gradually dropped references to seasonings and condiments as 'correctives', to render foods healthier. This accompanied a sharp fall in the importation and use of spices, first in France, and slowly elsewhere in Europe. Two French cookery books are suggestive of this new trend, François La Varenne's *Le cuisinier françois* (1651) and Nicolas de Bonnefons's *Les délices de la campagne* (1654). Both works are associated with a new style of cookery, influential (though not always without local tensions) throughout Europe. They were intent on capturing the 'natural' flavours of foods, even if much refinement and elaboration (and expense!) was considered necessary to achieve this. Strident flavours and ingredients were replaced by complementary ones. When sugar and spices are mentioned, it is not as 'correctives' but on the grounds of 'taste'. Instead of being seen as essential ingredients in a dietary regime meant to maintain or re-establish health, sugar and aromatic spices were now used – or not – as a matter of personal taste.

On the strength of this evidence, Jean-Louis Flandrin argued that a relaxation of the links between cooking and dietetics occurred from the mid-seventeenth century. With physicians less concerned with food and diet, cookery was freed to pursue flavour alone. It became less worried about the maintenance of health through food. The seventeenth and eighteenth centuries witnessed what Flandrin called the 'liberation of the gourmet', which asked for 'new creations without regard for the "medical" properties of the food they were eating.'[73] Spicy foods and contrasting flavours were rejected in favour of the mild seasonings and silky, rich sauces that have characterized French cookery ever since.

Except that it was not so simple. Cooks and diners were still influenced by the prevailing medical philosophy, but the latter itself had also changed. The simplicity and 'naturalness' so often evoked by French cookery writers, especially during the eighteenth century, was just what the doctor ordered – and by doctor we mean Cheyne. Cheyne might not have approved of 'the French style of cooking', but his dietary advice had a great influence on the *nouvelle cuisine* of the 1740s.[74] Both physicians and cooks were writing in favour of lighter, less 'doctored' foods, espousing the same broader philosophy. It is not so much that cooks were freed from medicine as such, but that medicine and cookery followed parallel paths, which led more or less in the same direction, occasionally intersecting. Cooks, like the French François Marin, continued to display a knowledge of medicine in their published works.[75] Indeed Menon (for whom no first name is known) referred explicitly to 'the work of monsieur Lémery' as having been of 'great help' in his own 'observations on the knowledge and characteristics of foods.'[76] Menon presented his cookery books as health manuals, ascribing medical qualities to different dishes and ingredients.[77] Later in the century, a cook such as the Naples-based Vincenzo Corrado was concerned enough about the link between food and health to ensure the 1786 edition of his cookery book *Il cuoco galante* had testimonials from the likes of biologist Lazzaro Spallanzani. A few years earlier Spallanzani had demonstrated the chemical role of gastric juices in the process of digestion – although here he limits himself to a few pleasantries about the variety and imagination of Corrado's recipes.[78]

For their part, physicians remained concerned with diet as a factor in health and disease, even if they were much less concerned about the minutiae of menu planning, as we have seen in this chapter. As late as 1804, the physician Alexander Hunter claimed that 'no man can be a good physician who has not a competent knowledge of cookery'.[79] His delightful *Culina formulatrix medicinæ* was that rare thing: a cookery book which happened to contain dietary advice, all penned by a doctor. Hunter returns us to the world of the prince and the physician typical of the Renaissance court, with which we began Chapter 1: the latter dishing up dietary advice for the former. Likewise, three hundred years later, Hunter's stated aim was 'to be of use to gentlemen of the medical line, by laying before them a list of the most approved dishes served up at the tables of the great', allowing them to make their recommendations 'scientifically'.[80] That said, the 'observations' following each recipe tend to be exercises in wit and the advice more culinary than medical. From his time spent training in Rouen and Paris, the Scottish-born but longtime York resident brought Continental tastes to his recipe collection.[81]

There were many reasons why the elites of Europe ate as they did and indeed why food fashions changed, and among these were a range of medical and physiological ideas. The rationale – and the practice – is the subject of the next chapter. Following on from our overview of the changing discourse of medical dietetics and preventive medicine, in these first two chapters, we now turn to a more thematic approach, in order to examine how this discourse interacted with and impacted upon the changing foods and foodways of Europe.

CHAPTER 3
RICH FOOD, POOR FOOD: DIET, PHYSIOLOGY AND SOCIAL RANK

Introduction: Sumptuary legislation

Jean Bruyérin-Champier echoed a common preoccupation of his age when he noted, in 1560, that 'it cannot be doubted how everything that was created for necessity ended up by going beyond measure and what was invented to preserve health was transformed into gluttony'.[1] This was how Bruyérin-Champier began his discussion of sumptuary laws and the restriction of luxury in ancient Rome, although he must have had an eye on his own times, too. The period from the fourteenth to the sixteenth centuries witnessed great social mobility; and, partly in response to this, the ideology of the ruling elites was particularly attentive to defining the life-styles of the different social groups which made up society. The ways of eating, dressing and living of each group were scrupulously codified.

Sumptuary laws were the result. The point of this legislation was to control people's behaviour and consumption, with the expressed intent of reducing waste and ostentation. Laws limited what could be spent on wedding banquets and other occasions involving noble families, guilds and religious brotherhoods. This campaign against waste and ostentation was in part a moral question (as it was for Bruyérin-Champier); but even more, the sumptuary laws aimed to maintain the social hierarchy, making sure those below the highest echelons did not spend above their status, and so upset the social order. Food restrictions assumed an increasing place in the legislation during the course of the sixteenth century, influenced by the reforming climate of the Reformations.[2]

Two examples will suffice to give an idea of the nature of this legislation. The motives behind the sumptuary legislation passed by England's King Henry VIII in 1518, before his break with Rome, are made quite clear in the title: 'for the puttynge a parte the excessive fare and redusynge the same to such moderacion as folowyngly ensueth'. If a cardinal was permitted nine dishes at his dinner, an archbishop was only allowed eight, marquises seven, lords six, judges and sheriffs five, and so on down the line (strangely echoing the cumulative songs of popular culture, such as 'The twelve days of Christmas'). That said, when preparing a wedding feast, all were permitted to serve six additional dishes above their allotted tariff. The legislation also detailed how many birds, and of what types, could go into a single dish. Anyone who disobeyed the legislation, 'and so following their sensual appetite ... shall not only be reputed and taken as a man of evil order, contemptuously disobeying the direction of the king's highness this council, but also to be sent for to be corrected and punished at the king's pleasure'.[3]

In the Republic of Venice the legislation was less hierarchical in tone, but just as specific. In Venice, banqueting came under the authority of a special tribunal, the *Provveditori sopra le pompe*, founded in 1515. An edict of 1562 decreed that 'at each meat dish no more than one serving of roast meat and one of boiled meat is to be served, in which there are to be no more than three types of meat'. Game animals were prohibited. On 'lean' days (those without meat, like Fridays), at lunch, 'two sorts of roast [fish] and two of boiled [fish] and two of fried, with their respective starters, salads, dairy products and the other usual and regular things' could be served; but not fish like sturgeon or trout, lake-fish, or any pastries or sweets made of sugar. The edict specified that public officials were to enforce the law by inspecting kitchens, dining chambers and the activities of cooking staff.[4]

The status hierarchies that the sumptuary legislation strove to reinforce were closely linked to traditional physiological perceptions, as we shall see in this chapter. The foods mentioned and the way of serving them were all deemed as suitable for the elites, but not for those lower down, like artisans and tradesmen, even if they were well off. The sixteenth century saw both a rise in status of the urban bourgeoisie and attempts by the ruling elites to put limits to this. If the elites could not stop the bourgeoisie's economic advance, they could at least try and prevent them from behaving like the elites.

It was the objective that is historically significant here – what the elites were attempting to achieve and why – rather than the success or failure of the sumptuary legislation. Already by Bruyérin-Champier's time there were serious challenges to the Galenic understanding of the body which underpinned the food restrictions. Furthermore, the legislation was never going to succeed in practice, given the difficulty of enforcement.[5] Even the intentions backfired. As Montaigne put it, writing two decades after Bruyérin-Champier, 'The way by which our laws attempt to regulate idle and vain expenses in meat and clothes, seems to be quite contrary to the end designed... For to enact that none but princes shall eat turbot, shall wear velvet or gold lace, and interdict these things to the people, what is it but to bring them into a greater esteem, and to set every one more agog to eat and wear them?'[6] If this could be the reaction in the late sixteenth century, by the end of the early modern period the sumptuary legislation enacted with such vigour in countries like Bruyérin-Champier's France must have seemed like ancient history indeed.

Social 'quality' and 'carnivorous Europe'

A whole range of sources – correspondence, treatises of political theory, works of fiction, studies of animal husbandry, medical and dietary literature – all share an underlying characteristic: references to food and dietary behaviour have specific social classes, categories and groups in mind. The basic assumption is that one should eat according to one's 'quality': the presumed physiological characteristics and cultural customs of each individual in society. The idea was inherited from the Greeks and Romans, as we saw in Chapter 1. Naturally, this sort of system favoured the elites; after all, the expression 'people of quality' referred exclusively to them. As a means of maintaining health and treating disease, this use of diet was evidently their privilege alone, for it required much attention, time, learning – not to mention cost. And by the late Middle Ages a new factor began to enter into the equation, when a person's quality began to refer to their *social* quality as well. The individual's quality was also determined by their position in the social hierarchy, their wealth and, above all, their power. As far as the elites were concerned, this social quality was determined at birth and it became part of one's being, the very fabric of one's body. It was as fixed and clearly defined as the social order itself. Eating certain foods, prepared in certain ways, became more than a matter of habit and choice; it assumed an expression of social identity, which the elites felt obliged to follow in order to reinforce the social order.

This social motivation was accompanied by a physiological one. The wealthy and powerful – the nobility – ate refined foods and elaborate dishes because it singled them out as wealthy and powerful; but these were also the foods that best suited their 'complexions' (their physiological make-up). The urban and rural poor, common and rustic by nature, were left with common and rustic foods. Attempts by the poor to eat above their status were always a source of ridicule in the literature of the time, as we shall see below. Not only was medical advice consistent with this ideology; it contributed to it. As early as the 1340s the physician to the duke and duchess of Savoy warned, in a regimen he wrote for the couple, that anyone not eating the food of their social condition would suffer pains and disease. Giacomo Albini, the physician's name, affirmed that the rich should avoid heavy soups made of legumes or offal (such as tripe), which he believed were of little nourishment and hard to digest. The poor, for their part, must avoid refined and choice foods, which their rustic stomachs would find difficult to absorb.[7]

From the fourteenth century, medical knowledge thus reinforced the position of the elites. It was a time when the privileges of the elites were being threatened: by peasant revolts, by the rise of the urban bourgeoisie and by a rising tide of prosperity associated, rather paradoxically, with the tragedy of the Black Death, which came to Europe around the same time Albini was writing his regimen. Plague brought with it a sharp decline of population throughout the latter fourteenth century. Successive epidemics of plague reduced the population by somewhere between a third and a half of pre-plague levels. The immediate effects of this catastrophic mortality was that few people were left to produce the food, leading to famine and further death; however, over the longer term, there was a marked increase in the quantity, quality and variety of foods available to the average person. Because of the shortage of labour, working conditions improved, with an end to serfdom and wage rises.

Surplus income meant that more could be spent on food, with meat topping the list. Such was the shift that the social historian Fernand Braudel referred to the period 1350–1550 as the era of 'carnivorous Europe'.[8] Fresh pork and a huge variety of salted, smoked and otherwise cured pork products were more plentiful than ever. Writing in 1560, on the cusp of a downward shift, Bruyérin-Champier took for granted the French peasant's consumption of smoked pork lard, pork chops 'and, in general, the whole animal'.[9] Beef was also common. In Italy it was a cheap by-product of the ever-growing market for leather goods, such that the hides of the animals were more valuable than their meat. In Italian towns even people earning the lowest wages, such as street-sweepers and laundresses, could afford to eat meat often (a situation not matched again in Italy until well after the Second World War). Servants ate beef regularly, almost daily, and it was served three times a week in charity hospitals.

A certain amount of social mixing was the result, particularly within noble households. Just as they were given access to much the same medical provision, household members (including domestic staff) might share food from the same pot. The household of Richard Cholmley, courtier to Henry VIII from 1539, provides an example: 'Always like to have a great train of menials about his person', according to the family chronicler, in order to make an impression, Cholmley nevertheless permitted 'the idle serving men … going into the kitchen [who] would use their liberty to stick their daggers into the pot and take out the beef without the leave or privacy of the cook'. Such was Cholmley's generosity and largesse that 'there used to be as often as many as twenty four pieces of beef put in the morning in the pot, yet sometimes it so happened that but one would be left for Sir Richard's own dinner'.[10]

Outside the confines of the household, the response of the elites to this state of affairs was to reinforce their privileged position, by limiting access to power by non-noble groups. The result was a closure of ranks and exclusion of the 'populace' from the pleasures of the banquet (other than as occasional onlookers). The banquet became, for the elites, a way of celebrating themselves, of self-representation and social discrimination, a means for expressing and demonstrating power. Through the banquet, the prince showed his ability to organize a well-orchestrated table around himself, with the right people seated at his side, people who administer the tools of government, just as they eat the quantities of food elaborately prepared and served, by small armies of cooks and assistants.

With the Renaissance, ostentation became the defining mark of the tables of the rich and powerful.[11] Of course, a certain element of ostentation had always been present at their tables, but now it became an end in itself, the main feature. This ostentation was symptomatic of a deep social, political and cultural shift: a sign of the increasing separation, the increasing distance, between the ruler and the ruled. As a result, the banqueting table ceased to be the site of social cohesion around the leader it had been in the Middle Ages and became more and more the site of separation and exclusion.

When the nobleman and ruler of Bologna, Giovanni II Bentivoglio, celebrated the marriage of his son with Lucrezia d'Este in 1487, he had a grand banquet organized in the city. As the chronicler of the event Cherubino Ghirardacci wrote, 'Before the dishes were served, they were first carried with much pomp around the square in front of the palace to show them before the people, so that they could see so much magnificence for themselves'.[12] Needless to say, the 'people' could only look. Bentivoglio's court was famous even then for its splendour and festivities, but they stood in stark contrast with the poverty of most of the city's inhabitants. The wedding banquet itself, as described by the chronicler, lasted seven hours, during which a dazzling array of elaborate and bizarre dishes were served. All of this was paraded in front of the eyes of the hungry populace before it was brought in to the guests. That said, many of these things even the guests would only have looked at, rather than eaten. Not even the most gourmandizing of appetites would have been able to sample everything. The dishes were not served one after another, in succession, but brought in and placed on display together, in groups, with each guest choosing from these according to his or her own preferences. Above all, guests were expected to admire – just like the populace – the abundance and magnificence of the dishes, and to be amazed by the sheer spectacle of the meal, like a theatre (Figure 3.1).

Various routes allowed this banqueting style and associated cookery to spread from the Renaissance courts of Italy throughout the rest of Europe, as Philippe Meyzie has

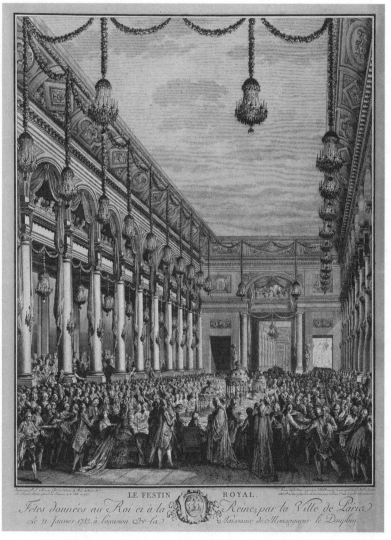

Figure 3.1 'Le festin royal': banquet given by the city of Paris to celebrate the birth of the dauphin. Engraving by J.-M. Moreau after P.-L. Moreau, 1782 (Wellcome Library, London).

suggested.[13] The publication and translation of numerous cookery books, by the likes of Bartolomeo Scappi and Bartolomeo Sacchi (better known as Platina), was one way. Another involved political and social connections, such as the contribution made by the Angevin and later, Aragonese, kings of Naples and Sicily to the transmission of this cuisine to Spain and the French Valois court.

Elite dining styles and medical theory: I

Some of the earliest printed regimens were written by court physicians. As participants in courtly life, they were not overtly critical of its alimentary excesses: that would have been biting the hand that fed them. But they did try to ensure that lip-service was paid to Galenic advice, even if courtly cuisine was in the process of developing an aesthetic pretty much opposed to dietary theory. In 1515 there was still enough common ground for the physician Michele Savonarola to produce a dietary manual for the Este court in Ferrara, where he was court physician. The short work combined medical and culinary concerns, outlining 'all the things which are commonly eaten; which are unfavourable and which beneficial; and how they are prepared', to quote the title.[14]

This harmony was not destined to last. Consider the court of England's Henry VIII, which abounded with the latest regimens and dietetical advice. When it came to physical exercise the king was duly active, but when it came to diet he was a man of gargantuan appetite (with a taste for red meat) and an ever-expanding girth, with predictable consequences for the state of his health and well-being which the court medical practitioners were obliged to deal with.[15] His sumptuary legislation long behind him, Henry's obesity became the subject of ridicule by Catholic propagandists, who linked his unrestrained gourmandizing to his break with Rome.[16] But Henry and his court were in no way unique, such that during the sixteenth and early seventeenth centuries the most persistent dietary critiques revolved around princely courts. The medical writers of the dietary manuals no longer considered themselves aspirants to this uppermost culture, as they were less and less connected to courtly patrons. They increasingly disassociated themselves from the luxurious eating style and symbols of courtly refinement and rejected the most extravagant foods. They had nothing to lose in making these condemnations, and perhaps they were just a little chagrined at finding themselves excluded.[17] How much notice the elites took is another matter.

The prevailing image is that of courts 'addicted to ... voluptuousness and bellychere', happy 'to wallow in their disordered and lascivious appetites, tendryng and cockeryng their wanton carcasses', as do 'a great many princes and potentates who live without checke at their pleasure and ease'.[18] These harsh words were written by Guglielmo Grataroli, an Italian Protestant physician exiled in Switzerland. Gluttony and perverse tastes, combined with sloth, typified the condemnations of medical writers. Magnificent fowl such as peacocks, swans and pheasants were stereotypical foods served at court, but increasingly condemned by dietary writers as tough and difficult to digest, as were large fish like sturgeon and aphrodisiac foods or anything overly expensive, especially when done to excess. And if individual foodstuffs were condemned, so too was the banqueting of which they were a part: surfeit, inebriation, a harmful variety of foods, and expensive and unhealthy dishes eaten without order late into the night.

The dietaries provided moral lessons aplenty of courtly banqueters unable or unwilling to restrain their appetites. In Thomas Moffett's late sixteenth-century regimen they all seem to revolve around European dukes. Writing on chickens, then a rare luxury, Moffett related their reputation for 'stirring up lust' this way: 'For which purpose Boleslaus duke of Silesia did eat thirteen cock chickens at a meal; whereof he died, without having his purpose fulfilled'. And Moffett warned his readers about strawberries thus: 'Let every man take heed by Melchior duke of Brunswick how he eateth too much of them, who is reported to have burst usunder at Rostock with his surfeiting upon them'. Elsewhere, Moffett mentions 'Switrigalus Duke of Lithuania [who] never sat fewer then six hours at dinner and as many at supper', although we can only imagine what happened to him.[19] Closer to real life, and to demonstrate that not only dukes might be subject to such urges, the family of cardinal Bernardino Spada put his death down to his gorging on snails in autumn of 1661, 'ignoring the capon and other substantial foods'.[20] More famously, the death of emperor Charles VI in 1740, according to Voltaire, was caused by 'an indigestion of mushrooms that caused him an apoplexy; this death of mushrooms changed the destiny of Europe'.[21] In this case, rather than a surfeit of mushrooms, the cause may have been eating poisonous ones.

Medical advice and social rank

In his section on chickens, Moffett also made another significant point. They were 'so pure and fine a meat' that 'no man I think is so foolish as to commend them to ploughmen and besomers'.[22] Such food would corrupt in the strong stomachs of peasants and sweepers before being digested. As light foods, as well as luxuries, chickens were best suited to the more delicate stomachs of the social elites. Advice originally meant to distinguish hot constitutions from weak and cold ones had, by the end of the sixteenth century, become a matter of social distinction, if not outright prejudice. In his autobiographical discussion of his own regimen (1576), the polymath Girolamo Cardano wrote, 'I am especially fond of the wings of young chickens'.[23] Centuries before 'Buffalo-style chicken wings', what is today virtually a waste product of battery farming was then available only to, and suitable for, the elites.

But let us return to Moffett. Perhaps no more prejudiced than his medical colleagues, just more detailed, Moffett makes frequent class references with regard to foodstuffs. Rye was suitable 'for labourers, servants and workmen, but heavy of digestion to indifferent stomachs'. Herring 'give none or a bad nourishment, saving to ploughmen, sailers, souldiers, mariners, or labouring persons, to whom gross and heavy meats [foods] are most familiar and convenient'. Conversely, there was 'no meat so wholsom' as pheasant, 'but to strong stomacks it is inconvenientest, especially to ploughmen and labourers, who eating of phesants, fall suddenly into sickness, and shortness of breath, as Pisanellus hath wittily (and perhaps truely) noted'.[24] The wit in Pisanelli's reference to the dire effects of pheasants on peasants is lost on me, but Moffett evidently appreciated it.

Just as certain foods were deemed unfit for peasants, so others were deemed unfit for the elites. A whole range of foods was banned from 'high table' on the basis of their association with those who worked. It would seem that with price rises in fresh food, peasants were more and more constrained to eat sausages and preserved or salted meats – if they were able to eat meat at all – and salted fish. Fresh meat became more of a luxury item, and indeed, dietary manuals of this time welcomed no other form. Likewise organ meats were now off limits to elite palates, in part because they were considered difficult to digest and in part because they were considered edible only by a certain class of people. Moreover, a number of foods previously eaten by all ranks in society were now consistently stigmatized in the dietary manuals: porridges, gruels, pottages and beans.

This perception developed partly because the diet of the poor got worse during the early modern period. And, as the lower classes became more impoverished, their diet became more distinctive. The foods they ate became more obvious symbols of poverty and to eat these foods became a clearer act of debasement, especially for those who should have been able to afford better.

The late-medieval diet had been relatively varied for all parts of the population, with a large proportion of this derived from meat and other animal products, fats and wine, as we have seen. But this relative prosperity could not last forever. By the early 1500s, Europe's population had more or less recovered from the Black Death. Plague had not gone away, of course; but local populations recovered faster and more fully from epidemics than they had previously done. Increasing population put a strain on resources. Wages stagnated, and then fell, in relation to the cost of living. Grain prices kept rising, with the result that bread eventually became so expensive that there was little to spend on other foods. Consumption on meat and wine by the poor and middling classes dropped from the middle of the sixteenth century and cereals, always the cheapest source of nourishment, came to dominate the popular diet, at the expense of other foodstuffs.

In response to rapidly growing demand for cereals, new lands were put under cultivation. In the Low Countries, the building of dikes and drainage canals allowed agriculture near the coast. New staple foods were also developed in response to the increasing demand, such as rice. Grown in Spain, where it had been introduced by the Arabs, it spread to parts of northern Italy and the Low Countries. Another new foodstuff was buckwheat. Not actually new, having been in Western Europe for some two centuries, but it was in the sixteenth century that the use of buckwheat spread throughout much of Europe: the Low Countries, Germany, France and northern Italy. The European encounter with the New World also brought two new products, maize and potatoes, whose impact will be discussed in Chapter 7. Finally, there were also a few improvements in agricultural techniques, such as more efficient ploughs and better irrigation.

Yields remained low, however; and, in any case, none of these developments was enough to counter Europe's population expansion. For example, the population of

Castile doubled between 1530 and 1591, going from three to six million.[25] During this time Castile went from being a net exporter of wheat to a situation where it was forced to import it, buying from English and Dutch merchants. Meat also increased in cost, due in part to the expansion of cereal cultivation, at the expense of pasture, combined with population increase and decline of salaries. It has been estimated that in Germany meat consumption went down from a high of 100 kg per head of population in the fourteenth and fifteenth centuries to a historical minimum of 14 kg between the eighteenth and nineteenth centuries.[26] Butchers were forced out of business. Braudel gives the example of the small French town of Montpezat whose only slightly declining population supported 18 butchers in 1550, 10 in 1556, 6 in 1641, 2 in 1660 and just one in 1763.[27] Formerly, veal had been for the master and beef for the servants; but by 1650 the real distinction was between those who ate quantities of meat (any meat) on a regular basis, and those who did not. The effect was particularly pronounced in southern Europe, whereas in parts of northern Europe the decline in meat consumption was less marked, such as Hungary, Poland and England.

Declining meat consumption was not lost on contemporaries. Gilles de Gouberville, a country squire in Normandy, wrote in 1560 (in his journal), 'In my father's day people ate meat every day, the servings were large and wine was drunk like water. Today everything's changed; everything is dear, the diet of the best off peasants [today] is worse than that of the servants of yesterday'.[28] We find the same sentiment expressed in a Swabian source from 1550. If the statement is a commonplace, it is because it reflects a widespread perception. Frenchmen reminisced for a time when King Henri IV was supposed to have said that he wanted the people of France to dine every Sunday on stewed chicken (*poule-au-pot*). Whether the king said it or not, it evoked an image of well-being dimly remembered by his oldest subjects and later inscribed in village traditions as part of a lost golden age.[29]

There was a positive side to this, though one no doubt appreciated more by the medical writers than by the peasants themselves. Medical writers of the sixteenth and seventeenth centuries tended to envy the peasants their simplicity, which spared them the harmful effects of overly rich and sophisticated dishes. Bruyérin-Champier went so far as to compare peasant foodways to those of all people during a long-gone 'golden age': 'virtuous in flavour, honest and close to nature'. 'Indeed [peasants] live and content themselves with their cereals, their fruits and the produce of the land'. This regime rendered them 'virtuous and honest, such that in the countryside we see men living longer and in more robust health'.[30] As physician to two French kings (Francis I and Henri II), perhaps Bruyérin-Champier should have got out a bit more.

Access to fresh meat defined early modern elites, in their own eyes as much as in the eyes of others, serving as a point of social distinction. Elite institutions like the French convent school of Saint-Cyr insisted on meat – beef, veal and mutton – as a standard part of the fare for the aristocratic girls in their care. And when hard times came or when the demands posed by an increasing sweet tooth during the eighteenth century competed with meat in the convent's budget, they simply made do with more game meats.[31] A cycle of rising prosperity in the late eighteenth century provided a taste of this aristocratic model for a broadening sector of the population. Meat consumption rose once again, towards the end of the early modern period, and especially in northern Europe. In Zurich, an inquiry of 1772 reported that 'several years ago' 1,400–1,500 bullocks were enough to feed the city each year, whereas 2,600–2,700 were now needed. The same trend was evident in Paris, where annual per capita meat consumption rose from 51 to 61 kg during the second half of the eighteenth century.[32]

Our daily bread

Nothing evinces the divide between rich and poor in early modern Europe more than bread. At once unifying, in that it was eaten (or at least desired) by everyone, it was also divisive. So important was bread, in both the reality and the imaginary, at all levels of society, that one could recount the history of Europe and its people through bread. As the staple par excellence, imbued with religious symbolism, it reflects the ideologies, beliefs and aspirations of the entire period. In Christian art, particularly in Catholic art, Christ distributing bread to his disciples at the Last Supper is considered one of the most exalted subjects; and the highest form of bread for early modern painters was *risen* bread, not the unleavened bread commanded by Moses which Jesus would have eaten during Passover.

According to the regimens, the best bread was made of hard wheat, well milled and sieved, made into a dough properly salted, kneaded, well risen, before being well baked in an oven and cooled. Anything of mixed flour, containing too much bran, was thus inferior, as was anything unsalted, unrisen or burnt. This view went back to the ancients; but what was new, right from the start of the early modern period, was an increasing concern with establishing a hierarchy of bread. Regimens differentiated between the kinds of cereal used, as well as the corresponding elements of society to which they were best suited physiologically. If barley bread could still be praised in the late fifteenth century, by the seventeenth century it was generally lumped together with bread made of 'inferior cereals' like rye, oats, millet and spelt. This is the context for Samuel Johnson's famous dictionary definition of *oats*: 'a grain, which in England is generally given to horses, but in Scotland supports the people'.[33] The description reveals both Johnson's low opinion of the Scots and his low opinion of oats. As this suggests, there was also a geography of bread. Two main European regions existed (with substantial overlap, it has to be said): one in which the idealized bread was white, made from wheat, well risen and cooked (France, Italy, England and part of Spain), and another where bread was dark and contained rye and sometimes spices (Poland, Germany and most of central and eastern Europe) (Figure 3.2).

The Spanish, for example, considered bread – preferably wheat bread – the central component of their daily food intake. Although they also ate meat, fish and vegetables, they could only conceive of these as supplements to bread, not as substitutes for it. Hence their utter amazement when, in the New World, they came face-to-face with people who 'did not know what bread was'.[34] Here, Spaniards could find themselves surrounded by

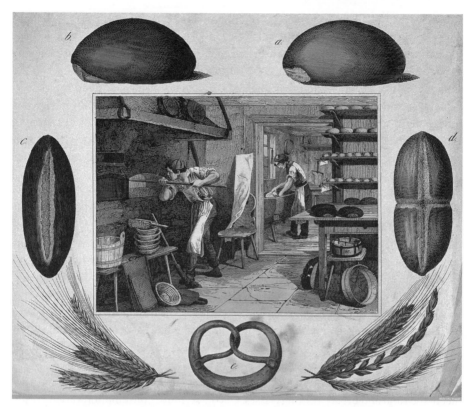

Figure 3.2 Bakers and bread types. Coloured etching, late eighteenth century (Wellcome Library, London).

fish and fruit but still starve for the lack of wheat bread. Travelling in South America in the late eighteenth century, the Spanish soldier and naturalist Félix de Azara was regarded as 'unique in Europe' because he omitted bread from his diet, although in his case it was due to a wheat intolerance.[35]

Geography intersected with class. Dark or inferior bread was not just what a peasant could afford; it was also what was judged best for his rustic constitution, as the doctor-agronomist Charles Estienne, edited by Jean Liébault, suggested:

> The bread that is made of wheat meale whole and intire, as from which there is nothing taken by temze [sifting], is fit and meet for hindes [agricultural labourers] and other workefolkes, as delvers [tillers], porters, and such other persons as are in continuall travell [labour], because they have neede of such like food, as consisteth of a grosse [coarse], thicke, and clammie iuice, and in like manner such bread fitteth them best, which hath no leven in it, is not much baked, but remaineth somewhat doughie and clammie, and which besides is made of the meale of *secourgeon* [barley flour], of rie mingled with wheat, of chesnuts, rice, beanes, and such other grosse sort of pulse.

And perhaps there is an element of truth in this advice, to the extent that the hungry have always sought out heavy foods, which give a welcome sensation of satiety. The elites, by contrast, were recommended white bread: 'made of the flower of the meale, being the purest and finest part thereof, [it] is good for idle and unlaboured persons, such as are students, monkes, canons and other fine and daintie persons, which stand in neede to be fed with food of light and easie digestion'.[36] Just over a century later, the advice was little changed, although the gloss put on it was more positive and the medical reasoning behind it quite different. The German iatromechanic physician Friedrich Hoffmann praised Westphalian pumpernickel bread, made from rye, as the ideal nutriment for those engaged in hard physician labour.[37]

Medical theory reflected social reality: over the course of the early modern period the quality of bread actually declined in may parts of Europe. For instance, in the late 1400s farm workers in the Languedoc region of southern France were eating white bread with their meat and consuming liberal amounts of olive oil and red wine. Three generations later, meat rations had fallen drastically, wine and olive oil consumption had also dropped, and white bread had been largely replaced by dark loaves, made mostly with barley and rye.[38] In Geneva, where once the flour sold at market had been exclusively wheat, this was now seconded by spelt flour: an indication that cereals considered inferior were becoming increasingly common among the middling ranks of society. At a time when culinary choices were rapidly multiplying for the elites, the popular diet was becoming much less varied, nutritious and plentiful.

Bread consumption also went up, becoming a more significant proportion of the daily diet of the rural and urban working classes. Of course, bread consumption varied greatly from place to place, from year to year (according to price) and from season to season (given that supplies are scarcest in spring). Overall, however, it has been calculated that from the fourteenth to the sixteenth centuries daily average bread consumption was around 500–600 grams per person – assuming there was no famine, of course. By the seventeenth century consumption had increased to around 800 grams, and this would get still higher during the eighteenth.[39] All the sources we have, which are necessarily fragmentary, suggest the predominance of bread and other cereals in the diets of European peasants, something like 80 per cent of all caloric intake.

This dependence on cereals explains why famines had such calamitous effects, particularly during the seventeenth and eighteenth centuries. During famines town governments would do their utmost to buy in extra supplies of flour, to keep the inhabitants from rioting. In the countryside there was no such provision, however, so the rural poor would flock to the towns in the hope of finding food, dispensed by religious charities. The towns would be overwhelmed, and would have to take drastic measures. In 1693, for example, the Calvinist city of Geneva had 3,300 refugees, welcomed there for religious reasons, half of whom were receiving poor relief. When that year's harvest proved particularly bad, these refugees were asked to leave the city. Although many of them were elderly, women or children, who had no other place to go, Geneva's city council decided to cancel all forms of poor relief, hoping this would force them to leave the city before the onset of winter.[40]

The predominance of cereals in peasant diets was much more pronounced than in the diets of the elites. The elites could afford more and better cereals than the peasantry but they ate less bread because they could afford other foodstuffs. And the bread they did eat was different than the bread eaten lower down the social scale. Bread was a social marker, effectively dividing European society into the haves and the have-nots (albeit with various gradations of 'haves-less' in between). The bread of the elites was white, that of the peasants generally dark. There were a handful of exceptions to this: for instance, Sicily and Provence were rich in wheat and so the peasants here benefited. Otherwise, the lower down the social scale, the darker the bread became, a bread hierarchy mirroring the social hierarchy. At the lower rungs it contained more bran (the hull of the grain), which made it darker and rougher, and frequently this wheat flour was mixed with cheaper flours, like barley or rye, to make it go further. So common was this that it had its own name in English: maslin. Depending on the region, flour made from chestnuts, chick-peas or broad beans might be added to wheat flour, especially in times of dearth.

In 1617 the Bolognese writer Giulio Cesare Croce represented the distinction between 'wheat bread' and 'bean bread' in the form of a literary disputation between the two categories, pitching town against country. 'I reside in the cities', boasts Wheat Bread to Bean Bread:

> In the minds of kings, emperors
> Princes, dukes and marquises
> I appear, and have graces and favours among them.

'Go back to dwelling in your lairs', Wheat Bread tells Bean Bread: 'you are so dark/ Wretched to digest, coarse and hard / ... go back outside, among the peasants'. Wheat Bread continues:

> And whoever still persists in tasting you,
> For three days seems to have a rock on his chest,
> So much does your food irritate and harden.
> And in passing through, and dropping out below,
> He who knows says so, whether or not there is suffering,
> And if one remains weak and weary.

For his part, Bean Bread boasts of feeling 'much better among the peasants./The peasants know how to knead me better/... [they] make me big, fat, round and even'. The two agree that each should stick to where he is best appreciated, Wheat Bread in the town, Bean Bread in the country.[41]

It has even been suggested that the poor quality of the bread kept the peasants who ate in a state of stupor, a 'collective vertigo' in Piero Camporesi's words.[42] Some of the grass weeds that grew in the wheat fields are mildly hallucinogenic, such as darnel. Other grasses were added on purpose to extend flour, such as vetches (a small legume), poppy seeds, lupins and broad beans. The bread may have been heavy and unsavoury, but whether it was hallucinogenic because of that, is another matter. That said, we can document one serious disease that did occur because of bad bread, and that is ergotism, which results from eating rye which has been tainted with the ergot fungus. Ergotism causes hallucinations, burning sensations, gangrene and even death.

A final difference between the bread of the peasants and the bread of the elites, not generally mentioned in contemporary sources, was freshness. While the elites ate bread fresh every day, the peasants baked theirs once a week, or once a fortnight, in order to save on scarce firewood, labour and duties payable to the landlord for use of the oven. In certain Alpine valleys bread was baked once or twice a year, in huge loaves with a thick crust. In the Dauphiné mountains it was baked into large loaves which dried so hard they needed to be cut with a hatchet before being dunked in the soup. Eating hard, stale bread was no easy task, but it helps explain the watery soups that so often accompanied it. This combination of bread and soup, and the large pots to cook them in mentioned in peasant inventories, gives an idea of monotony. If European peasant diets did not have the variety of elite diets, the ingredients that went with the bread or into the soup can be extremely varied. Understanding what accompanies the bread is essential to understanding rural diets.

Another solution was to cook the flour mixture, unrisen, in the hearth, resulting in a sort of flatbread, all too often burnt on the outside and raw on the inside. Of course, Europeans consumed cereals in other ways too, which in some regions were more common than baking. A small amount of whatever grain would be roughly crushed, cooked in a liquid (such as water or milk), with minimal fuel, to provide a nourishing meal. Such were frumenty, gruel, porridge, hasty pudding: the variety of names in English alone suggesting the prevalence of this type of dish. If Galen (echoed by Johnson) had viewed oats as fit only for beasts of burden, Thomas Cogan confidently boasted of their consumption in Northern England, alongside barley, much to the benefit of the local population.[43] (Mind you, Cogan seems much more enthusiastic about their use in ale.)

What can explain the shift in favour towards oats? It was due in part to Cogan's willingness to question Galen in the light of his own experience of English diets, a theme we shall revisit in Chapter 4. But it was also due to a shift from the use of whole oats in Galen's time to hulled oats by Cogan's time. These had been only 'recently invented by doctors', according to Bruyérin-Champier (1560). 'Rich and poor alike consume them often during Lent', he notes. Bruyérin-Champier is very careful to distinguish – unlike Samuel Johnson writing two hundred years later – between whole oats, about whose use he follows Galen, and hulled oats, of which he is quite favourable. Indeed Bruyérin-Champier describes an oatmeal porridge he Latinizes as *avenatus* that was 'appreciated at the most elegant tables'. 'Cow's or goat's milk is added [to shelled oats], or the milk of sweet almonds, as well as sugar, which gives it a most agreeable taste, so that it is absolutely delicious and very healthy to eat'.[44] The way had been prepared for the French physician Louis Lémery to view oatmeal porridge as 'a food very pleasing to the taste, and very wholesome'. By no means suited for labourers alone, it agreed 'at all times, with every age, and all sorts of constitutions', in Lémery's words.[45]

By the end of the eighteenth century a Scottish physician felt bound to recommend a return to such dishes, which had been largely abandoned, at least in England, replaced by a diet of buttered white bread and tea. As far as William Buchan was concerned, the 'lower orders' ate far too much bread, which was the principal cause of their poor health, for too much bread filled up the alimentary canal and dragged the 'nutritious juices' of other foods along with it.[46] A case of too much of a good thing? Not really, in Buchan's view. The dream of the European poor had come true in England: that of being able to subsist on white bread. This was a problem: not because it did not suit their constitutions, as would have been argued in previous centuries, but, Buchan argued, because white bread contained less nourishment and because it was the milling and baking of white bread which were the most open to fraud. This was made worse by what Englishmen and women ate with their bread. 'The French consume vast quantities of bread', Buchan noted; 'but its bad effects are prevented by their copious use of soups and fruits, which have little or no share in the diet of the common people of England'.[47] Indeed, French medical writers regarded only stale bread as potentially harmful, which when eaten in large amounts could cause potentially fatal indigestions.[48] But the English, to return to Buchan, usually ate their bread with salted meat or, worse still, with tea, which 'the lower orders make a diet of'.[49]

What had formerly been deemed suitable only for labourers was now, at least in Buchan's view, the best of all: 'The best household bread I ever remember to have ate, was in the county of York. It was what they call *meslin bread*, and consisted of wheat and rye ground together .... This bread, when well fermented, eats light, is of pleasant taste, and soluble to the bowels'.[50] Buchan is writing from personal experience here, but he is writing *for* the 'lower orders'. So it turns out that the best breads for working people are those made with mixed cereals. The rationale for Buchan's recommendation was different, now based on mechanical and environmental health ideas, as well as enlightened physiocratic theories about how to feed the most people. Yet the general advice remained the same as that offered by Galenic doctors three hundred years earlier. 'For the more active and laborious', Buchan recommended 'a mixture of rye with the stronger grains, as pease, beans, barley, oats, Indian corn and the like'.[51] Better even than mixed bread was a return to the porridges, hasty puddings and vegetable soups of the past.

'Grosse Meate is Meete for Grosse Men': Vegetables and legumes

Buchan also had great things to say about leeks. 'The leek is not so generally used any where as it deserves to be', Buchan wrote; 'there is no ingredient goes into soup that is more wholesome or that gives a better flavour'.[52] Once again, he had the food of the poor in mind here. The medical opinion of leeks three hundred years earlier was much more negative; but the difference is more apparent than real, since they share a viewpoint based on class. The words of this section's title are those of the Manchester schoolmaster Thomas Cogan, writing à propos of leeks in 1584.[53] Cogan uses a fine bit of word-play to convey the idea that their coarse texture rendered leeks hard to digest, which in turn made them suited only to the strong stomachs of equally coarse people. Medical theories had changed over three centuries but the lucky eaters of leeks remained the poor. In his 1583 dietary, Baldassare Pisanelli describes many vegetables, in addition to the leek, as fit only for 'those who labour a lot', 'for rustic people', 'to give to peasants [*villani*]': cabbage, radishes, broad beans and beans.[54]

Vegetables and legumes were closely associated with the peasant consumption of cereals and seen in similar terms by medical authors. Vegetables were mostly consumed in the form of a pottage, anything from a thin soup to a thicker stew, the liquid of which was usually flavoured with roots and herbs, and wherever possible, a small piece of meat, usually salt-pork, and accompanied the consumption of bread. Dried legumes were classed as cereals in the regimens and, like cereals, also went into the making of soups, porridges and bread. In mountainous areas of Europe – in Spain, France, Italy, Germany and elsewhere – stands of chestnut tree were carefully managed and their fruit took the place of legumes as the staple foodstuff of the poor. It was eaten like a legume, either fresh or, when dried, was used the rest of the year, boiled, roasted, cooked in stews or turned into a flour (which could then be made into a coarse heavy bread on its own, or mixed with wheat flour). The familiar winter sight of sellers of roast chestnuts in many of our cities is all that remains of a once-thriving trade in chestnuts, transporting them from southern Europe to northern European ports.

When it comes to legumes, we should distinguish between Old World beans, which existed from antiquity, and New World beans. The beans grown by Europeans before the sixteenth century were the broad bean (fava) and the black-eyed bean (or black-eyed pea). Prior to the Columbian exchange, the black-eyed bean was called *phaseolus* in Latin, and this, rather confusingly, was the name applied to all the New World species of bean when they arrived in Europe.[55] This is a sign of how quickly and how easily New World species of bean entered the European food chain (something we shall return to in Chapter 7). Beans were a very important food, particularly for the poor, and for everyone during Lent and on other holy days when no meat could be eaten. When dried, they could last through winter and be boiled into soups, mashed or cooked into other dishes. Although legumes were one of the most frequently eaten foods during the early modern and modern periods, medical opinion was hostile to them, as we have seen. They were considered a 'gross' (heavy and coarse) foodstuff, difficult to digest and the cause of flatulence. Only labourers were thought to have stomachs strong enough to digest them, to the extent that 'bean-eater' became an abusive label.

There was one leguminous exception, enthusiastically eaten by all ranks, and that was the pea. For Pisanelli, peas were 'pleasing to the taste, stimulate the appetite, cleanse the chest, ease a cough and provide good nourishment'. For Giacomo Castelvetro they were 'the noblest of vegetables'.[56] And as this suggests, social distinction managed to find a way in. The poor ate peas out of necessity and they were invariably dried. They were then cooked with water as needed, a dish known in England as a 'pease pottage' – but every region of Europe had its variant. The resulting mush could also be used to bulk out flour in bread-making, as Cogan remarked: 'the bread which is made of [peas] is unwholesome, yet it is much used in Leicestershire'. (I have been unable to verify this.)

Cogan concludes, 'But I leave it to rustickes, who have stomaches like ostriges, than can digest hard yron'.[57]

If rustics had their peas-bread and pottage, the elites had something entirely different: fresh, shelled, green peas. This was part of Europe-wide turn towards vegetables by the elites, that began in Renaissance Italy, which we shall explore further in Chapter 6. Cardano wrote that, in Lombardy, peas 'are greatly esteemed among nobles and have risen to the most lavish banquets of princes'.[58] The court of King Louis XIV of France was mad about fresh peas, from the moment a courtier named Audiger brought a hamper back from Genoa, in January 1660, and presented it to the king and his courtiers, to the attempts by royal gardener La Quintinie to raise out-of-season green peas in the glasshouses of Versailles.[59]

The rage for vegetables suggests how fashions in food were quicker to change than medical opinions. In the regimens, ideas about particular foodstuffs tended to withstand the decline of Galenism and its replacement by chemical or mechanical medicine. Lémery – who used the language of essential, volatile or pungent salts, earth and phlegm, and oils – nevertheless reached the same conclusion as the Galenists about a wide range of foods. Lémery's foods that are heavy, nourishing, windy and so suited 'to those who have a good stomach' are the familiar ones: chestnuts, beans, millet, radishes and turnips, for example.[60] At least Lémery's sense of experimentalism spared the leek (as Buchan would later do). 'We do not find, though much used amongst us', Lémery concluded, 'that [the leek] produces all those ill effects that are attributed to it'.[61] Gone is the preoccupation with rank and a direct association between the 'quality' of the person and their digestive ability of their stomach, pervasive one hundred years earlier. If Lémery's elites still get to have fresh green peas to themselves, this is probably due to a question of supply and demand: 'the smaller and greener they are, the better their taste; and thus they are serv'd to the tables of people of quality, and such as are for nice eating'.[62] In Lémery there is no sense that light foods like chicken or pheasant were harmful to strong stomachs, as had once been the case, but they were instead recommended as suitable for all.[63]

Just bread and beans?

It is tempting to take from the preceding discussions of bread and beans that urban and rural labourers ate a drab, unvaried and unchanging diet, leaving them constantly hungry or under-nourished. To a certain extent this is true. There is no doubting that the behaviour of the rural and urban poor was shaped by a culture of hunger and that a reliance on cereals put the poor at immediate risk in case of harvest failure. However, this *vision misérabiliste*, dwelling on an assumed peasant wretchedness – so beloved of demographic and social historians and followers of the *Annales* school of the 1950s and 60s, with its emphasis on food quantities and calorie-counting – may have gone too far to counter the previously held rosy ideal of peasant self-sufficiency. As Florent Quellier has suggested, popular diets were much more varied, more open to the outside and more dynamic than is often assumed.[64] Their diets remained embedded in the culture of hunger while being open to variety and new flavours, and were never entirely cut off from the usages of the rest of society. Other sources of nourishment – derived from gifts, harvesting and gleaning, poaching and petty theft, the keeping of small kitchen gardens – supplemented peasant diets.[65] Variety also came in the form of the many feast days and celebrations, which served to offset the reality of hunger, albeit temporarily.

Two examples of such possibilities are the important place of mushrooms in peasant diets, free for the taking (with a bit of expertise), and the domestic production of cheese. In his *Traité des champignons* (1793), the French physician Jean-Jacques Paulet noted how in Tuscany, and in particular around Florence, 'the inhabitants of the countryside were particularly well-versed in the knowledge of these plants', bringing some three hundred different varieties of mushroom to market. Aside from Tuscans, the Europeans who ate the most mushrooms were Hungarians, Poles, Bavarians 'and Germans in general'.[66] Mushrooms were enjoyed by rich and poor alike, throughout the period, despite the dangers posed by accidentally ingesting poisonous varieties. If Pisanelli had warned that 'they are never good at any time [of the year], age or for any complexion, because they do more harm than good', he nevertheless had to admit that 'they are highly esteemed at table, because they generate appetite and take on all the flavours given to them'.[67] After two centuries of mycological investigations, identifying and classifying safe and dangerous mushroom varieties, Paulet could afford to be much more enthusiastic.[68] Paulet noted how mushrooms evidently contained 'a juice capable of nourishing'. Curiously, Paulet's preference for the whiter varieties suggests an ongoing prejudice against dark-coloured foodstuffs, one in contrast with clarity and brightness promised in by the Enlightenment.[69]

Cheese, produced domestically, also had an important place in European peasant diets and, like mushrooms, added both variety and nourishment. As the physician Louis Guyon put it in the sixteenth century, 'cheese is good for workers, labourers, soldiers and others hardened to labour because it takes a long time to be digested and prevents hunger from returning quickly; which is why the poor use it instead of any other fare or food and why, of the diverse quantities of fat and aged cheeses that are found, they devour them like everything else and are not made ill by them'.[70] Cheese was part of the peasant imagination, a stock element of the Land of Cockaigne. 'Bread and cheese, curds and whey/The bumpkin eats the live-long day', went the rhymes of the Dutch *Kerelslied* (Peasants' Song).[71] It was also part of peasant reality. Small-scale domestic production brought in much-needed income and augmented the family diet. It has been estimated that at the turn of the sixteenth century, half of all rural households and up to one third of urban households in Holland produced butter and cheese – though how much was sold and how much was consumed at home is another matter, given the market for Dutch cheese, especially throughout northern Europe (Figure 3.3).[72]

The rustic associations of cheese help explain why the elites were advised to avoid it. When the hot-tempered Bolognese painter Guido Reni was sent, by one of his patrons, an entire round of 'cheese of Piacenza brought up to him by two porters',

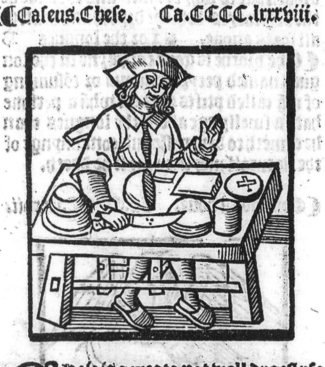

Caſeus.Cheſe.　Ca.CCCC.lrrrbiii.

Cheſe is a meate not well dygeſtyfe and doth grete harme to them that hath a harde lyuer and mylte. Cheſe moch eaten dooth encreaſe the ſtone in the bladder / therfoze ſayth the excellent mayſter Conſtantyne. The cheſe is not good eaten foz relygyous perſones dwellynge in mo⸗

Figure 3.3 'Caseus. Chese'. Woodcut from Peter Treveris, *The grete herball whiche gyueth parfyt knowlege and understandyng of all maner of herbes and there gracyous vertues*, 1529 (Wellcome Library, London).

alongside another cheese 'specially ordered from various far-off lands', Reni sent them back with the words that 'this was a gift worthy only of he who bore it' (referring to the porters).[73] Such was the elite revulsion for cheese in an age when putrefaction and fermentation were not clearly distinguished that entire books could be written against it. In his 'medico-philological' treatise 'on the vileness of cheese', the Frankfurt physician Johannes Peter Lotichius blamed cheese – 'a foodstuff so foul and putrid that only its colour distinguished it from excrement' – for a myriad of diseases.[74] Martin Schoock's shorter study of the aversion to cheese is less hostile in tone, perhaps not surprisingly given his origins: the Dutch professor of logic was unable to explain this phenomenon and put it down to individual idiosyncrasy.[75] Both books were academic exercises, scholarly disputations whose evidence derived from classical and humanist sources, and need to be taken with a pinch of salt. But even so, there was near-universal agreement that the harder, drier and more aged the cheese, the more difficult it was to digest and the less suited it was to anyone but a labourer. Thomas Moffett explains why: 'for it stayeth siege [excrement], stoppeth the liver, engendereth choler, melancholy and the stone, lieth long in the stomack undigested, procureth thirst, maketh a stinking breath, and a scurvy skin'.[76] Pietro Andrea Mattioli, who appears to have been Moffett's source here, went even further, arguing that the only good use for hard cheese was as a treatment for the gout: to be applied *outwardly* to painful areas.[77]

And yet these were precisely the sorts of cheeses appreciated by the elites of Europe. The German agronomist Konrad Heresbach wrote in 1568 that 'in our dayes, the best cheeses are counted the Parmasines [Parmesans], made about the ryver of Po, esteemed for theyr greatnesse and daynetinesse', of which he recommends buying 'above threescore pounde'.[78] Given that their advice was so consistently ignored, and on such a massive scale, the popularity of parmesan, and cheese in general, put physicians in a bit of a quandary. The surgeon-empiric Leonardo Fioravanti admitted to a great liking for what his medical knowledge suggested he should avoid, including 'the miraculous cheeses' of Parma and Piacenza, as well as certain rustic mountain cheeses. As Fioravanti wrote in a letter of 1568: 'there is no group of people in the world who believe less in medicine than do we doctors, and in the towns there are no men more unregulated than we, because the things which we prohibit the sick we ourselves eat without fear'.[79] Moffet had the answer. After asserting that 'dry cheese hurteth dangerously', and explaining why this is so, he goes on to praise parmesan. This is no contradiction, Moffett suggests, explaining how this particular cheese manages to maintain the characteristics of youth while it ages: 'the Parmisan of Italy ... by age waxing mellower and softer, and more pleasant of taste, digesting whatsoever went before it, yet is itself not heavy of digestion'.[80]

The advice changed little over the years. From his chemico-mechanical perspective, Lémery agreed that cheese was highly nourishing and difficult to digest, and so most suited to labourers and best avoided or eaten moderately 'by old folks, and nice persons us'd to an idle life'. He recommended cheese that was neither too young or too old as being 'the wholesomest', which parted from Galenic advice, and concluded that 'Roquefort, Parmesan, etc. are for the nicest tables'.[81] As with mushrooms, so with cheese: what for the labouring classes was a dietary necessity was for the elites a matter of choice and distinction.

Without denying the impact of food crises and periods of dearth, it is evident that hunger was not a permanent reality in European peasant diets. Nor was drabness. In addition to the presence of mushrooms and cheese, the rapid assimilation of chilli peppers in various places, such as Spain and Hungary, testifies to the search for flavour and colour. Salt pork and salt beef likewise gave flavour to peasant dishes, as did the savoury tang of cured vegetables like sauerkraut. If soup and gruel tended to dominate, peasants also employed other cooking techniques: roasting over charcoal, baking in the embers, barbecuing and stewing.

Here is where kitchen inventories come into their own as a source for the historian. Kitchen equipment in peasant households in the southwest of France between 1700 and 1850 provide evidence for the use of spits, metal frying pans and pie dishes (*tourtières*). Indeed 90 per cent of households here had a frying pan.[82] In New France the metal *tourtière* was common enough in households to bestow its name on the foodstuff itself – a case of the container giving its name to the contents – a meat pie seasoned with cinnamon and cloves.[83] In modest English households, tinware utensils occupied a similar place, as basic commodities, from the second half of the eighteenth century.[84]

Peasants were connected to broader economic and commercial developments, just as there were different kinds of peasant. As a result, European peasant food culture should not be reduced to a single, static model, any more than that of the elites should be. Differences existed according to one's place on the hierarchy, from the simplest field hand to the yeoman farmer, and according to geography, ranging from the cereal-growing plains, to the mountains and the urban hinterlands. These differences are evident in relative openness to the markets, although this tends to increase everywhere in Europe from the eighteenth century. Thus we find the vineyard labourers of Bordeaux consuming Irish salt beef and Newfoundland cod, and eating cheese imported from Holland in preference to their own. Peasants begin to consume what had previously been luxuries, such as coffee, like the Savoyard peasants who roasted their coffee in the cooking pots used in cheese making: a sign of the perfect adaption of a new, exotic product to traditional peasant culture.[85] As with an implement, so with food: if the elites turned novelty into a value and a necessity, ordinary cookery did the opposite, passing change and innovation off as the familiar, putting new ingredients into old dishes.[86]

The inroads made by foreign goods are most evident in port towns, where the range of products was largest. By the eighteenth century coffee with sugar or milk formed part of the breakfast of artisans and journeymen in the port of Gdansk. Sailors' wives in the Courgain district of Calais drank tea, as one doctor bemoaned in 1777, up to four times a day![87] The foodways of urban labourers were potentially more varied than those of the countryside and their consumption patterns differed both from the urban elites and from rural inhabitants. People of the towns took many of their meals outside the home, or at least purchased ready to eat dishes. In cities like Paris inhabitants rarely had cooking facilities or a chimney, at the most a stove, according to household inventories. Stocks of food were also rare. Throughout Europe the modest urban artisan or labourer had to purchase food and drink from a range of different shopkeepers and pedlars. In Lyon, for instance, there were twenty-seven trades in the food sector in 1597, from orange-pedlars to tripe-dealers.[88] Many if not most food-pedlars were women. Formal and informal economies interacted, as shops competed with street hawkers and peasants who came into town to sell their produce.

Elite dining styles and medical theory: II

However varied the dietary habits of the poor may have been, it was those of the elites that were most defined by change. Elite dining preferences underwent a dramatic shift during the seventeenth century, reflected in changes in their attitude towards the nature of food preparation and consumption. The banquet gave way to the dinner party. The site of this change was not Italy, but France. And it was not at the royal court – which remained quite conservative in its dining style, retaining Renaissance banqueting habits of baroque ostentation and variety – but among the aristocratic high society of Paris.[89] This was the world of the *salon*, a regular cultural gathering of people under an inspiring host, often a woman. During the seventeenth century the salon evolved into a well-regulated practice that focused on and reflected enlightened public opinion, by encouraging the exchange of news and ideas. The rigid hierarchy of rank was discarded, in favour of more open conversation.

The same thing happened at dinner parties, also favoured by the same social groups and for the same cultural purposes. The key feature of the Parisian dinner party was that it abandoned the hierarchical seating plan of the court, favouring instead an arrangement that placed people in close proximity to one another *around* a table of moderate size. Gone was the high or low end of the long, narrow, trestle table, replaced by diners sitting shoulder to shoulder around a square or round table. This stressed the formal equality of everyone who sat down, where all diners were served or had access to the same dishes and where they would serve themselves more than had previously been the case. Guests ate and talked in a more convivial atmosphere than previously. Their dinners were also more private occasions than the Renaissance banquet.

As a result, traditional-style banquets came to be associated with institutional settings (the dining halls of schools), ceremonial occasions (guild banquets) and of course the royal court (where tradition continued to reign). The success of the dinner party also changed the dimensions of the cook's job. Once the ceremonial aspects of meals diminished, so too did the emphasis on creating spectacular visual effects with food. Moreover the total number of dishes the kitchen was expected to prepare, relative to the size of the group, went down. From the diner's point of view there was actually more variety, since all diners had access to all dishes. Moreover the attention to detail and the use of exacting techniques went up. Nicolas de Bonnefons took six pages to explain how properly to prepare *bisque*, a layered, thickened pottage made with pigeons, that was considered an elegant dish, served on festive occasions. De Bonnefons advised very small servings, since pigeon bisque was a dish 'to be tasted, not one to fill up on'.[90] The dish was symptomatic of the quest for 'natural' taste by the elites, from the second half of the seventeenth century onwards. It represented a new standard of luxury. The same rank of people who had previously spent large amounts of money on imported spices, now turned to a conspicuously natural and delicate style of cookery. Labelled 'modern' by its proponents, to set it apart from the traditional cookery of the Renaissance, it developed first in France and soon became fashionable throughout much of Europe.

The trend ran parallel to medical theories advising restraint, moderation and simplicity as much at the table as at the sick bed. Medical writers like the French Paracelsian Joseph Du Chesne criticized excessive artifice at elite tables, although he also suggested that a total lack of correction, such as among the poor, might be just as dangerous.[91] Du Chesne argued that the best and healthiest results occurred when reason and art were combined. He exhibits a gastronome's appreciation for different regional foods, usually simply prepared, where the main ingredient is allowed to shine.

More than a 'liberation' of cookery from medicine, seventeenth-century cookery mirrored changing medical philosophies, as the Galenism of the Renaissance gave way to chemical and medical approaches. Renaissance culinary styles were rejected. The general trend is evident in the verb 'season'. Like *assaisonner* in French, 'to season' an ingredient or dish had meant to temper or balance food, in the Galenic sense: to make it ready for eating, as well as to impart flavour to it. Now the verb lost the former connotation, as flavour became the more important consideration. To quote Du Chesne à propos of *assaisonner*: 'to make [foods] more agreeable and flavourful to the taste'.[92] The *way* foods were seasoned also changed. The strong flavours, heavy spices and acidic tastes (of vinegar or verjuice) of Renaissance cookery were increasingly replaced by an increasing use of butter, cream, gravies and sauces. As in cookery, so in medicine. In his chapter on 'the things necessary for preparation, sauces and seasoning of foods', Du Chesne (1620) lists salt, sugar, pepper, ginger, cloves, nutmeg, cinnamon, saffron, as well as honey, oil, vinegar and verjuice. Just over eighty years later the focus has shifted to butter, of which Lémery (1705) says, 'it is in use everywhere. There is almost no sauce in France which does not contain it'.[93] Spices were still used, but their number was increasingly limited to black pepper, cloves and nutmeg, with other spices such as cinnamon relegated to sweet dishes.

Medicine was called on to justify this shift in elite cookery. When the physician Jacques-Jean Bruhier re-edited Lémery's *Traité des alimens* in 1755, he added much of his own, including a completely rewritten introductory chapter. It gives us an indication of what has changed over the half century from the book's first edition. Originally, Lémery criticized as 'pernicious' the use of seasoning simply to make foods more attractive, so that we eat more; but he went no further.[94] In Bruhier's edition the seasonings, too, are unhealthy. Bruhier praises the then influential Dutch physician and chemist Herman Boerhaave, and his opposition to condiments of any sort, arguing that they harmed even the healthiest people.

> Unfortunately, seasonings are now used only to pander to taste, to stimulate the appetite, or to put it better, to produce a false one, given that nature itself possesses sufficient *irritamenta gulae* [incitements for the palate]. Now what is more pernicious than this practice? Given that, according to the celebrated Boerhaave, seasonings abounding in acids, salts and spices harm even the healthiest of people by their dominant acrimony, damaging the small vessels which make up the tissue of the parts most necessary to life, and weigh down the body rather than nourish it, by stimulating it to take on a quantity of food in exceeding its needs.[95]

This trend is evident in de Bonnefons's *Les délices de la campagne*, first published alongside his *Jardinier françois*. De Bonnefons sought to capture and maintain the 'true' flavour, smell and taste of the main ingredient in a dish. A cabbage soup should taste entirely of cabbage, leek of leeks and so on.[96] It was no longer necessary to alter the natural properties of ingredients in order to make them healthy; it was enough to bring out the properties of the foods themselves. That said, there was nothing simple or natural about the 'natural taste' advocated by Bonnefons. Rather, considerable refinement and artistry, not to say cost, went into creating distinct but complementary flavours.

Medical concerns were certainly present in de Bonnefons, but in a diminished measure and in a different guise. This shocked one traditionally minded contemporary who complained that the new cookery was so much 'sauce rather than diet'.[97] The new French sauces were indeed not only different in consistency and taste: smoother, often rich in fats, made with cream, butter, bouillon or wine. They were also different in function, no longer intended as dietary correctives to the main ingredient, but a means of bringing out its perceived 'natural' characteristics. But then, this was just what was increasingly perceived of as healthy and digestible.

Increasingly during the seventeenth century Frenchmen and women travelling abroad would remark on the overpowering use of spices. This suggests how much their food habits had changed at home – changes that had yet to make their way further afield. At the eastern end of Europe, Gaspard d'Hauteville, resident in Poland for some twenty years, wrote in 1686 that 'their sauces are very different from the French' and he noted how the Poles 'add lots of sugar, pepper, cinnamon, cloves, nutmeg, olives, capers and raisins'.[98] And to the west, when Madame d'Aulnoy visited Spain in the 1670s and 1680s, she complained about a dinner served on St Sebastian's day, 'so full of garlic and saffron and spices' that she could not eat any of it. On another occasion she commented that the fish pie would have been quite tasty 'had it not been full of garlic, saffron and pepper'.[99]

At the same time, elite tables throughout Europe were becoming more French. Through this process the habits of the European elites were brought closer together, sharing similar tastes and points of reference. The means varied.[100] It might be a single individual. For instance, in 1768 the young Danish king Christian VII travelled to France, including a stay at Versailles. Back in Denmark, the Danish court adopted the rules of the *service à la française*, with increasingly sumptuous table decoration and elaborate place settings. Books, too, might have an impact. Beginning with *Le cuisinier français* of 1651, the printings and translation of French cookery books are testimony to the diffusion of French cuisine throughout Europe. But it is groups of people who had the most impact. One such group were the French ambassadors abroad. As ambassador to Naples from 1760 to 1765, Aymeric Joseph de Durfort entertained at his grand receptions with goods brought in from France, including wines from Graves and Champagne. There were sporadic attempts to buck this trend, as in the English counter-model of a more sober and plain cookery against the overly sophisticated and luxurious French one; but by and large the French model was unstoppable. The result was, in the words of the cosmopolitan Parisian Louis-Antoine Caraccioli, 'there is but a single table among the greats of Europe, the same style of dining. At all the courts only this exquisite delicateness is known, bringing as much pleasure to see the dishes as to taste them'.[101] Meanwhile, lower down in society, throughout Europe, national and regional models continued to hold sway.

Conclusion

Compared with the complexity of Renaissance court cookery, modern cooking in the delicate style was straightforward, even simple; but it was also a highly refined form of conspicuous consumption. Perfectly ripe vegetables and fruits were highly prized because they were short-lived and fragile; when served out of season they became signs of exclusivity, requiring special, painstaking treatment by armies of gardeners and domestic servants. In the course of the eighteenth century, cookery based on fresh farm and garden products would become indelibly linked to the ideal of the simple and virtuous life as imagined by Jean-Jacques Rousseau. But, in reality, the modern style of delicate cooking, as developed first in France, was expensive and exclusive. Its appeal was wholly dependent on access to an abundance of raw materials – that were seasonal, perishable and most readily available to the aristocratic landowners whose estates produced them.

Medical ideas about class and constitution persisted throughout the early modern period. Chemical and mechanical theories about the digestive process and the workings of the body may have tempered the Galenic precept that the rich and poor should eat differently because their bodies had different consistencies, but the impact on dietary advice was limited. In 1785 the British military surgeon Andrew Harper was still recommending that the children of poor people be fed only 'plain and substantial food', avoiding 'rarities'. This was to prevent their stomachs from becoming 'too nice' (delicate), which would only be against their own best interests, as they were 'likely to live hard'.[102]

CHAPTER 4
REGIONAL FOOD: NATURE AND NATION
IN EUROPE

Introduction

Pity the poor colonists in the English colony of Virginia: during a period of scarcity, the inhabitants of the Jamestown settlement were instructed by their leader, John Smith, to eat as the natives did, foraging in the forest for food. Smith told them that if they could get it past their mouths, their stomachs would digest it. But the colonists replied that they would not eat 'savage trash'.[1] The colony suffered terrible food shortages, notably during the 'starving time' of the winter of 1609–1610. In October 1613 the Spanish ambassador to England, Diego Sarmiento de Acuña, informed King Philip III of Spain that the Jamestown settlers were 'sick and badly treated, because they have nothing to eat but bread of maize, with fish; nor do they drink anything but water – all of which is contrary to the nature of the English'.[2] Writing some forty years later, John Hammond agreed. In a short tract designed to encourage settlement, Hammond stressed the 'fruitfull' nature of the colony, 'apt for all and more then England can or does produce; the usuall diet is such as in England'. He added that 'it was only want of such diet as best agreed with our English natures, good drinks and wholesome lodgings were the cause of so much sicknesses, as were formerly frequent'.[3]

The settlers' reluctance to consume and cultivate maize was partly to blame. In their minds, the novelty might feed them but it would certainly lead to disease. At a time when wheat was the most common 'corn', and when 'corn' simply denoted any cereal or grain, the English colonists were extremely suspicious of this New World plant. Smith may have had no problems with maize, having travelled further afield than the colonists and having gained an appreciation for the health and strength of the Indians, but the colonists did not agree. Forcing them to eat it was tantamount to equating them with Native Americans, with whom maize was already closely associated. Maize may have been fine for 'the barbarous Indians, which know no better', as the apothecary and botanist John Gerard wrote in 1597, but it 'nourisheth but little, and is of hard and evill digestion'.[4] Of course, dietary novelty worked both ways. It was observed of the Algonquians that when they 'change their bare Indian commons for the plenty of England's fuller diet, it is so contrary to their stomachs that death or a desperate sickness immediately accrues'.[5]

The Spanish had been grappling with this dilemma since Columbus first 'sailed the ocean blue'. When he returned the following year, 1493, to the small colony he had established on the island of Hispaniola (modern-day Haiti and the Dominican Republic), he found not a trace of the colonists. He blamed the unfamiliar air and water of the Caribbean and was confident that mortality would cease once settlers could avail themselves of 'the usual foods we eat in Spain'.[6] Likewise the Portuguese, in the torrid climate of Equatorial Africa, depended on shipments of wheat flour, wine, olive oil and cheese from Europe: 'If the ships which bring these goods did not come', wrote a Portuguese pilot around 1540, 'the white merchants would die, because they are not accustomed to negro food'.[7] If there was little Europeans could do to change the new climates they faced overseas, they could at least try to control what they ate and drank.

Why was diet, and in particular dietary consistency, so important to Europeans? This chapter has three aims. We shall examine why diet was so closely linked to national 'temperaments' and 'natures', and why changes in diet could affect the health of both the nation and its inhabitants. And we shall explore what happened to such ideas when Galenism, with its emphasis on the role of diet, lost ground to newer and different medical visions of the body and its place in the natural world, before being revived towards the end of the early modern period.

The 'attractive virtue' of foods

A direct link existed between food and the body. An 'attractive virtue' or power bound together the qualities of the eater and the eaten. In the definition of Christopher Langton, 'every part of the body draweth to it such iuyce as is mete and convenient to nourishe it, and that iuyce, which is sooneste made like, is most convenient for nowrishment'.[8] Langton was writing while still a medical student, which may explain why his words have a ring of the textbook about them. Suffice it to say that the products of different locales were environmentally adapted to meet and suit the needs of the local inhabitants. (A similar argument was made about class, as we saw in the previous chapter.) Classical dietary theory held that individuals were best nourished by foods to which they were most accustomed, and these were most often the foods that grew in their region. With long use, they become most assimilated into people's bodies. It followed that a shift in this pattern would upset the body's own equilibrium, resulting in ill health. This held true even if one's usual food was not particularly good. As the anonymous author of the *Régime de vivre* put it, 'The meat [food] that one is accustomed to eating, whether in and of itself it is bad or harmful, is nevertheless better and more suitable for the body than good meat to which it is unaccustomed'.[9]

The formative influence of diet applied as much to nationalities as it did to individuals. In a work that was eventually translated into French, Italian, English, Latin, German and Dutch, the Spanish physician Juan Huarte de San Juan explained the basic Hippocratic and Galenic principles concerning the fundamental effects of environment and diet on the body. It was all down to the body's 'temperature', otherwise known as temperament, character or constitution. People's 'temperatures' differed from one another 'by reason of the heat, the coldness, the moisture, and the drouth [dryness], of the territorie where men inhabit, of the meats [foods] which they feed on, of the waters which they drink, and of the aire which they breathe'. This applied both to individuals and entire nations.

'The difference of nations, as well as in composition of the body as in conditions of the soule, springeth from the variety of this temperature'. We know self-evidently by experience, Huarte goes on, 'how far are different Greeks from Tartarians, Frenchmen from Spaniards, Indians from Dutch, and Æthiopians from English', in terms of their vices and virtues, their wit and manners. The Spaniards differ among themselves for the same reason.[10] The effects of climate and diet on national and regional bodies are expressed as given, mentioned here only in passing, for Huarte's real purpose is to explore the link between body and mind, talent and temperament.

Huarte cites Plato, Aristotle, Hippocrates and Galen in his discussion of national differences, but his own times played a role, too. For this was the age – the sixteenth and seventeenth centuries – that saw the rise of the nation-state. With this process came the idea of national particularities, indeed national stereotypes. Spanishness, Frenchness, Englishness and so on were all both bodily *and* political conditions, each accompanied by its own 'constitution'. In both political theory and physiology the word 'constitution' was used to describe the basic make-up of the body and the tendency for one segment or humour to predominate, sometimes to a dangerous degree. In politics, regulations, laws and good government could keep these tendencies in check; regimen exercised this same control over the individual body. Typical of this close link between food and nation, the prominent and savvy court physician Laurent Joubert wrote a treatise on 'the qualities and virtues of all the foods eaten in France, and the way to make healthy use of them', entitled *Matinés de l'Ile d'Adam*. Alas, the book was never published and has been lost.[11]

At a time when most people's primary identification tended to be with their particular town or region, rather than with their country, national stereotypes had nevertheless already formed. As we shall see, dietary writers had a strong sense of nationally based eating habits, sometimes warning against the 'strange' tastes and customs of neighbouring countries. Parallel to this, distinct regional cooking patterns emerge in the culinary literature, with recipes increasingly labelled 'French', 'German', 'Spanish', 'Italian' and so on. The development of notions of culinary nationalism and chauvinism has a history, closely linked to perceptions of the nation and its place in the world.

The dietary manuals of the fifteenth century, in continuity with late medieval cookery, embraced the exotic and the novel, as Ken Albala has demonstrated.[12] Italian regimens of the fifteenth century expressed a cosmopolitan and international outlook, virtually free of criticism of foreign cultures. Food and other stereotypes were certainly mentioned, as were regional variations in available food products. Writers referred to geographic distinctions like butter versus olive oil, or wine versus beer, habits which had separated northern and southern Europeans from antiquity. However, there was none of the fear of foreign contamination that we shall see in some later works: few warnings to avoid foreign foods and to stick to what was native.

This openness and relative lack of xenophobia continued in some parts of Europe, such as the Italian and Spanish peninsulas. This was due in part to a perceived continuity in Mediterranean regions with the ancient world. Here, ancient dietary advice continued to chime with local practice. This is most evident in Francisco Nuñez de Oria's *Regimiento y aviso de sanidad* of 1586. Nuñez devotes a lengthy chapter to 'the different diets of peoples', but his sources consist primarily of ancient authors like Pliny, Plutarch, Pomponius Mela and Caesar, with a spattering of Nuñez's contemporary Jean Bruyérin-Champier to bring things up to date.[13] For Nuñez de Oria there existed a clear continuity with the ancient world, to the point that it is not always immediately clear whether he is referring to the ancient world or his own times. And despite the rise of Spain as a nation-state during this period, complete with overseas empire, and despite his references to the French physician Bruyérin-Champier (to whom we shall return below), there is no pro-Spanish gloss to his geographical survey of culinary habits. Nuñez de Oria's comments remain neutral, indeed almost generic. Thus of the Laplanders, he says simply that they are 'exceedingly proud and rustic, they have no fruits, not apples, wine or autumnal produce. They are great archers and bowmen, living by killing wild beasts and wearing their furs'.[14]

This regional equanimity is evident even in three Italian regimens devoted to particular cities, a curious regimen sub-genre rooted in the Hippocratic notion of place. While extolling the virtues of their chosen subjects, these city-centred dietaries do not lose sight of their vices and are not afraid to praise foreign influences when appropriate. Tommaso Rangoni's advice to Venetians on the maintenance of their health recommends they eat bread made by German bakers, enticed to the city for the purpose. Of course, Venetians were open to the outside world, 'living within a sea full of goods', as Rangoni put it.[15] The Veronese Bartolomeo Paschetti, who spent the last thirty years of his life in Genoa, similarly entitled a book for the people of his adopted city. It takes the form of the discussion among a group of Genoese gentlemen, moderated by a doctor (Paschetti), in which the Genoese are actually singled out on only a few occasions, and not necessarily in a complementary fashion. Their taste for luxury, for instance, makes them prone to be short-lived.[16]

Alessandro Petronio's dietary recommendations for the inhabitants of Rome, despite its particular Roman focus, are remarkably open to foreign influences – especially when it comes to wines, it has to be said. Petronio was no ordinary doctor, being personal physician to the pope and director of the city's main hospital; and Rome was no ordinary city, since, as the seat of the papacy, it was quite international, home to 'a great multitude of different people, natures, habits and occupations'.[17] But even so, Petronio is open to a wide range of culinary influences and writes without a trace of chauvinism. In one case, what might seem like a boast comes with reservations. Thus Petronio claims that the foods of Rome are such that outsiders can eat more of them and more often than they are accustomed to. But this is not necessarily a good thing: being lighter, the city's foods provide less nourishment and mean that people do not live as long as elsewhere. 'By contrast', Petronio continues, 'when nourishment is firm and solid, as in Spain, there they live much longer'.[18] Petronio's Rome is a welcoming place, assuming the visitor follows a few simple rules. Those visiting the city 'from very cold places, as are Flanders, Germany and England, and especially during spring and summer, should avoid strong wines or at least drink them with large amounts of water'. The good news is that they can eat 'common foods without harm, and even in abundance, but they should avoid salty things'.[19] The only group that occasionally gets singled out in Italian dietaries is the Jews, as we shall see in the next chapter.

Renaissance dietary authors from the patchwork of German and Dutch states might be fearful of strange foreign foods and they might promote native customs even if they flew in the face of humoural theory; but even they never lashed out against foreign customs per se.[20] The criticisms of German doctors were confined to the dangerous fashion for expensive foreign spices. Ulrich von Hutten, along the lines of Paracelsus, looked longingly back to a time when Germans 'did not desire such goods, but used only those things which grew locally': to a golden age when 'their food was raised in the soil and air of the Fatherland'.[21] A hundred years later the Dordrecht physician and town councillor Jan van Beverwyck wrote a treatise in support of 'indigenous' Dutch ingredients, the land being a 'storehouse of fertility'.[22] By this time the Dutch had their own quite successful trading company bringing spices back to Europe and triggering a 'Dutch market for rarities'.[23] But, van Beverwyck asked, why drink the new foreign beverages when there was good old Dutch beer? This might sound narrowly jingoistic, but van Beverwyck's concept of the indigenous was as much pro-European as it was pro-Dutch. European plants and animals, he argued, were best suited for European bodies: 'since they live under the same sky with us, and in the same soil, and they consume the same food, known to us, and they assume a nature harmonious to our own nature' (Figure 4.1).[24]

There was thus a trend for German and Dutch medical authors to extol the virtues of the local against the exotic and luxurious, but this rarely degenerated into a suspicion of other European regions. That was largely confined to some French and English writers. The early influence of Paracelsus, with his stress on the efficacy of local ingredients, is partly responsible; but there was much more to it. The process of state-building, the religious differences brought about by the Protestant and Catholic Reformations, and the many wars fought during the period came together to bring about a heightened awareness of cultural differences and food prejudices. Both France and England were nation-states which already had a pronounced sense of national identity; they also happen to be the two countries which most often generated commentaries openly hostile to the food habits of their European neighbours. And they did not stop there. They also had a tendency to criticize or ridicule food habits of regions on the fringes or adjacent to their own states. For the English, this meant the native Welsh, Scots and Irish; for the French, this meant German food habits (particularly, their *drink* habits), but also such regions like Brittany and Normandy.

Take *De re cibaria*, the 1560 treatise by Jean Bruyérin-Champier, court physician to King Francis I, which examines food habits from around the world from the standpoint of traditional humoural theory. Bruyérin-Champier considers wine drinking a sign of refinement and civilization, typical of the French: Germans who live closest to France, he says, tended therefore to be more urbane and placid than the barbaric beer-drinking Germans to the north.[25] But Bruyérin-Champier's praise does not extend to *all* the French. He notes that the diet of fish, dairy products and fruit drinks among the Bretons, Normans and Flemings gives them leprosy and he considers the Gascons a nation unto

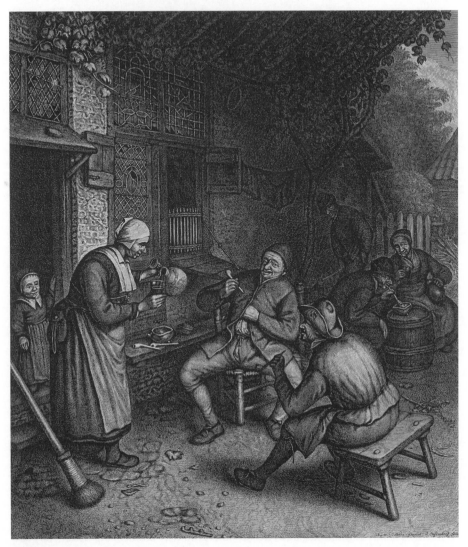

Figure 4.1 'Good old Dutch beer': tavern scene. Engraving by J. Suyderhoff after A. van Ostade, seventeenth century (Wellcome Library, London).

themselves. As for Spaniards resident in France, enamoured of but unused to the rich French diet, they are always farting and belching, and become more obese 'even than the Swiss'.[26] Bruyérin-Champier provides the reader with a stereotyped survey of who eats what and where, which gets harsher in its condemnations the further it travels from France.

Mind you, the English physician Andrew Boorde has something awful to say about nearly every foreign people, masked as wit. After leaving the Carthusian Order, and following a medical education in Montpellier, Boorde became a spy for Thomas

Cromwell. These experiences shaped his *A Compendyous Regyment or a Dyetary of Helth*, published in 1542, and his *Fyrst Boke of the Introduction of Knowledge*, published five years later. What follows are some of his versified national food stereotypes.

On the Irish:
I do love to eate my meate [food] sytting upon the ground,
And do lye in oten strawe, slepyng full sound ....
I do use no potte to seeth my meate in
Whefore I do boyle it in a bestes skyn;
Then after my meate, the brothe I do drynk up,
I care not for my masser, neyther cruse nor cup.

On Icelanders:
And I was borne in Islond, as brute as a beest;
When I ete candels ends, I am at a feast.
Talow and raw stockfysh, I do love to ete;
In my countrey it is right good meate;

On Flemmings:
'Buttermouth Flemyng' men doth me call;
Butter is good meat, it doth relent the gall.
To my butter I take good bread and drynke;
To quaf to moch of it, it maketh me to wynk.

On the Aragonese:
And I was borne in Aragon, where I do dwel.
Mesyle baken [maslin bread], and sardyns I do eate and sel,
The whych doth make Englyshe mens chykes lene,
That never after to me they wyll come agene.[27]

This same mixture of proud nationalism and insularity is evident in the attitude towards medical remedies. From the late sixteenth century onwards, for perhaps a hundred years or so, the more English these were the better. Writing in 1580, the physician (and later churchman) Timothy Bright affirmed that 'English bodies, through the nature of the region, our kinde of diet and nourishment, our custome of life, are greatly divers from those of strange nations, whereby ariseth great varietie of humours and excrements in our bodies from theirs'. The result was that 'the medicines which help [foreigners] must needes hurt us'.[28] The French royal physician François Aignan argued the same, and more, for France. Chapter ten of Aignan's 1696 treatise bears the unambiguous title: 'That God bestowed on every town and on every province all that is necessary for medicine, without the help of foreign countries'.[29]

Contrast this proudly localistic medical world view with that of a Spaniard, the physician-botanist Nicolás Monardes. His openness to the possibilities ushered in by the wide array of plants arriving from the New World is made clear in his *Historia medicinal de las cosas que se traen de nuestras Indias Occidentales*, published in three parts (in 1565, 1569 and completed in 1574) and widely translated. The title of the English translation leaves no doubt, eloquently proclaiming: *Joyfull News Out of the New Found World*.[30] Born the year of Columbus's second voyage (1493), Monardes kept an extensive garden in Seville, which just happened to be the port of entry for all Spanish ships arriving back from the New World.

Monardes was writing from a Galenic perspective, but even an important early French Paracelsian could combine a local perspective on food habits with a global one, without necessarily denigrating the latter in favour of the former: Joseph Du Chesne (Quercetanus) shared Monardes' eye for 'rare and beautiful things'.[31] The most influential French chemical physician of his day, Du Chesne was open-minded when it came to identifying and describing food habits, past and present. He was clearly proud of his Gascon origins, followed by those of France in general, as is evident in the lengthy chapter on diet in his *Le pourtraict de la santé* of 1606.[32] And yet, the rich and varied dietary details Du Chesne provides demonstrate a geographer's fascination for the foreign and an anthropologist's open-minded acceptance of difference which is unusual for the period.[33]

Natural qualities and the risks of foreign travel

As a native of Gascony who practised first in Lyon and then moved to Geneva, where he spent many years and became Calvinist, before returning to France to live in Paris as physician to King Henri IV, one wonders how Du Chesne would have coped with the different cuisines he was obliged to consume. The Hippocratic importance of 'airs, waters and places' was certainly not lost on Du Chesne, but given his general curiosity, one suspects he would not have regarded change as a threat. His chemical approach to diet may also have given him a different perspective on how foods were assimilated into the body. For the Galenic physician, however, this was quite a different matter – and quite a serious one. The advice was to keep to native customs and avoid dietary change, especially if this meant foreign food habits. That was fine if one kept to one's own land; but what if one had, or wanted, to undertake foreign travel?

The dangers of travel were not limited to highwaymen, unscrupulous innkeepers and poor roads. The traveller's very body was at risk when he left his native soil. In 1575 Hieronymus Turler, Saxon lawyer and enthusiastic traveller, nevertheless warned the two young German students for whom his book was written, that, like plants uprooted and planted in different soil, they might 'grow out of kinde'. Changes to 'the nature of the soil, influence of the heavens, and goodnesse of the aire, and that diverse maner of nourishment' caused plants to lose their 'naturall qualitie', colour and taste. Likewise in people, a change in the diet and air 'that compasseth them' brought about a change in their very constitution and temperament, leading in turn to a change in behaviour and interests. 'By this means', concluded Turler, 'a Dane is transformed into a Spaniard, a Germane into a Frenchman or Italian, namely by daily conversation, use of life and custome'.[34]

In the short term, sudden changes to air and diet upset the body's equilibrium and normal pattern, risking illness. In the long term, prolonged exposure could lead to changes in one's very self. The master of Manchester grammar school, Thomas Cogan, wrote of an English gentleman who, after travelling 'in forrayne countries', returned home, 'as it were despising the olde order of England, would not begin his meale with potage, but instead of cheese would eate potage last. But wise Englishmen I trust will use the olde English fashion stil'.[35] And they would know what this 'English fashion' was, thanks to a first spate of cookery books printed in England at around this time.

Italy posed special attractions, and special dangers, for Englishmen. During the sixteenth century the states of Italy were in the aesthetic vanguard of Europe, with Renaissance culture enthralling visitors and invaders alike (the latter including the Spanish and French). This culture was exported throughout the continent, in food just as in learning, art and architecture. European elites began to cook more vegetables, especially artichokes, asparagus and mushrooms (as we shall see in Chapter 6); they began to serve meals and carve meats the Italian way; and, in a more general sense, the Italian Renaissance aesthetic began to pervade the overall flavour of aristocratic dining.

Travellers were especially susceptible to this influence. William Thomas, author of the first English history of Italy, was forced to admit that he had lost a taste for 'the heaviness of flesh or fish'. 'Before time [I] could in maner brooke no fruite', Thomas writes, 'and yet after I had been a while in Italie I fell so in love withall that as longe as I was there, I desyred no meate more'.[36] At least Thomas seems to have confined his aberrant behaviour to Italy. English literature of the period, especially plays, abounds in examples of Italianate fops who affect strange fashions. This was the start of the fashion for the 'grand tour', accompanied by a real concern that good English customs and diet would be debased as a result.

Dietary change was just as much a concern for those who migrated from one part of Europe to another. To what extent should one adapt? This was a particular concern of religious orders like the Jesuits, whose members were drawn from all over Catholic Europe. In May 1556 Revd Adrian Adriaenssens, a native of Antwerp and rector of the Jesuit college in Louvain (modern-day Belgium), wrote to Ignatius Loyola, founder of the Order, to ask his opinion on the quality of the meals that should be served in the Louvain college. The puzzle came about because the community was composed of people of different 'nations', who were accustomed to different types of food. Loyola replied that it was a good idea 'to get accustomed to the more common and more easily obtainable food and drink, especially if one enjoys good health'. In terms of drink, Loyola added, this meant that 'one should get accustomed to beer, or even water, or cider, where this drink is in common use, and not make use of imported wines, at greater expense and with less edification'.[37] The reaction of the college's French, Italian and Iberian Jesuits to Loyola's advice is not recorded.

If dietary change posed a very real health threat to Englishmen embarking for the continent, or for wine-drinking Jesuits in Belgium, think of those Europeans who ventured to the New World. To continue the missionary thread, when the Franciscan Junípero Serra was about to leave Cadiz for the New World, a confrère wished him the following: 'Brother John, you are going to the Indies: God keep you from losing sight of bread'.[38] The missionaries' first thought was towards the saying of mass, which had to consist in the consecration of hosts made from wheat and wine made from grapes. From their Huron outpost in New France, the Jesuit Francesco Bressani plaintively wrote, '[W]e have passed whole years without receiving so much as one letter, either from Europe or from Kebek [Québec], and in total deprivation of every human assistance, even that most necessary for our mysteries and sacraments themselves, the country having neither wheat nor wine, which are absolutely indispensable for the Holy Sacrifice of the Mass'.[39] In New Spain, a Nahuatl translation of the Lord's prayer included the words 'May you give us now our daily tortillas' and the eucharist might be referred to as a 'blessed little tortilla'.[40] Such translations made sense at a devotional and literary level; but that is as far as it went. When it came to the mass, Catholic doctrine had it that only wheat bread could undergo transubstantiation into the body of Christ.

Missionaries like Bressani and his brethren considered self-sacrifice a fundamental part of their activity among the Native Americans and this notion of penitence included having to share the Huron diet of maize, fish and water.[41] The sudden and prolonged change in diet and environment was the explanation for high rates of disease and death in the New World experienced by the first groups of European settlers, as we saw at the start of this chapter. Nuñez de Oria stated flatly, 'going to the Indies is contrary to the human constitution'.[42] The suggestion in this case was the opposite of Loyola's: to keep as much to known foods as possible. The differences between old and New World were too great, so that dietary consistency would necessarily serve as a necessary bridge between the two. This was partly responsible for the widespread need Europeans felt to reproduce the familiar landscape in the New World, complete with Old World plants and animals. It helped introduce security into an insecure world – and no world was so insecure than the new one, certainly for the early colonists.

Recreating and keeping to the familiar was easier said than done in the early years of European settlement. What about over the longer term and the generations that followed? From a Galenic point of view, if the food people ate helped to determine their natures, then it followed that the children born of Europeans in the New World be constitutionally similar to their forebears if they continued to eat the same foods (thus easing their worries about the threat of a physical and moral transformation into natives). So thought the Spanish physician Diego Cisneros. Comparing Spaniards and creoles – people of Spanish heritage born in the Indies – Cisneros wrote that 'where there is such similarity in diet the complexion and natural temperament cannot alter'.[43] Just how much New World food was admissible remained a moot point. The avocado, it seems, was safe: 'a very good fruit and healthy for Spaniards'.[44] Staple foods like maize remained more problematic, as we shall see in Chapter 7.

Of course, diet was not the only factor determining a person's nature. Differences in climate would also play a role, so that creoles were bound to differ somewhat from the European-born. Juan de Cárdenas – who enthusiastically praised the wit, speech and comportment of Mexican-born Spaniards as more accomplished than that of Old World Spaniards – also defended their particular diet and way of life. For this, Cárdenas has been styled as one of the first defenders of creole legitimacy.[45] Nevertheless he identified inhabitants of the Indies as being most susceptible to certain types of disease – such as the French pox, stomach aches and strong menstrual pains – due primarily to the high heat and humidity.[46]

As we shall see in the second half of this chapter, despite the shift in medical philosophies that would come after 1650 the New World remained a sort of test case, for it placed Europeans – and people who continued to see themselves as such – in a radically different environment. As Trudy Eden has demonstrated, eighteenth-century accounts agreed that Anglo-Americans ate 'English' foods, but tended to eat much better than their counterparts in England. Colonial writers praised the virtue of the inhabitants' middling way in dietary matters, in keeping with the latest medical advice, as offered by doctors like George Cheyne.[47]

Domesticating Galen

The colonists' reference points remained European, even while the dietary advice, and especially the medical theories underpinning it, had changed significantly. How had this come about? To answer this, we need to return briefly to the late sixteenth century. The dietary nationalism of European regimens did not consist merely in criticizing what was perceived as strange and different. In addition, and more importantly, it served as a catalyst for change within dietary theory. When it came to applicability, the classical tradition had one limitation: it dealt with a Mediterranean climate and roughly the same range of Mediterranean foods. When this classic theory was applied to very different regions, with their different climates, it was bound to cause difficulties. The result was a defence of national food customs, especially in areas north of the Mediterranean, however much these customs went against Galenic doctrine. A propos of the aubergine, a recent fashion in England, but which rarely ripened fully in the English climate, John Gerard wrote, 'I rather wish English men to content themselves with the meat and sauce of our owne country, than with fruit and sauce eaten with such peril; for doubtlesse these [aubergines] have a mischievous qualitie, the use whereof is utterly to bee foresaken'.[48]

But everywhere in Europe we see local habit, preference and experience beginning to carry as much or more weight than the specific advice of Galen or Hippocrates (who could not have known of these local or changing habits). Galenism was 'modified and domesticated', in the words of literary historian Thomas Olsen, to suit new contexts.[49] Even someone as rooted to the ancient tradition as Nuñez de Oria, albeit in his case more Arabic than Galenic, writes favourably of the Spanish love for mixed salads ('with more colours than the rainbow'), the consumption of which in other parts of the world is said to cause leprosy.[50] Guglielmo Grataroli (our Italian Calvinist living in Basel) loosens classical strictures against foods like duck, sea-going fish swimming upstream and cheese, which may 'without daunger be eaten', he comments.[51] All of these would have been common foods in Grataroli's adopted Basel, as Albala has suggested.[52] And the proud Gascon Du Chesne waxed lyrical about the onions, leeks and garlic of his native region.[53]

The paradox is that it was Galenism itself that made this domestication possible. This is because Galenic ideas had always supported the notion that the foods best for us were the ones which best suited our 'natures' (as we saw at the beginning of this chapter). Galenic theory might have favoured wine over ale, but it was consistent with that same Galenic theory to argue that 'ale for an Englysshe man is a naturall drynke', as Boorde did.[54] And he meant 'naturall' quite literally, as being consistent with their 'natures'. Conversely, Boorde regarded beer (made with hops), which had just arrived from Holland, as 'a naturall drynke for the Dutche man', but harmful to Englishmen, likely to give them the inflated 'faces and belys' of the Dutch. It was therefore quite in keeping with Galenic theory to argue that for the Scots, because of their harsh climate and plenty of exercise, their diet of oatcakes was ideally suited to them – even though the diet would be harmful to anyone else. Likewise, the more delicate Italian soil and mild climate produced foods more suited to the constitutions of the Italians. What people ate locally created a 'second nature' in them. This allowed them to eat foods that might ordinarily harm people from elsewhere.

Among English authors, the domestication of Galenic advice is most evident in the changing attitude to beef. Galen had not been keen on beef, because it was heavy and so prone to cause melancholy and the diseases associated with it. One of the earliest writers to praise English beef was the Anglo-Welsh historian Thomas. In *The Pilgrim* (1546), a purported dialogue between Thomas and several Bolognese nobles, he writes of the 'common people' of England surviving on 'flesh, fowl and fish' the way Italians depend on 'fruits and herbs'. The reason was down to climate. 'For like as the subtle air of Italy doth not allow you to feed grossly, so the gross air of England doth not allow us to feed subtiley', Thomas explains. In support, Thomas tells them a contemporary proverb: 'Give the Englyshman boeffe and mustarde'.[55] Thomas presents beef production and consumption as one of England's recent economic and cultural achievements, part of its newfound identity: a food of substance in keeping with the people's forthright and vigorous nature.

For Cogan, English beef was not only better than that encountered by the ancients; it was more suited to the climate of the country and the temperament of its inhabitants. Had the ancient writers 'eaten the biefe of Englande, or if they had dwelt in this our climate, which through coldnesse (*ex antiperistasi* [the Aristotelian process by which one quality heightens the force of another, opposing quality]) doth fortifie digestion, and therefore requireth stronger nourishment, I suppose they would have judged otherwise', Cogan remarks. Cogan stresses 'how well it doeth agree with the nature of English men'.[56] Thomas Moffet concurred, writing that 'there is not a better meat under the sun for an English man'.[57] Indeed, Moffet, whose *Health's Improvement* abounds with regional commonplaces, even goes so far as to condemn veal for the English, which was normally preferred over beef. For Moffet, veal 'flesh is but a gelly hardened' if the animal is too young. Veal is better suited to Italians, with their hotter climate: 'yet in our country it falls out otherwise through abundance of moisture, so that howsoever sound bodies do well digest it, yet languishing and weak stomacks find it too slimy and can hardly overcome it'.[58]

The reality was a bit more complicated. The English were eagerly growing and consuming fruit during the sixteenth and seventeenth century, which went against both Galenic wisdom and the accepted stereotype the English increasingly had of themselves as meat-eaters.[59] It was a stereotype that all sorts of writers – medical authors included – seemed to accept, if not to foster: the meat-eating, plain-speaking Englishman versus the politic and wily Italian/Frenchman/Spaniard (delete as appropriate). As Jean-Louis Flandrin noted, English travellers abroad tended to judge the culinary standards of a country by the quality of its beef, in the way that French and Italians might use bread as a measure (or indeed vegetables).[60]

The rich Spanish stew known as *olla podrida* provides another example of a dish praised in its native land while being criticized just about everywhere else. The Spanish golden age playwright Pedro Calderón de la Barca made the dish the star of a short farce, *La mojiganga de los guisados* (The farce of the stews).[61] In the play, Sir Stew (Don Estofado) defends challengers to the title of 'princess of stews', which is eventually won by his wife, Lady Olla Podrida. She praises her noble ancestry and boasts, 'My dowry is large: bacon, cabbage, chick peas, aubergine, cardoons, onions and garlic'. By Cervantes' time *olla podrida* was well known enough to be one of the dishes ordered removed from the table of Sancho Panza by his court physician (as we saw in Chapter 1).[62] And the doctor was not the only one to have reservations. Writing in 1603, the Roman physician Scipione Mercurio considered the dish – at the time also fashionable at Italian courts – one of the most harmful dishes imaginable: 'a food fit to kill man'.[63] Mercurio actually spelt it *putrida* (putrid), which allowed him to affirm that its putrefying perniciousness in the stomach was evident in its very name. The actual etymology of the word *podrida* is from the medieval Spanish *poderida*, meaning 'heavy', although this would not have been much better in Mercurio's mind (or indeed of most medical authors). The dish was still being criticized 150 years later by doctors like Giuseppe Pujati (1768), because of its complexity and mixing of diverse ingredients, even if the motivation was no longer the 'qualities' of the ingredients but their chemical compositions.[64]

Elsewhere, the Strasbourg physician Melchior Sebisch (Sebizius), despite being an orthodox Galenist, welcomed condiments, such as horseradish, used solely for pleasure and taste, not to 'correct' a dish.[65] His father, also a physician (and also Melchior), had an interest in horticulture, translating the horticultural *Maison rustique* into German.[66] Sebisch the younger wrote approvingly of Alsation dishes that would have sent Galen spinning in his grave: sauerkraut, beer, oatmeal pottage and pork, that most unhealthy of meats. Sauerkraut, in particular, provided Sebizius with a quandary, for there was no Latin word for it. But the use of vinegar as a means of preserving foods like cabbage, from Alsace eastwards through to Poland, provided the sour and acidic qualities of central and eastern European foods which so struck French visitors.[67] In any case, Sebisch was a healthy seventy-year-old when he published his dietary *De facultatibis alimentorum* in 1650, and would live another twenty-five years, so the local dishes and seasonings could not have done him any harm.

Pork's healthiness was praised even more in Spanish America. Pork was particularly abundant there, with lard replacing the more expensive olive oil in colonial cooking. Nuñez de Oria was the first to praise the pork of the New World, as 'more delicate, tender and healthy' than Old World pork.[68] The Englishman Thomas Gage reported on the presence of hogs in Cuba, so numerous that they were used to supply ships on their return to Spain, and the transformation in medical knowledge that came about as a result. He makes the challenge to Galenism quite clear. 'My selfe chanced to take physicke there', Gage recounts, 'and whereas I thought that day I should have a fowle or rabbet after my physicks working, they brought me a boyled peece of fresh young porke, which when I refused to eat, they assured me it was the best dish the doctors did use to prescribe upon such daies'.[69] Worried that the pork would 'open his body' – presumably the last thing Gage wanted after taking his medicines, which were probably purgatives – his doctor in Havana insisted 'that what porke might worke upon mans body in other Nations, it worked not there, but the contrary; and so he wished me to feed upon what hee had prescribed, assuring mee that it would doe mee no hurt'.[70]

Mediterranean food preferences – including a penchant for veal and kid, for olive oil and vinegar, for figs and raisins – either lost validity or were tempered with newer fashions. It can be argued that this process of domesticating Galenism may have contributed as much as any factor to the gradual abandonment of classical authorities on the whole. Once the specific applications of classical theory lost significance, the foundation was bound to collapse. Eventually custom became more important than physiological doctrine.

Not content with garlic and onions: Nation in the new medical ideologies

Writing in 1642, in his lively guide for Englishmen travelling abroad, James Howell made a new use of an old word. Thus, when he comes to his description of Holland, Howell remarks that the 'humour of the people' is 'patient and industrious'.[71] Humours are no longer bodily fluids, but one element in a list of 'comportments, fancies and inclinations' in which the peoples of Europe differ.[72] They are not a cause of all the rest. As a result, one could separate diet from temperament – now 'humour' – as Howell does in his discussion of the differences between the French and the Spanish.

The French and Spanish 'differ not only *accidentally* and outwardly in their clouthing and carriage, in their diet, in their speaches and customes', according to Howell, 'but even *essentially* in the very faculties of the soule and operations thereof, and everything else'.[73] Howell was not only well travelled but a proficient linguist, so he spoke from experience, but with a lightness of touch. His comparison between the French and the Spanish stresses their contrary habits: 'Go to their diet, the one drinkes watered wine, the other wine watered; the one begins his repast where the other ends; the one begins with a sallet and light meat, the other concludeth his repast so; the one begins with his boyled, the other with his roast'. In attempting to understand the contrary natures of the two peoples, he refers to various 'philosophicall authors' and Hippocratic notions regarding the 'qualities of the clymes and influences of the stars', which, since they differ in the respective countries, it is quite natural that 'the temper and humours....But for Howell this influence can only be indirect and accidental, for their cultural differences are far greater than their different climates would allow.[74]

Nor is Howell particularly worried about the foods the English traveller will eat abroad and the inherent risks to his health, as an earlier author in the Galenic tradition might have been. In Spain, the heat might be a danger – the traveller 'must take heed of posting in that hot countrey in the summer time, for it may stirre the masse of bloud too much' – but, after France, he will find that 'the Spaniard drinks better wine [and] eates better fruits'.[75] With the Grand Tour in full swing, Howell thought 'forrein travell' a good thing, a 'moving academy' for the mind, especially beneficial for islanders, 'cut off (as it were) from the rest of the citizens of the world'.[76] Far from being 'undone' by foreign foods, the real risk for the English traveller was that when he returned home he was overly enthusiastic in 'commending the wines of France, the fruits of Italy, or the oyle and sallets of Spaine'.[77]

The changes in environment occasioned by travel might still cause worry, now explained in chemical terms; but fears about food were no longer about the risk to one's nature. They were reduced instead to the level of individual preferences and tastes. The Bolognese priest Sebastiano Locatelli, who travelled to France during the mid-1660s, was an enthusiastic eater of local food while there: a breakfast of ham, salted meat and hard-boiled eggs was regarded as 'a sacrifice for the sake of economy'.[78] Of course, the perceived differences between Italian and French food were not as great as those between English and French food. Moreover, by the mid-1600s French power and cultural influence was at its highest, and culinary literature flowed from French printing presses. But even so, Locatelli commented on the difficulties in acclimatization. In Lyon, he suffered a terrible headache – Locatelli was prone to this – and reported, 'It is said that the influence of climate alters most nourishment in the blood. I willingly believe it'. It took two months for Locatelli to become accustomed to the air of the place and for 'the whirlwind in my head' to subside. Aside from his headache, the 'first effect that foreigners feel of their visit [to France]' is what Locatelli refers to as 'stomack flux' – still the bane of travellers the world over. He says that the best solution is to avoid eating the fruit at first, however good it might be. Ever the optimist, Locatelli found the purge welcome, 'since I am naturally predisposed towards constipation'.[79] The episode does give Locatelli the chance to praise French veal and chicken broths, widely given as a remedy to the sick.

Where books of travel once cautioned a wariness of the foreign, it was now those people reluctant to embrace it who found themselves ridiculed. A Dutch physician and writer, Olfert Dapper, poked fun at the man who was 'merely content with garlic and onions, the kind that grow before his own door, and does not look around to see whether there are also people living on the other side of the mountain, who enjoy cinnamon and sugar'.[80] Travel fed the mind and the body, broadening one's horizons and one's waistline.

Chemical and mechanical philosophies eliminated the uniqueness of each human body. 'Nature' became but a matter of taste and orientation. Whether foods were chemically fermented in the body (according to the iatrochemical model of digestion) or simply nourished the machine (in the iatromechanical model), diet was less the cause of one's 'nature', and more a manifestation of it. This did not mean that national stereotypes disappeared: far from it. In a dietary treatise that is Galenic in structure, modelled on Pisanelli's, but chemico-mechanical in content, Louis Lémery managed to get a few chauvinistic words in. In his 1702 *Traité des aliments*, Lémery says this of cattle-rearing: 'The French, whose country abounds in necessaries, also make use of several sorts of animals, which they prepare and dress in so delicate a manner, and with so fine and agreeable a taste, that it may be said, they have refined cookery, and do therein, as they fancy they do in everything else, excell all nations'.[81] Lémery likewise agrees with previous French and English authors who praised the consumption of beef as healthy, in contrast to Galen; but he does not add anything to this view that reflects his new medical ideology, other than to say that beef 'contains much oil, volatile salt and earth' and is particularly suited to 'young bilious people'.[82] The same pattern is evident in his comments on the effects of beer, which makes people fatter than wine and makes them more drunk. So far, so French: the only difference with previous Galenic dietaries being that the explanation of beer's 'principles' is couched in the chemical language of the time.[83] As we noted in Chapter 2, Lémery's medical ideology may be new, but his conclusions are anything but.

National stereotypes lived on, whatever the medical theory. Towards the end of the seventeenth century another French doctor, François Pinsonnat, wrote without a shadow of doubt or irony that 'the Italians are naturally more inclined towards repose and sensual pleasure than other nations'. Pinsonnat's compatriots, by contrast, normally work hardest of all, 'more than the Italians, the Spanish and all other nations'.[84] According to another author, 'the diversity of regions makes men of different customs, humours and ways of life'. This explained why northern peoples ate more than southerners, 'why the Spanish and Africans bear hunger with less impatience and uncomfort than most Italians, and why they better than the French, and why the French of the south more easily than the English and Germans'.[85] It was no longer a matter of the foods people ate determining their natures, but the climate, which in turn determined food preferences. Climate was the justification Andrew Harper offered for the Englishman's fondness for meat in his health manual of 1785, although he was convinced that Englishmen ate far too much 'animal food'. It resulted in a 'putrescent crassis to the blood', causing obstructions and nervous diseases (Figure. 4.2).[86]

Harper's view demonstrates the influence of both George Cheyne, earlier in the eighteenth century, and William Buchan, closer to Harper's own time. Indeed we can use Buchan's best-selling health guide as our guide to changing medical ideas regarding food and nationality. In William Buchan's *Domestic Medicine*, first published in 1769 and frequently republished thereafter, there is as much continuity as change when compared to the regimens of earlier centuries. The continuity – although it is much more a revival – is evident in the importance Buchan gives to the six non-naturals,

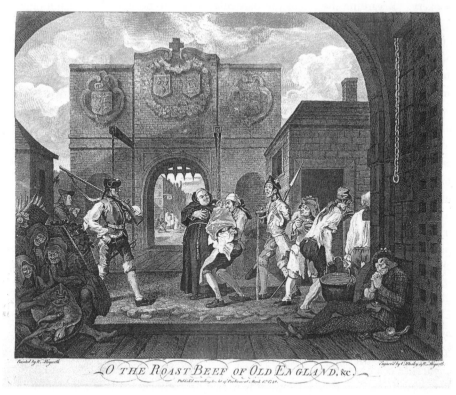

Figure 4.2 'O the roast beef of old England'. Engraving by C. Mosley after W. Hogarth, 1848 (Wellcome Library, London).

which also give structure to the first part of the book. As described in Buchan's chapter 'On aliment', still fundamental is the notion that what we eat affects our bodily make-up. 'There is no doubt but that the whole constitution of body may be changed by diet alone', Buchan writes. He stresses how 'the preservation of health depends upon a proper regimen of the diet'. Proper diet can also be used to treat diseases and infirmities. Buchan also reminds us to avoid 'great and sudden changes in diet'.[87]

All of this advice would have been familiar to the readers of sixteenth-century regimens. Gone, however, is the Galenic approach consisting of detailed advice concerning individual foodstuffs. It is not Buchan's intention to 'inquire minutely into the nature and properties of the various kinds of aliment in use among mankind; nor to show their effects upon the different constitutions of the human body'. This is replaced in Buchan by an insistence on moderation and simplicity as general rules.[88]

As Buchan remarked, in an essay added to his manual at the very end of the early modern period (1797), 'Habits are indeed obstinate things, especially those which relate to diet'.[89] At the same time, taste now reigned supreme over every other consideration, such that man now 'devours the productions' of every climate, rather than just his own. And if the foods 'do not suit his palate or agree with his stomach, he calls in the aid of cookery'.[90] Regarding the English in particular, a new trend is visible, beginning with Cheyne and culminating with Buchan: a new attitude to meat consumption. What was once a boast of medical writers, 'the great quantity of animal food devoured by the natives', is seen instead by Buchan as the main cause of the high rates of consumption and scurvy in England. Rather than highlighting a link between meat-eating and a direct and down-to-earth nature, Buchan points to 'the choleric disposition of the English [which] is almost proverbial', their high meat consumption inducing 'a ferocity of temper unknown to men whose food is chiefly taken from the vegetable kingdom'.[91] Buchan relates a number of food stereotypes, generally approvingly: high bread consumption among the French, boiled barley among the Dutch, oatmeal hasty pudding throughout Britain, potatoes in Ireland, roasted onions among the Turks, leeks in Wales, sauerkraut in Germany.

Tastes and preferences should not be taken for granted, especially when they result in poor food choices, as in the English reluctance to eat soups. The explanation for this poor choice, Buchan explains, is said to lie in 'custom': 'but how customs arise is not so clear a matter'.[92] This broader question is one which earlier writers of medical advice left to one side, assuming regional and national customs to be 'natural', that is, in keeping with the place and its people. For Buchan this is not, or at least no longer, the case.

Since Buchan was well known, and published, on both sides of the Atlantic, let us end where we started this chapter: with Europeans (and their descendants) seeking to find their place in the New World they had so significantly reshaped. By the end of the eighteenth century, differences between themselves and Native Americans and African slaves (and their descendants) were increasingly ascribed to race, a factor Buchan does not consider. Underlying racial differences were held to be stronger than diet in determining people's natures. This is the subtext of Thomas Jefferson's *Notes on the State of Virginia*, written in 1781 and published six years later.[93] Jefferson was not a doctor, of course, though he was certainly well educated: and perhaps this allowed him to take quite a different view about the role of diet, custom and nature from that espoused by Buchan. Nor is his work a regimen. However, Jefferson's study concerns us for three main reasons. First of all, Jefferson merely lists the local flora and fauna, along Linnaean lines; he does not describe what foods people eat and how, whether Native Americans or European inhabitants, as authors in previous centuries might have done. Secondly, he does not ascribe much of a role to the environment in explaining differences between animal or human species, warmed as they were by 'the same genial sun' and with 'a soil of the same chemical composition'. 'A Pygmy and a Patagonian', Jefferson wrote, 'derive their dimensions from the same nutritive juices'.[94] And finally, as this point suggests, the role of diet had changed. It was more a question of the quantity and quality of food affecting bodily size and strength; the rest was down to race. Jefferson doubts whether people's 'bulk and faculties' depends 'on the side of the Atlantic on which their food happens to grow, or which furnishes the elements of which they are compounded'.[95] For Jefferson, Indians were a separate race of the species 'Homo sapiens Europæus', with some similarities between them, whereas Africans were a separate species, with differences like colour that were 'fixed in nature'.[96]

Conclusion

As the vast gulf separating Buchan and Jefferson suggests, the end of the early modern period saw significant disagreement over the relationship between diet, nature and nationality. If Jefferson proposed, rather controversially, an entirely new racialist take on the subject, Buchan's approach was more traditionally 'medical'. But even with Buchan, his stress on the role of taste in his own time signals that a great shift had taken place since the time of the Galenic revival at the start of the period.

In Galenic medicine the link between food, nature and nation was tightest: what you were determined what you ate and what you ate determined what you were. That was the surest way to health; any change in this custom was bound to cause serious health problems. This belief also fostered a fear of difference, for what was foreign became, at the very least, a source of ridicule, or much more likely, a threat to one's very nature. At the same time, Galenism allowed for the introduction of new foods, when they were considered particularly suitable for the natures of certain nations. If Galen had only known of our beef, say, he would certainly have approved of it, the argument went. In this way, medical authors could sanction the changes in national diets that were already taking place. What should not have been healthy became healthy. And this was just as well, given that the diets of Europeans were changing in significant (and different) ways; indeed, we must not lose sight of the changing nature of national food cultures, avoiding commonplace notions of their unchanging nature.[97]

It could be argued that it was the very flexibility and adaptability inherent in the Galenic system that weakened its place in the medical knowledge of the seventeenth century. In any case, the shift in medical philosophies towards the chemical and the mechanical rendered what one ate much less problematic. It severed the direct link between nature and nation, turning foodways into a matter of taste and fashion. Humours went from being bodily fluids, the fabric of one's body, to particular habits and behaviours; nature was more about tastes and inclinations. As a result, travel to foreign lands, and the changing food preferences that resulted, might make you a laughing stock back home, but they were not going to change the very fabric of your body. In eighteenth-century Europe national stereotypes flourished as they used to be in the sixteenth century, but they were now put down to climate rather than diet. Finally, with Buchan, along with the return of preventive medicine in the doctor's armoury, we see a return of the link between diet and nature, between what one ate (for better or for worse) and the make-up of one's body. Even Buchan cannot dismiss the dominance of taste in dietary choices, which so preoccupied many of his contemporaries. Taste in foods was now seen as a reflection of national characteristics, not a determinant of them. But it is Jefferson who turns the issue on its head, by proposing race as the main determinant of nature, not diet or even climate.

CHAPTER 5
HOLY FOOD: SPIRITUAL AND BODILY HEALTH

Introduction

It is often assumed that particular food practices, abstentions, rules and taboos are characteristics of other religions, absent from Christianity. When viewed from the perspective of history this is quite untrue.[1] Indeed St Benedict of Norcia, in his monastic rule of the sixth century, developed a clear ideal of dietary discipline for his monks, but one that was also pragmatic. His rule encapsulates the themes of dietary abstinence, but within a flexible framework, that are the focus of this chapter. The rule's key dietary prohibition forbade the consumption of four-legged animals, as Benedict did not regard red meat as necessary to the diet of a normal healthy adult. Thus from very early on in the monastic tradition asceticism and the avoidance of certain foods were closely linked. Moreover, Benedict envisaged only a single daily meal. At the same time, flexibility was built in: two cooked dishes would be provided at that meal, so that individual monks could choose that which most suited their state of health, and a third dish of vegetables or fruit could be added. Individual monks could also be offered larger portions or more bread if they were performing heavier manual labour than usual, at the abbot's discretion. Special provisions were also made for the elderly and the young. Finally – and this is just as important as the Christian tradition of self-denial – Benedict affirmed the goodness of preparing and eating food. He instructed the cellarer to look on all the monastery's cooking utensils 'as upon the sacred vessels of the altar'.[2]

Fast-forward to the seventeenth century, nothing exemplified the difference between Catholics and Protestants than attitudes towards religious fasting and enforced abstinence. When it came to fasting during the forty days of Lent, Protestant Europe, no longer constrained by decrees emanating from Rome, produced treatises in praise of the free consumption of meat. One of these was written by a Dutch Calvinist headmaster, Arnold van den Berghe (Arnoldus Montanus). The author of several works on theology, history and geography, Montanus's 'Diatribe on the consumption of meats and the Lent of the papists' delivers exactly what it promises.[3] For their part, Catholic authors denounced Protestants for being meat-eating gluttons, never having to curb their appetites and renounce it, if only temporarily. They printed treatises in defence of Lenten fasting. Paolo Zacchia's *Il vitto quaresimale* (The Lenten diet) is typical, methodically dismissing medical warnings against fasting and providing a detailed and legalistic survey of what can and cannot be eaten.[4]

To appreciate these attitudes and the seismic shift that occurred, we need to understand Christian dietary practices before the Protestant and Catholic Reformations. The chapter will then go on to explore the impact of the Reformations on ideas about abstinence and the place of the individual; changing medical theories about the effects of fasting on health; and the shift in Christian dietary habits and views about them, which occurred during the eighteenth century.

Diet and the Christian calendar

Prior to the Reformations, Europe was united in the way its dietary habits and food culture were influenced by Christianity. In the previous chapter we touched on the meaning given to bread in European culture, eaten as it was by Christ at the Last Supper. When Christ said 'this is my body', and 'this is my blood', these words were interpreted in a very literal sense. Christians quite literally consumed the body and blood of Christ when they participated in the Mass, which had the power to wipe away sins and gain access to everlasting life. Small wonder that bread itself was more than just 'the staff of life', but also pointed towards the afterlife.

Religious belief and practice infused food culture in another way: that of calendrical habits and customs. Certain days of the year were imbued with special practices. These were the holy days, the days of vigil and celebration scattered throughout the course of the year. Bearing in mind that there were no regular weekends off from work or the public holidays of today, these feast days were the only occasions when people could avoid working and let off steam. Together, these feast days and celebrations provided what Florent Quellier has called 'des espaces compensatoires de la faim': times and practices which offset the reality of hunger.[5]

Even the smallest village had its patron saint. In addition to offering divine protection for the village, the particular saint was also the occasion for a holiday, and holidays of course mean food, so that a particular foodstuff often became associated with the occasion. Some of these food associations have little to do with the saint in question and more to do with the time of year when it was celebrated. Thus eating goose or drinking new wine for the feast of St Martin (11 November) had nothing to do with the life and miracles of St Martin of Tours. In northern Europe goose came into season around then, and the year's new wine was considered ready for drinking, after the grape harvest two months earlier. Both became linked to St Martin.

Saints' holidays were 'fixed' feasts, in the sense that they happened on the same day every year. Christmas was the most important of these fixed feasts, following the fast of Advent (marking the 'coming' of Christ). Customs associated with Christmas varied greatly from place to place throughout Europe and it is difficult to determine when many of them originated. Many of them are probably nineteenth century in origin, like many of our most favourite carols, but they probably had pre-modern antecedents.

More important than Christmas, from a liturgical point of view, was the feast of Easter, celebrating the resurrection of Christ. Easter was a 'moveable' feast, its timing depending on the phases of the moon (after the vernal equinox), so that it could be set for anytime between 22 March and 25 April. Then and now, Easter was associated with eggs. This was partly as a symbol of resurrection and rebirth, following Christ's death, but was also due to the fact that one was allowed to eat eggs again following the fasting of Lent, during which eggs were forbidden. In Scotland and northern England 'pace' eggs (from 'paschal') were exchanged in celebration, a convenient way of using up the glut of eggs accumulated during Lent. Lamb was also served at Easter, once again, partly because of its association with Christ (called 'the lamb of God'), and partly because Easter falls during the lambing season.

Easter introduces us to a third crucial relationship between Christianity and food culture in Europe: the pattern of feast and fast, fat and lean, celebration and abstinence. Easter Sunday was a period of celebration and rich dining – a return to meat. This is rendered most explicitly in the Hungarian word for Easter, *Húsvét*, which literally means 'meat-taking'. This only makes sense when we recall that the forty days that preceded Easter was an extended period of strict fasting, known as the 'great fast', *nagyböjt*, in Hungarian. Lent re-presents the forty days Christ spent in the wilderness fasting, when he was tempted by the devil. During Lent all healthy individuals were expected to abstain from all animal flesh and animal products (milk and butter, in addition to eggs). Only one meal was allowed. People were allowed to eat fish, however, and this is how fish took on its association with periods of abstinence, called 'lean' days in the English of the time. In terms of food culture, fish was opposed to meat, and the two were kept clearly separate, never served at the same meal.

For those who lived adjacent to Europe's coasts or along its waterways, acquiring fish could often be done quite economically. But away from the coast, only the better off could afford fresh fish. For most Europeans, 'lean' days meant buying and eating dry, salted or pickled fish, such as stockfish or herring. Lake and river fishes also underwent similar treatment in order to satisfy distant markets. The most important fish of all was the cod, either dried or salted, sourced in particular from the Grand Banks of Newfoundland. These became the site of ongoing disputes between Basques, French, Dutch and English mariners and fishermen throughout the early modern period, all to satisfy the European market for fish, dictated by devotional concerns. Fished and salted hundred of miles (or more) away from where it was consumed, at all levels of society, the consumption of salt-cod throughout Europe, even in areas where fresh fish was readily obtainable, is an example of both effective and organized commercialization. Salt-cod consumption even bucked religious trends, increasing during the eighteenth century despite the decline in the number of fast days. It also reminds us how it was often necessary to buy goods in order to feed oneself in early modern Europe (Figure 5.1).[6]

That said, apart from the fish, for most Europeans their Lenten diet of grains, vegetables and legumes was not that different from what they might have eaten on most days outside of Lent. This was for two reasons. First of all, because most Europeans could not spend more for their everyday fare. And, secondly, because Lenten-type fasts applied to many other days during the course of the year. As mentioned, Advent was also a period of fasting, and so were all Wednesdays and Fridays, as well as the evening

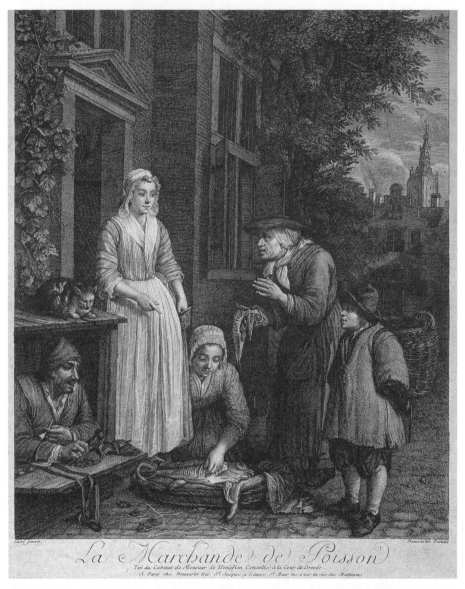

Figure 5.1 'La marchande de poisson' (The fish seller). Engraving by J. Beauvarlet after A. Carré, eighteenth century (Wellcome Library, London).

before any liturgical celebration (known as a 'vigil'). In all, some 150 days a year were set aside as fasting days.

Along with the fast, came the feast. One of the wildest periods of the Christian year were the few days preceding the start of Lent, a celebration known as Carnival. Derived from the Latin 'carne vale' (good-bye to meat), it culminated on Shrove Tuesday, known as *Mardi gras* in French ('fat Tuesday') and explicitly as *húshagyó kedd* ('meat-abandoning Tuesday') in Hungarian. There was much eating, drinking, parading and mayhem; but it all came to an abrupt end the following day with Ash Wednesday, marking the beginning of Lent. Carnival was more than just a food fest. During it, normal social rules and conventions were subverted: wives got to boss their husbands around, apprentices played tricks on their masters, local notables were mocked by the populace. It was a time when people could vent their frustrations and let off steam, knowing that come the next day, everything would return to normal. Although it was a period of rebellion and misrule, Carnival actually reinforced the social order and the usual patterns of subordination.

The impact of the Reformations

Both the Protestant and Catholic reformers were agreed in their disapproval of Carnival, and made attempts to reform if not eliminate it; but they took different stances regarding the practices of fasting and abstinence. Their reactions had in common the medieval theme that fasting did not have merit in and of itself, but had a greater purpose of helping gain salvation, when prescribed to the individual as appropriate and necessary. However they differed in how to apply this in a reformed religious climate. The Catholic Church clung to the significance and practice of fasting, and the rules that buttressed it. For most Protestant reformers, private, voluntary fasting might be seen as a useful devotion, and the occasional public fast a useful way of ordering the body politic, but that was as far as it went. Otherwise, Protestants were expected to maintain simple, abstemious habits throughout the course of the year. As a result, in half of Europe the cycle of feast and fast was definitively broken. During the seventeenth century fasting would be a matter of individual choice for most Protestants, although a similar development is evident among some Catholics during the eighteenth century, as we shall see.

In 1522, Huldrich Zwingli defended a member of his Zurich congregation, accused by the civil magistrates – who enforced fasting regulations – of eating sausages with his workers during Lent. The man, a printer, justified his actions to the court by stating that he had an unusually large amount of work that Lent. In response to the case, since the man just happened to be Zwingli's printer, Zwingli prepared a lengthy sermon in which he defended the principle that Christians were free to eat any foods at any time, even during Lent. One of Zwingli's points was that those people who are most vociferous in defence of fasting tend to be from the leisured classes, able to compensate the meat and other prohibitions with the pleasurable consumption of alternatives such as fish.[7]

For Protestant reformers, the problem of forced Lenten observance was made worse by the ecclesiastical practice of purchasing indulgences and dispensations. For example, one could obtain the right to eat butter during Lent by payment to the church, and although this was meant to be on health grounds, the practice was open to much abuse. Doing without butter or pork fat during Lent was particularly difficult in northern Europe, where it meant having to make use of much more expensive imported olive oil. Martin Luther argued that most people could not afford the dispensation and were forced to use olive oil during Lent:

In Rome, they make a mockery fasting, while forcing us to eat an oil they themselves would not use to grease their shoes. Then they sell us the right to eat foods forbidden on fast days…but they have stolen that same liberty from us with their ecclesiastical laws…Eating butter, they say, is a greater sin than to lie, blaspheme, or indulge in impurity.[8]

Luther was referring to the fact that early Christians had no food prohibitions. St Paul considered less important what went into a person's mouth than what came out of it, in the form of evil words. And it is indeed curious that those countries which used butter in cooking, as opposed to olive oil, are almost identical to those that broke away from the Catholic Church in the sixteenth century, as Jean-Louis Flandrin first suggested.[9] That said, we might argue that in the case of England, Henry VIII had more than butter on his mind when he broke with Rome.

The humanist Desiderius Erasmus pointed out the contradiction of a gastronomy dedicated to making the most out of lean days, the refined dishes developed during periods of fasting to make up for the absent meat. In the same year as Zwingli's defence, Erasmus, who had a dispensation to eat meat on health grounds, wrote a controversial letter to the humanist bishop of Basel on 'the prohibition of eating meat'. In it, Erasmus asked whether it was opportune to insist on lean days given that kitchens were more active on fast days than on regular ones, preparing more refined foods and at much greater expense. The result was that while the poor suffered hunger the rich dined with even more luxury than normal.[10] Erasmus's assertion is supported by the high number of recipes in Italian, French and Spanish cookery books dedicated to fast-day cooking.

Erasmus went further in his 1526 critique *Concerning the Eating of Fish*, which consists of a dialogue between a fishmonger and a butcher, which begins in satirical mode.[11] The two men argue over who would fare better if everyone was freed from observing Lent. The fishmonger thinks that meat would be less valued if it was not forbidden, while the butcher is sure that if the church allowed meat it would be in conformity with basic dietary principles condemning fish consumption, since cold and moist fish causes diseases in cold months. They go on to accuse one another, the butcher claiming that fish stinks, the fishmonger that butchers pass off cats and dogs for rabbits and hares. The debate then turns into a theological discourse on how the laws and fasts of the Old Testament were abrogated by the New Testament, although a multitude of food restrictions somehow arose nonetheless, Erasmus remarks. This sort of critical questioning was still possible on the eve of the Reformation. Erasmus was able to be critical of church practices without breaking with the church, while for Luther only a definitive break would do.

This does not mean that Protestant reformers dismissed fasting altogether. Luther was opposed to what he regarded as the arbitrary rules surrounding fasting, but held that fasting had its uses. It served to 'kill and subdue the pride and lust of the flesh', he wrote, adding, 'If it were not for lust, eating would be as meritorious as fasting'.[12] For John Calvin, all foods were clean, without temporal exception; but fasting was nevertheless important in preparing the individual privately for prayer, as well as promoting humility, the confession of guilt, gratitude for God's grace and, of course, disciplining lust.

Importantly, for Calvin fasting also had a public, community function. The organized fast, ordained by a pastor, would help assuage the wrath of God, thus combating the ravages of plague, famine and war.

These were more than theoretical discussions; through their stomachs, people's souls were at stake. The Reformation had a very real impact on what people ate. If Protestants rejected the Catholic belief that fasting was a path to salvation, they retained it as a devotional practice that served to bind the community. For Catholics, fasting remained an individual act; for Protestants, it was a public and symbolic one. But if Protestant reformers modified the nature of fasting, they certainly did not abandon it as a practice – at least not at first. Indeed, during the sixteenth century England and Scotland enacted far more laws enforcing abstinence from red meat during Lent than did France.[13] But then, in the middle of the seventeenth century, the English parliament replaced the medieval pattern of fasts with a single weekly fast-day, on Wednesdays. Even this was repealed in 1649, leaving England with no accepted or enforceable rule of fasting. King Charles II made one last-ditch proclamation on Lenten fasting in 1664, but this decade also saw the last prosecutions for breaches of the injunction. Henceforth the decision to fast or not, and when, would be a matter for the individual.

Fasting regulations aside, the Reformations had a profound effect on attitudes to food, especially in terms of attitudes towards luxury and excess. This campaign against luxury can be found in *both* the Protestant and Catholic Reformations and is especially evident and widespread during the sixteenth century. For example, the Swiss Protestant reformer Calvin and his followers advocated a return to the practices of the early church, which, in terms of food, meant an austerity and guilt-ridden attitude towards the pleasures of the flesh. Personal simplicity and distrust of elegant food flourished among Calvinists. Just as Calvinists considered all righteous people to be 'saints', so they expected them to act as such. They enforced this morality by different means, resulting in a kind of permanent sobriety and abstinence, not unlike that practised by some religious orders during the middle ages.

Among Counter-Reformation thinkers there was also a new attitude towards food. François de Sales, Catholic bishop of Geneva, offered a new kind of straightforward religiosity to lay people, providing examples of how people could be devout in their everyday lives, without having to follow the kind of heroic devotions and mortifications of the Catholic saints, or even those of monks and nuns. In his *Introduction to the Devout Life*, first published in 1619, de Sales wrote about food and appetite, as a way of talking about conjugal relations. Food was a necessity, in order to maintain life, which made eating (i.e., sex between husband and wife) a virtuous and praiseworthy act. It was a question of degree. 'As those who eat from the duty of mutual conversation should eat freely and not as it were by constraint, and, moreover, should try to show some appetite, so the marriage debt should always be rendered faithfully, freely, and just as if it were with the hope of begetting children'. By contrast, to eat 'merely to satisfy the appetite, is permissible, but not praiseworthy', and 'to eat, not from mere appetite, but to excess and immoderately, is more or less blameworthy, according as the excess is great or small'. However important and pleasing, food (sex) should not be allowed to become an obsession.[14]

Fasting and abstinence

Since the Middle Ages, monks and nuns had offered an example of asceticism to Christian Europeans. We have seen this with regard to the rule of St Benedict. Some orders, like the Carthusians, went further still, living a perpetual Lenten fast, never touching meat or animal products. This ascetic tradition had a long history in Christianity, the point being to mortify the flesh in an effort to strengthen the soul. The aim of this sort of asceticism was not to hasten death (since suicide was the destruction of God's creation, it was considered the supreme sin); rather, it aimed to chasten the body, ridding it of its appetites. Asceticism, considered a positive virtue that brought one closer to God, was the polar opposite of gluttony, one of the seven deadly sins. Just as overindulging brought with it the threat of eternal damnation, so self-sacrifice promised the reward of heaven.

It is quite possible that generations of extremely austere monastic men and women virtually starved themselves to the point of death following years of rigorous abstinence. For nuns in particular, this kind of devotion through self-denial provided a source of power and agency in a male-dominated world, which one social historian has called 'holy anorexia'.[15] Being a monk or nun provided people with this sort of opportunity for heroic asceticism; but even in more 'normal' conditions, monasticism allowed people to live and eat in a unique way. It allowed male and female religious to live as Jesus did, in comparative simplicity, among like-minded brothers or sisters, and devote one's life to prayer and other acts of devotion.

Originally at least, monks and nuns lived in relatively isolated communities, eating simple, communal meals. But as many of the orders prospered and became wealthy, like the Benedictines, their habits often imitated the local aristocracy, from whose ranks the monks might be drawn. The image of the fat, fun-loving friar became a popular stereotype, one the Protestant reformers railed against. The Catholic reformation responded to this state of affairs not by disbanding the monasteries, as the Protestants did, but by reforming them. Various orders, like the Franciscans, returned to their stricter, original observance. Nonetheless, substantial differences between religious orders remained throughout the early modern period, from the simple Franciscans and Poor Clares, on the one hand, to the wealthy Benedictines, on the other, as their rules attest.

And in fact most religious orders adopted a middle ground. Balancing sound nourishment with moderation was especially important for those active religious orders founded during the period of Catholic renewal. One such was the Society of Jesus, or the Jesuits as they were commonly known, founded by Ignatius of Loyola. The Jesuits were not technically a religious order, since they were not monks or friars in the tradition of St Benedict or St Francis, but an order of ordained priests. Their focus was on teaching and missionizing throughout the world, and for this they needed to be healthy and well-nourished. If the Jesuit curriculum represented a new and modern pedagogical model, followed in their hundreds of boarding schools across the Catholic world, when it came to feeding their members and those in their care, the Jesuits initiated a new dietary style. It was shared, if not imitated, by other active religious orders of the time.

As Jacques Revel first noted, this *modèle alimentaire* was in keeping with the spirit of the Counter-Reformation.[16] This is not to say that it was austere and frugal, which it certainly was not. Rather, it set a new standard that negotiated a course between courtly sumptuousness and refinement, on the one hand, shared by some aristocratic religious orders, and the simplicity and sameness of the strict monastic diet, closer to peasant cookery, on the other. It took ingredients and dishes from both. The Jesuit style followed a regular pattern of three courses – *antipasto, minestra/porzione* and *pospasto* – not unlike the dining habits of privileged, lay sectors of Italian society. Within a standardized meal plan the 'Jesuit diet' allowed for choice by the individual, offering different options at the same meal. It also allowed, indeed encouraged, people of different status to be served special foods. Diet could thus be tailored to individual needs and constitutions, as recommended by the medical knowledge of the time, always a concern of Ignatius (as we saw in Chapter 4). The emphasis was on both the quantity and variety of foods, considered necessary to fuel the social elites in leading the sort of active life the Jesuits valued so much. It was a dietary style that remained little changed from the beginnings of the Society of Jesus in the mid-sixteenth century to its suppression in 1773.[17]

Despite these differences, Catholic monasteries, nunneries and religious institutions continued to provide opportunities for heroic asceticism throughout the period. Even within the well-nourished Jesuit environment, there were individual Jesuits like Luigi Gonzaga (soon canonized), who favoured a much more rigorous and self-sacrificial approach to diet. Gonzaga, a student at the Jesuits' Collegio Romano in the 1580s, survived mostly on bread and water, apparently never eating more than an ounce of food at a time.[18] Heroic asceticism, enough to be regarded as saintly, was also possible within the Catholic Church hierarchy, which had previously been the source of such vehement criticism from Luther. There are numerous examples of saintly figures who opted to live a perpetual fast. Archbishop Carlo Borromeo of Milan, despite being a cardinal of the Catholic Church and a Milanese patrician, heir to vast estates, eschewed all creature comforts, according to contemporary hagiographers.[19] When Borromeo was not depicted among the poor and plague victims, providing assistance, he was represented alone at table, in solitary devotion, with bread and water his only nourishment. Other Catholic saints went even further than this. Not content merely to eat the very minimum, they actually sought to punish their appetites. The eighteenth-century Franciscan Giuseppe da Copertino abstained from even bread and wine, and sprinkled his plate of simple herbs or beans with 'a bitter powder' – a sort of anti-condiment. This became his regimen, so much so that when he had to eat meat because ordered to do so by his superior, 'his overcharged stomach immediately rebelled and rejected the meat', according to his hagiographer.[20]

Heaven knows what the monastery's doctor made of it all. If the influential priest and educational reformer Jean-Baptiste de La Salle (1703) felt it was necessary to subjugate one's taste, few medical authors endorsed heroic acts of dietary asceticism.[21]

Never mind that forcing oneself to eat what one did not like, for the sake of one's soul, as de La Salle recommended, was a view harsher than anything de Sales would have advised a hundred years earlier; from a medical standpoint it was believed to harm the body. It went contrary to the medical notion that individual tastes and preferences were a guide to the body's needs. And if regular monastic abstinence found little medical favour, extreme cases of saintly self-deprivation were that much worse. This was because, medically speaking, a constantly hungry body was believed to devour itself, in its search for nourishment, literally wasting away.

Physicians and fasting

People had a responsibility for their physical health that went beyond their immediate well-being. As the town physician of Frankfurt, Joachim Strupp, put it in 1573, 'we should honour bodies not as our own, but as God's image'. As God's creations, formed in his likeness, all people were obliged to care for the well-being of their bodies and souls, which the Lutheran Strupp regarded as the basis for all social activity.[22] In a Christian society, the personal reformation of the body and social order went hand in hand.

Doctors almost universally exalted a regime of moderation and generally condemned excess, whether that meant too much or too little. Although they might disagree on just what constituted excess, they agreed on the somewhat paradoxical notion that overeating was actually less nourishing than undereating. This requires some explaining. Galenic physicians recognized that young, healthy, robust and well-exercised people could, and should, eat more than older, sedentary, more delicate people. The former simply had the power to 'concoct' (digest) greater quantities of food. But when one exceeded the body's digestive power by overindulging, the process was spoiled. Food that remained undigested could never be put to good use by the body. Rather, it was believed to 'corrupt' there and cause all sorts of harm, physical and mental. The food decayed in the body, generating heat and fumes, which filled our head, dulling our vision and thoughts, as well as causing intense weariness. The flesh then absorbed this corrupt matter, and, paradoxically, the body wasted away, since it received no assimilable nutrients. This is the origin of one apparently strange comment that gluttons did not increase in bodily size.[23] According to the same theory of digestion, eating less food actually supplied the body with more nourishment. The body could 'concoct' all of it, and quicker, and so supply the body's needs. Hence the saying, which existed in a variety of European languages, that 'whoever eats less, eats more'.[24] Moderation was not just religious advice, for the good of one's soul; it also made practical medical sense.

In the same vein, 'moderate' fasting was considered healthy, for it acted like a good purge or blood-letting on the body, ridding it of excess. Weekly religious fasting allowed Christians to purge body and soul together and was, according to one doctor, more effective for health than medical purges.[25] The English physician Andrew Boorde, whose national peregrinations we followed in the previous chapter, was a great supporter of it, at least in theory, writing that 'abstynence is the chefyst medyson of all medysons'.[26] In practice, however, Boorde found the Carthusian dietary rigour of his own vows overly restrictive, and petitioned to leave the Order (although an accusation of being 'conversant with women' may also have had something to do with this). Fasting should be occasional. 'Seasonable abstinence is wholsome', wrote the French physician Jean Fernel, 'and most profitable is that evacuation which is made by fasting. For it worketh gently and without any violent forcing either of the body of the humours, and without bringing into the body any unnaturall quality, it proceedeth softly and by degrees'.[27] By contrast, 'immoderate' fasting was considered harmful, forcing the body to eat itself. 'Because both the nourishment and the superfluous humour being spent', Fernel wrote, immoderate fasting 'wasteth also the very substance of the parts, which is the seat of heat; at length it cooleth the body and diminisheth and impaireth the strength'.

For this reason, doctors were never particularly keen on long periods of abstinence or severe fasting. Not that Renaissance writers openly expressed this; they might mention that abstinence could be more dangerous than overindulging, but none openly criticized religious fasting. However, by the time of the Reformation, Protestant authors had no qualms condemning the practice of extensive fasting, now associated with the excesses of the maligned Catholic Church. For them, there was a big difference between temperance or moderate abstinence, on the one hand, and outright self-mortification, on the other.

On the positive side, Henry Mason, chaplain to the bishop of London, wrote in support of moderate fasting. People complained 'that fasting breedeth winde in the stomache, griping in the bowels, giddiness in the head, and faintness through the whole body'. But in fact quite the contrary was true: rather than 'an hinderance to their health', fasting was 'the only help either to recover or preserve it', Mason argued. He made his point based on personal experience. 'I can truly say', Mason went on, 'that though before tryall I feared hurt, by reason of my sickly and weake temper: yet after tryall I have found the quite contrary; my body more at ease, my spirits more free, and all my senses more fresh and lively'.[28]

On the negative side, and within the same Church of England, Thomas Moffet, English court physician and some-time member of Parliament, did not think fasting a good thing, perhaps because excessive fasting was so often praised by religious authors. Moffet put it this way: 'Maids and women are highly extolled for consuming their bodies with excessive abstinence; which being a thing against nature and Godliness (which forbiddeth us to scourge or mark, and much more to consume our bodies), it shall need no confutation at all'.[29] Excessive abstinence forced the starved body to feed on itself, threatening what God himself had created. Moffet may have had cases similar to the Swiss woman Apollonia Schreier in mind, who apparently survived for eleven months without food: cases that invited more wonder and suspicion than emulation (Figure 5.2).

Later Catholic medical writers were less than enthusiastic when it came to the Lenten fast. One of the problems was the prohibition against the consumption of meat, eggs and dairy products that resulted in a reliance on fish, and fish was simply too cold and

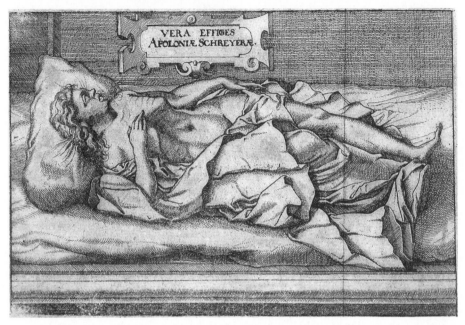

Figure 5.2 Extreme abstinence: Apollonia Schreier of Galz, near Berne. Woodcut from Paulus Lentulus, *Historia admiranda, de prodigiosa Apolloniae Schreierae, virginis in agro Bernensi, inedia… tribus narrationibus comprehensa*, 1604 (Wellcome Library, London).

moist in Galenic terms, prone to corruption in the body, to receive unreserved praise from dietary writers. Meat was necessary for a healthy body. Melchior Sebisch (Sebizius) warned readers that Carthusian monks, because of their predominantly fish diet, became phlegmatic, somnolent and fat. As a result, they suffered from diseases like apoplexy, paralysis, catarrh and arthritis.[30]

Few Renaissance physicians were enthusiastic about fish, but there are two notable exceptions. The first is the Milanese Girolamo Cardano, who devoted more space to fish than any other category of food in his *De sanitate tuenda*. This was inspired by both Cardano's engagement with the latest scholarly work on the subject and by the fact that Cardano was living in Rome when he wrote it, the centre of the Counter-Reformation.[31] The second is Ludovico Nonnius. Nonnius is best known today for having being painted by Rubens, but he was an important physician in his day. Born Luis Nuñes in Antwerp, of Portuguese-Jewish descent, the humanist Nonnius was extremely enthusiastic about fish and fish-eating. He published his *Ichthyophagia*, describing various species of fish and the health benefits to be derived from eating them, in 1616. Nonnius followed this up with his general dietary manual the *Diaeteticon*, in 1627. In it, he remarked that most people thought of fish as an unpleasant burden to eat, being forced to eat it during Lent. These negative connotations were reinforced by physicians, with their warnings against it. But Nonnius reminded readers that the ancients ate fish often, and only closer to his time did scholarly authority begin to turn against it. Against received wisdom, Nonnius argued that fish was among the healthiest of foods, especially appropriate for lawyers, students and others who get little exercise.[32]

No doubt Nonnius was also making a concession to the eating habits of his readership in the Spanish Netherlands, adapting Galenic theory to what was common dietary practice. Moreover, by the time of Nonnius's death fish was beginning to shed its Lenten associations of abstinence and find gastronomic approval. The influential French cook Nicolas de Bonnefons served fish and meat dishes at the same eight-course dinner, with the fish dishes receiving the same refined treatment as other foods.[33] It is a sign that ideas about Lent were beginning to change (but more on this below). Later still, we find a similar enthusiasm for fish, perhaps not surprisingly, in a Portuguese dietary, where discussions of different fish occupy over sixty pages.[34]

Other dietary prohibitions made Lent a time of necessary risk when it came to one's health. Only one main meal a day was allowed, even though doctors considered two to be healthy for digestion. A diet of fish and vegetables gave one quite literally *une face de carême* – a pale, glum and wearied countenance – as the French put it. Moreover, the sudden change in diet was a dangerous move away from the normal routine considered necessary for health. Finally, the prohibition of meat meant that people were tempted to eat more of what was allowed in order to feel full. In Lent of 1678 the Spada-Veralli household in Rome was observing Lent, eating 'leafy vegetables and foods of no consequence [*bagatelle*]'. Maria Veralli wrote to her husband Orazio Spada: 'Be careful not to eat too much since this undermines the complexion, since they [Lenten foods] are of little substance'. When Orazio complained of haemorrhoids, Maria ascribed them to 'these Lenten foods and the time of the year'. Fortunately, the family came through Lent with its health intact: 'I am pleased to hear that Lent has treated you so well that you are not suffering its after-effects'. But the end of Lent brought its own dangers in the feasting that followed it. In Maria's words to her husband 'Be careful over Easter, or the sudden change in foods will trouble you'.[35]

Nowhere in the Spada-Veralli correspondence do we get the impression that the family was reluctant to observe Lent; indeed quite the contrary would appear to be true. All of the hardships and risks were well known to Europe's Catholics. This does not mean they were resigned to their Lenten fates. On the illicit side, they could buy contraband meat. The eighty-two infractions in the French city of Lyon between 1658 to 1714, ranging from a few pounds of meat to entire animals, suggests a parallel trade in forbidden flesh.[36] On the licit side, they could seek a dispensation from the authorities. There must have been enough grumbling about lean periods, not to mention an increasing tendency for people to seek exemptions from Lenten observance on health grounds, that Paolo Zacchia felt the need to rebut each of the 'oppositions' to Lenten fasting and 'errors' committed in observing it in his 1636 treatise *Il vitto quaresimale*. For example, fewer meals, at set times, allowed us to exercise control over hunger and our appetites (including the libidinous), Zacchia wrote. Moreover, because Lent occurred during spring, when our bodies were full of superfluous bad humours and excess blood, the consumption of lighter and less nourishing foods was in fact good for our health, reducing our bodily heat. It cleared the mind to allow one to focus one's attention on spiritual matters, contributing to the health of the soul which was after all the main purpose of Lent.[37] The thrust of Zacchia's book is positive and constructive in nature, following the form of a traditional regimen but with an emphasis on which foods to eat, how to prepare them and in what order to consume them during Lent, so as not to endanger one's health.[38] The advice is at once practical and spiritual, given than Lent offers us the chance to take care of our bodies and our souls, Zacchia argues.

Outside of specifically designated days and periods of abstinence, and outside of particular spaces like monasteries, Christians were not expressly forbidden any categories of food. This distinguished them from their Jewish and Muslim neighbours. In a discussion of the rules relating to meat preparation, of which meats were best stewed and which roasted, Francisco Nuñez de Oria notes that most Spanish families ignored these rules; 'Turks and Moors', by contrast, paid much more attention to them, which is why they suffered from fewer fevers than Christians do.[39]

But in Nuñez de Oria's Spain such behaviour was being criminalized. Details of the dietary customs of Muslim converts to Christianity, the Moriscos, emerge from Inquisitorial trials against them. In Valencia it was customary for moriscos to bring their *cazuelas de carne*, meat stew-pots, to the Morisco baker for cooking in the oven. The details emerge from Inquisitorial trials against these Muslim converts to Christianity. In a trial from 1530 a man described only as 'Sancho's brother' was referred to as carrying a *cazuela*, complete with large chunks of meat seasoned in oil and oregano, on his head, bound for the bakery.[40] What could be deemed particularly Islamic about such activity? Certainly not the recipe or the fact of taking a pot for cooking in the baker's oven. It may have been the day or time of the year (say, on a Christian fast day) or the fact that he was a Morisco taking the pot to a Morisco baker (and thus evidence of an ongoing Muslim sensibilities) or the fact that the meat had been slaughtered in a particular way. In Valencia during the late sixteenth century, of the cases involving food, most accusations involved slaughtering meat in 'the Muslim manner' and fasting during Ramadan and not according to the Christian calendar.[41] What for Spanish Moriscos was a means of maintaining religious identity, for the Catholic authorities was an offence punishable by the Inquisition: lashes were administered, fines were imposed and butchers forbidden from practising their trade. The Moriscos were expelled from Spain in 1609, although their culinary contribution lived on.[42]

Few medical authors discuss Jewish food laws and rituals, but they do sometimes mention specific foods associated with Jewish communities. The most common of these was salted goose. Thus the Bolognese physician Baldassare Pisanelli believed that the consumption of goose, whose flesh had a 'bad odour' and was difficult to digest, explained why Jews 'are always melancholic, of bad colour and poor habits'.[43]

For the Inquisitors of Catholic Europe, ever on the lookout for Jewish converts to Christianity suspected of 'lapsing' into Judaism (and so known as 'Judaizers'), goose-eating was as sure a sign as circumcision. Thus in 1558 a suspected Judaizer of Montagnana was accused before the Venetian Inquisition 'that he routinely ate kosher meat [*carne sachatada*] and goose, according to the custom of the Jews'.[44] For European

Jews, the goose was an important resource in the domestic economy, just as raising a pig was for many Christian households. From foie gras to sausages and other cured meats, no part of the goose was wasted. Ghetto bakers in northern Italy even offered their clientele a delicacy, known as *ofelle* (and by a variety of other names): thin layers of pastry, moistened with verjuice, filled with foie gras, then fried in goose fat before being sprinkled with sugar and cinnamon, and then served crispy and hot.[45]

At least one Christian was grateful for being given the chance to try 'goose sausages in the hebrew style'. In 1573 Battista Gislato, court scribe for the Venetian Inquisition, testified that the converso Abraham Enriques Nunes offered him some: 'and so I took a slice and I found it to be of such a delicate and tasty consistency, that I asked for one as a present, and he kindly gave me it'. Gislato liked it so much that he later paid 16 *soldi* for one.[46] As this example suggests, the consumption of goose was not limited to Jews. French dietaries in particular outline they way goose could be prepared in order to make the heavy meat digestible and palatable.[47] But goose did become emblematic of Jewishness, both within and without the Jewish communities, as much as the hated yellow ring badge they were forced to wear in places in many towns throughout Europe.

Jews were also associated with another much-maligned foodstuff, the aubergine. Considered cold and viscous, the aubergine's Latin name *malum insanum* ('mad apple' in the English of the day) gives a fairly good idea of its low repute. In Spain, however, where it had been brought by the Arabs, the aubergine was widely eaten. In his 1554 commentary on Dioscorides, the Spanish medical humanist Andrés Laguna, himself of converso origin, related that 'in France and Germany, [the aubergine] is extremely rare. In Castile it is copious, especially in Toledo, which has exposed the Toledans to much mockery and derision'.[48] Nuñez de Oria discusses how the aubergine can be 'tempered', citing Arab authors like Avicenna, as well as 'Rabbi Moyses', or Maimonides.[49] In Spain, Jews, and in particular Jewish converts to Catholicism and their descendants, were sometimes referred to as *berenjenas* (aubergines) – and it was not meant as a compliment. In a 1508 census of Seville one woman resident of the San Pedro de Carmona quarter is listed as 'the Poor Aubergine'.[50] Inhabitants of Toledo, with a large population of conversos, were insultingly called 'aubergine-eaters' (*berenjeneros*). According to Lugana, 'after cooking it in water, they [the Toledans] fry it with oil and spices, and finally they eat it with walnut sauce'.[51] The aubergine-eating topos found its way into the literature of the day. Francisco Delicado's *Retrato de la Lozana andaluza* (1528) features a converso heroine who at one stage boasts about her talents as a cook – revealing her Jewish origins: 'And do I know how to make *boronía*? Wonderfully! And aubergine casserole? To perfection. And casserole with a nice bit of garlic and cumin, and a nice dash of vinegar. None could fine fault with anything I made!'[52]

Jews forced from Spain brought their taste for aubergines with them to Italy. Vincenzo Tanara, a Bolognese nobleman, gives a detailed entry about the aubergine's cultivation in his husbandry manual of 1644, bypassing the traditional medical advice against it. Tanara suggests that aubergines might do as family food on meatless days, 'as amongst the Hebrews they are a common food'.[53]

Fasting and health in the eighteenth century

If the Catholic Church continued to propose many of its saints as models of dietary asceticism throughout the early modern period, the everyday practices of Catholics were changing. There are many signs that the ascetic rigours of the Counter-Reformation were giving way to a more 'flexible' and individualized approach to devotion, which would usher in a shift in Lenten practices by European Catholics, especially during the eighteenth century. The Counter-Reformation had itself sown the seeds of this change in attitude by fostering a less legalistic understanding of penitential acts to achieve salvation, like fasting. Instead the Catholic Church stressed fasting as a spiritually driven expression of personal piety. One example is the devotion known as the 'Spritiual Exercises', introduced by the founder of the Jesuits, Loyola, and approved in 1548. Moderation in diet, so that one became 'master of oneself, both in the manner of eating and in the quantity of food eaten', was a feature of this structured set of prayers, meditations and mental exercises.[54] The 'Spiritual Exercises' lasted a month and could be undertaken at any time of the year, under the guidance of a spiritual director. They were certainly not intended to replace Lenten observance, but they did introduce a new way of practising abstinence, in a different devotional context.

When it came to Lenten observance, the Church now allowed consumption of previously forbidden foodstuffs – eggs, butter and cheese – in certain circumstances during Lent, such as famine or epidemics.[55] In Spanish America new foods stretched the boundaries of what was admissible. At the end of the sixteenth century the Jesuit missionary José de Acosta remarked that he felt 'some scruple' about eating manatee on a Friday, since, although classed as a fish, it looked and tasted so much like veal.[56] Another example comes in the form of the protracted debate over drinking chocolate, as we shall see in Chapter 7.

The churches seemed less concerned to enforce abstinence and warn against gluttony. By 1650, in England, for example, homilies against gluttonous eating were far less common than they had been. Lenten abstinence became a thing of the past. Fish consumption and the fish industry went into long-term decline in England, from which it never really recovered.[57] The absence of fish from English tables prompted the widely travelled Arthur Young to remark, 'Nothing provokes one so in a country residence, as a lake, a river, or the sea within view of the windows, and a dinner everyday without fish, which is so common in England'.[58] The thought was occasioned by a delightful supper of a brace of carp on the banks of the river Charente in France, where fish was still very much on the menu – and without any accompanying sense of guilt. Eighteenth-century French sermons and sermon manuals also showed greater indulgence to the sin of gluttony; indeed 'gluttony' itself underwent a shift in connotation. In secular circles, *gourmandise* was more and more about good taste and a refined palate.[59] From the church's point of view, gluttony was still considered sinful, as in the time of de Sales, but it was now considered a venial rather than mortal sin. The focus remained on excessive food consumption, which continued to be condemned, while opening the way for a limited amount of pleasure. In his influential *Theologia moralis* (Moral theology, 1753–1755), the southern Italian Alfonso de' Liguori wrote that it was not a sin to like eating, since it was impossible not to develop a taste for it.[60] In other words, the key figure in the Catholic Church's late eighteenth-century revival argued that, while it remained sinful to eat *for* pleasure, one could legitimately eat *with* pleasure. In this, as in much else, de' Liguori argued for a middle way between the rigours of Jansenism and a milder interpretation which divided the Catholic Church.

At the same time as the Catholic Church was becoming more flexible in its attitude towards food consumption, Lenten observance and fasting practices were becoming increasingly medicalized. In 1657 the Parlement of Paris gave physicians the authority to prescribe meat during Lent.[61] Priests had always been able to grant dispensations to their parishioners on health grounds. Legitimately exempt from fasting were all people under 21 and over 60, the sick, pregnant women, wet-nurses, pilgrims and the poor receiving charity. They were allowed to buy and eat meat and other prohibited foods, from butchers and other shops especially licensed for this. In France at least, the ecclesiastical exemption now had to be accompanied by a medical certificate. A person's religious obligations were now secondary to his or her physical needs and condition.

Fifty years later, medical discussions on the subject became heated when two high-ranking doctors from Paris's medical faculty published sharply diverging treatises on the subject. Philippe Hecquet wrote his 1709 work on Lenten dispensations to proclaim the moral bankruptcy of the Church and change the food habits of the French.[62] Hecquet bemoaned the high number of dispensations from Lenten observance. A strict Jansenist, Hecquet believed that in order to elevate the soul one must quell the needs of the body, which could only be achieved through strict fasting. Vegetables and fish were ideally suited to this purpose. This is where Hecquet's iatromechanical philosophy came in.[63] Because of their material composition, vegetables and fish were easily broken down through what Hecquet referred to as 'trituration': a grinding down that took place in the mouth and stomach wall, part of the more physical view of digestion that characterized iatromechanics. Far from being harmful, as most physicians argued, vegetables and fish were healthier than meat and helped prolong life, according to Hecquet.

This view was rebutted by Hecquet's colleague, Nicolas Andry. Andry's devotional bent was less rigorous than Hecquet's and he was also a follower of iatrochemistry, adopting a chemical view of the digestive process, which had fermentation as its key, as opposed to a mechanical one. For Andry, a diet without meat, with its superior nourishment, was harmful. Meat was healthier but one could have too much of a good thing, which was precisely why Lent was necessary. The Church had instituted a period of Lenten observance to foster a period of less nourishing food so as to reduce the passions of the body which came about from eating nourishing food.[64] If vegetables and fish were all that a body needed, Andry argued, then there would have been no need for Lent. Andry's defence of Lent also sought to put a positive face on Lenten observance, much as Zacchia had done, by detailing how a long list of foodstuffs might be prepared to render them healthier for the body, without sacrificing the refinements to which French diners were increasingly accustomed. Andry's exultation of the role of taste in this process was consistent with a less rigorous, more moderate interpretation of Lent and an increased emphasis on the role of the individual in determining appropriate fare.

While the debate over the nature of the digestive process raged on, chemical against mechanical, even Hecquet's defenders found it difficult to support his strict views on Lenten observance. European Catholics voted with their stomachs. In the years 1710 and 1711, over one-third of the residents of Parma's Jesuit Collegio dei Nobili, pupils and teachers alike, were exempted from Lenten observance.[65] The faithful increasingly sought dispensations, and these were less likely to be based on 'legitimate' health grounds, which compliant doctors were more likely to grant. Based on the records of the Hôtel-Dieu, Paris' main hospital, which was allowed to sell meat during Lent to people dispensed from Lenten observance on health grounds, Reynald Abad has shown how the quantity of meat consumed by Parisians during Lent rose significantly throughout the eighteenth century. Even taking population growth into account, the increase in Lenten meat consumption is particularly dramatic from the 1760s, prompting Abad to estimate that the five years from 1765 to 1770 alone saw a 40 per cent increase in the number of Parisians eating meat during Lent.[66] In 1774 the Hôtel-Dieu lost its monopoly to sell meat during Lent, which was extended to all licensed merchants. Parisians were reminded to conform to 'the laws of the church' when it came to dispensation; but in practice the authorities decided to 'leave the choice of fat or lean up to the individual stomach and the individual conscience', in the words of the dramatist Louis-Sebastien Mercier.[67]

The privileged elements of Parisian society lead the way, apparently eager to abandon the restrictions of Lent, their motives inadvertently highlighting the hypocrisy at the heart of these restrictions – even for those who followed them. For those who could afford it, Lenten asceticism was a thing of the past, replaced by a luxury which, while it respected the letter of the law, disregarded its spirit. As the *philosophe* Voltaire rhetorically asked in his *Philosophical Dictionary* of 1764, 'Why, on days of abstinence, does the Roman church consider it a crime to eat terrestrial animals, and a good work to be served sole and salmon? The rich papist who has five hundred francs' worth of fish on his table shall be saved; and the poor wretch dying of hunger who eats four *sous*' worth of pork, shall be damned'.[68]

This comment reflected changing dietary practices throughout Catholic Europe. The number of fast days observed by Catholics had declined significantly from its Counter-Reformation peak, as the example of eighteenth-century Spain suggests. The way these occasions were observed had also changed. In their fast-day observance, Spanish religious orders increasingly shunned dried or salted cod (*bacalao*) for fresh and daintier kinds of fish, if they could afford to (at a time when salt-cod was becoming more of a staple further down in society).[69] But this was nothing compared to Poland's bishops, if Jedrej Kitowicz's late eighteenth-century memoir is anything to go by. Using the excuse that their guests routinely included Protestants as well as Catholics, 'many bishops were offering open meat tables on fast days (as if the non-fast days were not sufficient, as if there was no fish or as if they could not afford it)'.[70] Even in traditional 'fish-dinners', Kitowicz says elsewhere, the fish might be cooked in a meat sauce, such as carp with a piece of bacon underneath, 'so nobody could see this treachery'.[71] The laity went further still. The meatless Christmas-eve vigil of one Polish aristocrat, in the mid-eighteenth century, was no sacrifice, including as it did 'enormous' pikes, 'broad' carps, flounder, small and normal-sized salmon, dried sturgeon imported from Lithuania, tench prepared in a 'special' way, stuffed perch, zander, long eels, oysters, frogs, snails and beaver-tail. The quantity of food served at the meal was huge, all of it cooked in a variety of different ways. Nor was there any abstention when it came to drinks, since the aristocrat, Klemens Branicki, kept a cellar 'known in the world'.[72]

Whether all of this is an indication of dechristianization is, however, problematic. After all, this same period saw the rise of Pietism in Germany and Methodism in England. John Wesley developed his own system of fasting which he hoped would spiritually invigorate the church and benefit the individual. For Wesley, spiritual and bodily health went hand in hand, through the pursuit of self-purification. As we saw in Chapter 2, Wesley was strongly influenced by the dietetical ideas of George Cheyne, with their strong moral element. In spiritual terms, limiting one's diet would help reign in the sensual appetites which harm body and soul: that 'we may be enabled to abstain from every passion and temper which is not pleasing in [God's] sight'.[73] Fasting, in particular, contributed to self-chastisement and aided in prayer. It provided a means by which divine grace affects the human soul. Wesley did not mean for meals to be sad and sombre affairs, however. While he decried 'variety and delicacy ', Wesley apparently enjoyed his food, and recommended cheerfulness, thankfulness and appropriate conversation at meals, 'every morsel a pledge of life eternal'.[74] This was an approach not dissimilar from that of the above-mentioned Catholic bishop and founder of a religious order de' Liguori. At the same time, Friedrich Hoffmann sought to achieve a synthesis between the scientific confidence of the Enlightenment and a fundamental Christian faith. In his own successful health guide of 1740, the Pietist Hoffmann suggested that a mind in God, well-cultivated reason and bodily health were together the source of 'true felicitousness'.[75]

Moreover, a moralizing strand permeates early modern views of diet: a constant, perhaps, rather than a trend. Thus at period's end we have a cautionary tale of dietary redemption in the form of Jean-François Marmontel's *Mémoires*.[76] Marmontel was a protégé of Voltaire, elected to the Académie Française in 1763 and who died in 1799. His life story takes him from a frugal but healthy peasant childhood in the Limousin region, with a diet based on dairy products and fruit, to the life of a successful author in Paris, characterized by courtly excess and the 'pleasures of the table'. When he is overcome by ill health, Marmontel resolves to take up a sober diet, and finds peace and calm as a result. In Marmontel's self-presentation, the 'Christian moral structures of sin, guilt, and atonement were transcribed almost unaltered into the corporeal domain in a secular language of eating', as Emma Spary has noted.[77] But we have been here before. Marmontel's account of bodily salvation through diet is simply a transposition of Alvise Cornaro's Renaissance Venice to the France of the *philosophes*.

Conclusion

What is without doubt is that religiously inspired food habits and preferences changed dramatically over the course of the early modern period. Attitudes towards asceticism were at their harshest, their most rigorous, in the century of the Protestant and Catholic Reformations, when they were in tune with Galenic notions of physiology. From the latter half of the seventeenth century, the asceticism and restraint associated with, and advocated by, the Reformations were losing cultural influence. Going too was any dominant medical rationale. The Catholic Church's flexibility allowed luxury in through the back door, for one could keep to the letter of the law by avoiding certain foods but ignore its spirit by dining extravagantly nonetheless. By the end of the eighteenth century Catholic Europeans were increasingly eating meat during Lent, where they had the chance; where they did not, they nevertheless aimed to eat dainty and luxurious foods. Over the early modern period, the Protestant Reformation had a role to play in the evolution of people's relationship with food and abstinence, as did the Counter-Reformation and medicine itself. Later, the secularism and individualism of the Enlightenment also led to changing attitudes, but just as important was a relaxation of observance requirements by ecclesiastical authorities throughout Europe and a changing, less legalistic notion of what should be required of the 'good Christian'.

CHAPTER 6
VEGETABLE FOOD: THE VEGETARIAN OPTION

Introduction

If ever there was an area of diet that illustrates the gap between medical advice and real food consumption, then that of vegetable foods must be it. Nor is there an area where medical advice changed more over the course of the early modern period. In 1550 the eminent and wealthy physician Tommaso Rangoni published a treatise with the very appealing and modern-sounding title of 'how to prolong human life to the age of 120'.[1] The book was successful enough to go through five editions over the next fifteen years – although Rangoni is perhaps more remembered today, at least among art historians, for his role as art patron, celebrated in a bust by Alessandro Vittoria for the facade of the Venetian church of San Giuliano.[2] In chapter 14 Rangoni deals with the dietary factors that most shorten a man's life. Mushrooms come first as a death-causing poison, and this is understandable, given the risks of eating poisonous varieties; but the chapter abounds with a variety of vegetables and fruits and the dangers they pose to human health, complete with the classical citations one would expect from a learned Renaissance doctor. Cabbage begets bad blood and the most noxious odours; garlic damages vision and causes pain, wind and vomiting; cucumbers are cold, hard to digest and generate corruption; aubergines generate blockages, headaches and haemorrhoids; cardoons and especially artichokes turn the blood black and turbid; and so on.[3]

Rangoni vilified foods like vegetables and fruits, perceived as qualitatively watery, viscous, cold and devoid of nourishment. This meant they had little 'sticking' power as they passed through the body, and so generated a watery, thin blood; this excess moisture got trapped in the membranes of the body and putrefied. The moisture had negative effects on the brain, compromising wit and intelligence, and in extreme cases leading to melancholy and related diseases. A Spanish doctor, Juan Sorapán de Rieros, put it quite simply: 'eating vegetables and falling ill are one and the same thing.'[4] Never was eating your 'five-a-day' more dangerous than in the Renaissance. As a result, many vegetables and fruits were seen as suitable only for rustics and labourers, who alone had the bodily heat necessary to counter their cold and moist qualities and the strong stomachs to digest them.

Historians, including myself, have really gone to town exploring the 'warning labels' that Renaissance physicians put on numerous vegetables, regardless of actual habits.[5] As a point of view so at odds with our own, it highlights the otherness of Galenic theory compared to that of modern biomedicine. And in fact, a selective reading of the Renaissance dietaries would easily confirm Rangoni's prejudices concerning the harmful nature of vegetables. Were the physicians so out of touch with the actual dietary practices of most of society and with the changing fashions among the elites? The answer is, no they were not. Jean Bruyérin-Champier admitted as much in his chapter devoted to cabbage. 'Its success continues so obstinately here [in France], where it adorns the tables of both the great and the poor, and medicine has not been able to dissuade people from regularly consuming it'.[6]

In the first part of this chapter we shall explain the apparent contradiction between medical advice and dietary practice in the sixteenth century, before exploring the European fashion for vegetables in the sixteenth and seventeenth, and ending with the popularity of vegetable-based diets in the seventeenth and eighteenth. As we shall see, vegetables pass from being considered sources of risk, best eaten in certain circumstances and in certain ways, to being sources of health, and best consumed over all else, during the course of the early modern period.

Dietary advice and actual consumption

The Renaissance medical attitude to vegetables is more complex than might seem at first glance. On the one hand, their virtual absence from many Renaissance dietary manuals can be explained by the fact that their authors did not really consider them as food. If they were not particularly nourishing, then they did not qualify as foods. But that did not mean that they were not used; rather, vegetables were seen as seasonings or correctives, whose role was to counteract an imbalance in the body or in another dish. Thus lettuce or spinach could be added to a dish to add moisture to it; chilli peppers could be added in to impart heat and dryness. On the other hand, the Renaissance dietaries that do discuss vegetables do so in a nuanced way, tempering risks with benefits, and offering cookery advice on how to counter the former.

This approach is most evident in the work of the Bolognese physician Baldassare Pisanelli. For instance, to return to cabbage, Pisanelli agreed with Rangoni that it was harmful to those of a melancholic disposition, especially during summer. However, Pisanelli suggested a 'remedy' to this quality, which was to boil the cabbage first in water, throw this away and then cook it in meat broth with fennel and black pepper.[7] He also distinguished between different members of the cabbage family. Pisanelli offered the same remedial suggestion for all of the vegetables and fruits in his lengthy section discussing them. If he agreed with Rangoni on the hopeless nature of cucumbers, as the coldest foodstuff imaginable, 'terrible at all times [of the year], for all ages and complexions', Pisanelli could at least see their virtue when used to treat fever sufferers. Leeks, likewise, 'the worst and most detestable and pernicious foodstuff that can be used', might at least be applied with benefit to haemorrhoids.[8] But these culinary rejections are exceptions. In all other cases, Pisanelli accompanied mention of a vegetable's harmful effects with 'remedies' to counter them, as well as enthusiastically identifying that vegetable's virtues.

When it came to garlic, that most rustic of vegetables, Pisanelli warned against its potential damage to the brain, eyesight and head, as well as to pregnant women. But he praised garlic for correcting the coldness and moisture of a salad, for drying poisons, clearing the voice, killing intestinal worms and improving coitus and urination. The 'remedy' for garlic? 'It can be cooked until it loses its bitterness – if this means it will lose some of its virtues, it will not have any of its defects – and then eating it with [olive] oil and vinegar or other dishes', Pisanelli suggested.[9]

The trick with vegetables was to identify their suitability. Pisanelli identified a few vegetables as 'good in all times of the year, for every age and complexion': fennel, asparagus, spinach, borage and chicory. However, most vegetables had to be eaten at a suitable time of the year. It was a question of balance. 'Heating' vegetables, like capers, cardoons, artichokes, carrots and radishes were best eaten in cold seasons, whereas 'cooling' vegetables, like lettuce, endive and squash were best eaten when it was hot. Secondly, suitability could be obtained through cooking. Spinach, slightly cold and moist in terms of qualities, should therefore be cooked 'in the pan in their own water and then seasoned with oil, pepper, vinegary juices and raisins'.[10]

Pisanelli's suggestions squared the circle between harsh warnings against and routine consumption of vegetables. The same practical advice helps to explain high fruit consumption during the same period, as Paul Lloyd has suggested.[11] The advice is neatly summed up in the medical saying, 'Raw pears a poison, baked, a medicine be'.[12] Properly cooked and seasoned, the elites could indulge in their passion for rare and expensive fruits, or even common ones. Later in the period, they could even be eaten raw (but we must not get ahead of ourselves).

Regimens, with their reservations about vegetables, are clearly not the most reliable source for evidence of actual consumption habits. In 1596 the English courtier and Italophile Robert Dallington noted that for poorer Tuscans, 'their chiefest food is herbage all the yeare through'.[13] In fact, he continues, 'herbage'

is the most generall food of the Tuscan, at whose table a sallet is as ordinary as salt at ours; for being eaten of all sorts of persons, and at all times of the yeare: of the rich because they love to spare; of the poore because they cannot choose; of many Religious because of their vow, of most others because of their want. It remaineth to believe that which themselves confesse; namely, that for every horse-load of flesh eaten, there is ten cart-loades of hearbes and rootes; which also their open markets and private tables doe witnesse.[14]

Other textual sources come in the form of agricultural treatises and herbals, both successful literary genres during the period. In an agricultural treatise printed in 1569, just twenty years after Rangoni's regimen, Agostino Gallo listed what were the then common garden vegetables.[15] These were grown for their usefulness and health-giving properties, which Gallo also details. They were cabbages, leeks, garlic, onions, fennel, carrots, squashes, turnips, radishes, peas, shallots, *erba sana* (all-good, a kind of wild spinach), artichokes and asparagus. From the point of view of plant husbandry, root vegetables were just as favoured as leaf vegetables, contradicting Galenic theory which saw the former as suitable only for rustics. In fact, Gallo, a merchant and landowner in Brescia, may offer a more accurate snapshot of actual consumption habits than the physician's advice. In addition to these common garden vegetables, in 'recreational' gardens Gallo lists plants grown for their flavour and for salads (lettuce, radicchio, tarragon, rocket, sorrel, borage and parsley), soups and other uses (mint, pennyroyal, chard and spinach). Finally, we have plants grown in pots to decorate gardens, like basil, marjoram and other 'kinds of lovely and sweet-smelling herbs'.

Konrad Heresbach, a German diplomat and landowner, painted a similar picture in his 1568 husbandry treatise. The work describes the cultivation methods for a wide variety of vegetables, giving their names in a variety of European languages, as the herbals of the time usually did.[16] A French source gives a similar picture. In 1600, Olivier de Serres described more than thirty plants that were highly desirable for the kitchen garden. De Serres, a Calvinist nobleman and horticulturalist, advisor to King Henri IV, described all of these plants in great detail, from roots to fruits, in book six of his *Théâtre d'agriculture et mesnage des champs* ('Theatre of agriculture and field management', really a complete guide to stocking and running a large estate).[17] The book's success is indicative of the increasing importance of cultivating and consuming vegetables in France during the seventeenth century, going through eight further editions during his lifetime (he died in 1619), and nineteen editions before 1675, in France alone. De Serre's enthusiasm for vegetables and fruits appears to have infected another member of Henri IV's court, the physician Joseph Du Chesne. His descriptions, even of root vegetables, are quite enthusiastic, detailing regional culinary uses and specific local varieties, while stressing their health benefits over medical warnings.[18]

On a much smaller scale, an English 'simpler', or herbalist, even waxed lyrical over the species of greens that could be collected by the side of the road or growing wild in fields. William Coles wrote that 'There is not a day passeth over our heads, but we have need of one thing or other that groweth within their circumference. We cannot make so much as a little good pottage without herbs [vegetables], which give an admirable relish and make them wholesome for our bodies'.[19] In his discussion of the 'alimentall' uses of plants, Coles chooses to ignore those commonly known and used as food, such as turnips and cabbage, to concentrate on 'those which are less known', like 'the tops of hops and turnips, running up to seed, [which] boyled and buttered, do eat like asparagus'. He mentions the buds of elder, nettle, watercress and alexander, which 'good women use to make pottage with in the spring time'.[20] Coles is unusual in his detailed interest in herbs and vegetables. He notes for example how colewort and cabbage were better once they had been touched by frost, which improved their flavour. He even comments on the way meat had come to the fore as superior nourishment in his time, while reminding his readers the ancient philosopher Pythagoras had lived on vegetables and lived longer than people normally did.[21]

We shall return to the importance of Pythagoras later on in this chapter. What is striking about vegetable consumption during the Renaissance is how it became fashionable among the elites. Vegetables had always been a mainstay of most people's diets and everyone ate at least some vegetables and herbs as a matter of course. But during the sixteenth century the Italian elites began to value them as perhaps never before; a trend that was destined to ripple its way through the rest of Europe. Plantsmen were stimulated to create new varieties, so that even the elites, ever in pursuit of luxury and trendiness, could find something to stir their fancy, to accompany their more traditional meat dishes. Root vegetables, the most humble of all, moved up the social scale. And even cabbage (again!) excited their curiosity. In 1519 Isabella d'Este, marquis of Mantua, sent some cabbage seeds to her brother, the duke of Ferrara, 'to eat in a salad'. These were followed by some actual cabbages, 'so he can give them a try'. Isabella helpfully explained to her brother how the stem had to be removed first, that they should be boiled briefly until tender and then seasoned with oil and vinegar 'like a salad'. 'Your Excellency will then see if this oddity is pleasing to him', Isabella concluded.[22] The previous day Isabella had sent the duke other 'strange things', 'that stimulate the appetite', in the form of artichokes and peas.[23]

The peas must have been a particular curiosity, given that it was only the end of February. Indeed what made vegetables attractive in Renaissance court circles was their novelty, in terms of new varieties of traditional plants, and their rarity, in being served up at unusual times of the year. Moreover, they were presented in elaborate ways, consistent with the banqueting style of the time, explored in Chapter 3. Giovanni Battista Vigilio's recipe 'to make a tasty and lovely salad', dating from the late 1500s, consists of fifteen edible plants, seven flowers, nine fruits and twelve seasonings. Vigilio's idea of a 'salad' – and the name that he gave to his gossipy chronicle of life at the Gonzaga court – was the 'mixing of diverse and various things'.[24] Vigilio's salad was a playful and ironic creation, so it was fitting that when the Spanish composer Mateo Flecha published the musical compositions of his uncle in 1581, which mixed different styles and humorous verses, he called them *Ensaladas*.[25]

Jean Bruyérin-Champier defines salads as 'mixtures of raw herbs and vegetables seasoned with oil, vinegar and salt', to which 'cooked vegetables are added' during winter.[26] He advises mixing 'the cold and the hot, the moist and the dry': for example, mixing rocket with lettuce, 'so as to temper the freshness of the lettuce and the heat of the rocket'. Even so, he was convinced that the 'use' of salads 'is little healthy when it is too frequent and abundant, such that we advise moderation in this area'. Salads, he added, 'are not intended for the pleasure of our palates but for the maintenance of our health: one must take them not as foods, but as medicines'. In other words, they served to balance other dishes and ensure proper 'concoction' in the stomach when consumed judiciously, in small amounts. However, Bruyérin-Champier warned, 'it is always the case that those who too often abuse herbs [vegetables], especially raw, are much more exposed to serious diseases, since the juice that spreads throughout the body is mostly harmful'. This 'juice' manifests itself in the bile we often vomit when we are sick, 'which in medicine is called *bilis porracea* [literally, leek bile]', evident proof of how harmful an excess of it could be.

Bruyérin-Champier singles out Italian courtly households as the worst offenders, each with its '*credentiarius* (doubtless after the credenzas on which the seasonings are set), whose main task is to mix the salads'. Italian medical authors were well aware of the growing fashion for salads, to the point of being victims themselves. One has the feeling that they are aware of waging a losing battle against elite tastes. Costanzo Felici singled out the way salads were eaten indiscriminately at different times of the day or at different points of the meal, and often with no other goal than to stimulate the appetite so that diners can eat more. And another Italian doctor, Salvatore Massonio, admitted – not without a sense of guilt – to greatly liking salad, but being troubled by the fact that, 'although so common that it is either eaten or at least known by everyone', salad is hardly mentioned by the ancient authors.[27]

The vegetable vogue in Europe

There was nothing new in the selection and development of new varieties of vegetables; this had been going on since classical times. But Renaissance Italy – 'the garden of the worlde' according to Heresbach – saw a concentration of this activity.[28] Italy's plantsmen produced new varieties which spread throughout Europe, adding to the stock of traditional ones – altering dietary and agricultural habits in the process. Vegetables became 'a sign of distinction and a delicacy'.[29] In England, the changes this brought about were dramatic enough to constitute a 'horticultural revolution'; in France, a 'vegetable renaissance', resulting in an increase in the variety of foods and the culinary potential of vegetables.[30] Medical authors often refer to the Italian origins of these plants, either explicitly or implicitly. Thus Francisco Nuñez de Oria mentions a particular variety of cabbage by its Italian name, *cappuccio*, which has pale green leaves and a compact form.[31] Bruyérin-Champier was more explicit, noting that 'in recent years we have been importing the use of many vegetables from Italy, regarded as very valuable, along with other luxury goods'.[32]

The trend towards more variety in the French kitchen garden, a major element in the work of de Serres, has even more pride of place fifty years later, in the work of cook and horticulturist Nicolas de Bonnefons, who recommended growing and eating a succession of ever-changing fresh vegetables throughout the year for elite tables. So, too, does the place of Italian plantsmen. Seven of de Bonnefons's named cabbage (brassica) varieties came from Italy.[33] And like de Serres, de Bonnefons procured seed for the rarer and newer varieties, such as 'what the Italians call broccoli' and cauliflower, from Italian sources – and he offered to do the same for his curious readers, for a price!

We first encountered de Bonnefons in Chapter 3, as the originator of a new style of cookery, in which vegetables played a prominent role. In his first book, *Le jardinier françois* (1651), de Bonnefons recommended forty-two kinds of vegetables, up from de Serres's thirty. The vegetables whose cultivation de Bonnefons described in *Le jardinier françois* were clearly related to their consumption at table. His section on 'cabbages' runs to several pages, in which he recommends planting about a dozen different types, all of which had distinct culinary uses.[34] This was indicative of a change in attitude towards the culinary potential of vegetables. In France, as had already happened in Italy a century earlier, vegetables came to be seen as worthy of sophisticated treatment, on a par with meats and fish (Figure 6.1).

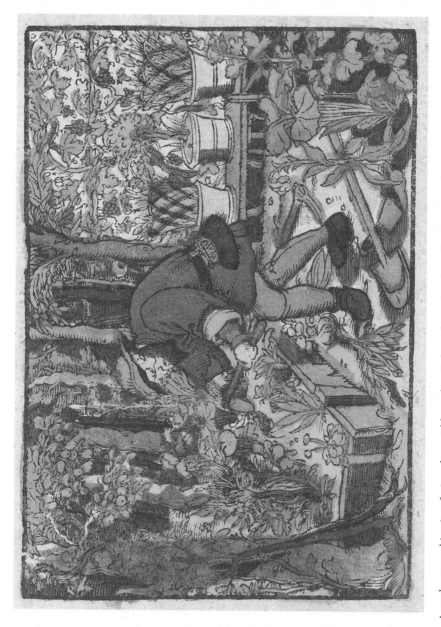

Figure 6.1 A gardener working in a fruit and vegetable garden. Coloured woodcut from Eucharius Rösslin, *Kreuterbüch, von natürlichem Nutz, und gründtlichem Gebrauch der Kreutter, Bäum, Gesteud, und Früchten, fürnemlich Teutscher Lande*, 1550 (Wellcome Library, London).

Contact with Italy was also crucial for the introduction of vegetables in the Polish diet. Polish abounds with Italian terms for vegetables; the words for artichoke, tomato, cauliflower, onion, asparagus, courgettes and chicory are all Italian in origin, as is the general term for greens and soup vegetables, *włoszczyzna*, literally meaning 'Italian things'. According to Polish tradition, these were introduced by Bona Sforza d'Aragona and her retinue, who came from Bari following her marriage to King Zygmunt in 1517. During her four decades in Poland Queen Bona's cooks prepared the Italian specialities of the time, importing the raw ingredients where necessary.[35] This may be just a convenient origin legend. Pointing to court account books, the historian Andrzej Pospiech has suggested that some of these vegetables originating in Italy were known in Poland as early as the fourteenth century: the result of commercial contacts with cities like Florence, Genoa and Venice, as well as the presence of Italian merchant communities in Crakow and Leopoli.[36] That said, the association remains with Italy.

Not everyone in Poland was so enthusiastic. One of the epigrams of the seventeenth-century nobleman and poet Wacław Potocki, from his *Garden of Rhymes*, pokes fun at the sons of Polish patricians who go to study in Italy, especially at the university in Padua. They are soon forced to return, complaining of being given only 'salad to eat' and never getting a decent portion of meat.[37] And in England, despite an increasing (and increasingly varied) consumption of vegetables there, at least by the upper classes, many English remained wary of 'sellets' and other vegetables. In a 1669 matrimonial dispute, a Londoner took her French husband to court, alleging cruel treatment. This included his leaving her 'meatless and very hungry', to quote from her deposition. He was, the wife went on, 'a Frenchman and useth the diet of herbs and other slight eating'.[38]

We can map the vegetable vogue among the elites of Europe by tracing the fortunes of the artichoke. It begins its life as variety of cardoon, itself a kind of thistle: the difference being that, with the cardoon, one eats the leaves, whereas with the artichoke it is the flower bud that is eaten. The artichoke was already being consumed in Naples in the fifteenth century, and from there travelled north to Florence, where it was first mentioned in 1466, and to Venice by 1480. Artichokes were first reported in Avignon in 1532, where they were called *carchofas* (after the Italian *carciofi*), and in Paris shortly after that.[39] Pisanelli described them as 'pleasing to the taste', but warned that they 'cause the genital member to stand erect' (a perception which may offer a clue to their popularity).[40] De Serres included the artichoke in his description of plants for the kitchen garden.[41] Fifty years later, de Bonnefons described it as 'one of the most excellent fruits of the kitchen garden', which he recommended 'not only for its goodnesse and the diverse manners of *cooking* it, but also for that the fruit continues in *season* for such a long time'.[42] These 'diverse manners' are presented in another work, where de Bonnefons provided a range of different cooking suggestions, according to whether the artichokes were young or mature, with special suggestions for the hearts.[43] In Germany, Heresbach remarked that what had started out humbly as 'a kinde of thistell', 'by the diligence of the gardner, [had been] brought to be a good garden hearbe and in greate estimation at noblemen's tables'.[44] Around the same time, the must-have for any self-respecting English gentleman was 'an artichoke garden'.[45] The English doctor Thomas Moffet remembered how they were once 'so dainty in England, that usually they were sold for crownes a piece; now industry and skill hath made them so common, that the poorest man is possessed of prince's dainties'.[46] Indeed Castelvetro, who details the different ways Italians prepare artichokes – including encased in pastry, 'delicious beyond belief' – nevertheless envies the English, 'fortunate enough to have [artichokes] all the year round' (Figure 6.2).[47]

A similar vogue is evident in fruit consumption. Far from having to hide or excuse their food preferences, doctors now wrote about them, as did the well-travelled Frenchman Nicolas Venette (1683). Venette, whose real name was Charles Patin, has been called the 'father of sexology' because of his treatise 'on the pleasures of the marriage bed';[48] but he also had something to say on the equally important 'use of tree fruits to maintain one's health or to treat oneself when one is ill'.[49] Venette's language and rationale are essentially a modified Galenism, but a century of food fashion from the time of Pisanelli has allowed a degree of enthusiasm about fruit. As was occurring with vegetables, fruit cultivation was experiencing a renascence, with new varieties and cultivation techniques, such that its products were considered

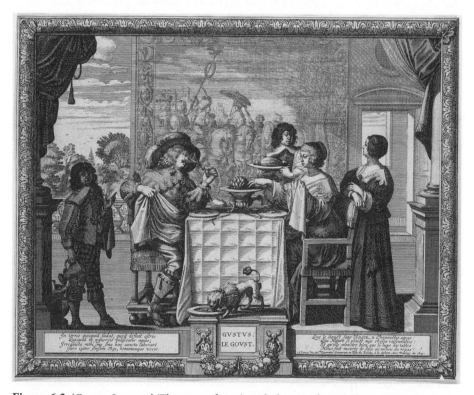

Figure 6.2 'Gustus. Le goust' (The sense of taste), with the prized artichoke as centrepiece. Engraving by A. Bosse after his painting *The artichoke feast*, c.1630–50 (Wellcome Library, London).

suitable for elite tastes and constitutions. This transformation is neatly summed up in the success of the peach, which goes from 'poison to passion', as Florent Quellier has documented.[50]

As with increasing vegetable consumption, changing elite preferences led the way, with medical writers forced to adapt their advice to these new foodways. As a result, doctors could now suggest that certain ripe fruits could now be eaten raw without endangering one's health. It might seem remarkable that a treatise like Venette's was evidently still considered necessary in order for one to know which fruits were best and which best avoided. Moreover, the advice itself remained the same. The sixteenth-century fear of melons may have been replaced by an eighteenth-century appreciation of them, but the advice on how to 'correct' their harmful qualities remained little changed – usually involving wine.[51] The rationale behind this shift is significant, based as it is on first-person observation. The Galenic suspicion of peaches, associated with the authority of the ancients, gave way to an enthusiastic appreciation of them, not only because new varieties had been developed but because medical writers observed for themselves that, far from having adverse effects, they might actually be beneficial to health. Thus Samuel-Auguste Tissot (1761) claimed that fruit could be used in the treatment of acute diseases, as 'persons of knowledge and experience will be very little, or rather not at all, surprized to see'. For instance, not only did fruit *not* cause dysentery, as had long been claimed, but it could prevent and cure it – all based on the personal experiences of Tissot and his patients over the previous decade.[52]

The 'herby diet'

At roughly the same time as the Italian elites were just beginning to adopt vegetables as the latest trend, one patrician was already reducing meat consumption as part of his diet. He was the Venetian Alvise Cornaro, who shifted to a frugal diet because of ill health and found himself much the better for it. It used to be claimed that Cornaro was born in 1464 or 1467 and died in 1566; but more recent studies have suggested that he contributed to his own longevity by increasingly exaggerating his age as time went on, claiming to be 56 in 1540 but 95 twenty-five years later.[53] In any case, he published his short book on 'the sober life' in 1558.[54] Soon, *Della vita sobria* was 'in everybody's hands'.[55] It became widely known outside of Italy when the Flemish Jesuit and moral theologian Lenaert Leys (Leonardus Lessius) translated it into Latin and published it alongside his own work, the *Hygiasticon*, in 1613. Cornaro's diet and his own longevity were frequently mentioned in European health guides when they wanted to impress upon their readers the virtues of moderation, temperance and simplicity. However, it was rarely more than a mention – not surprising, given Cornaro's claims that his recommendations would do away with the need for physicians and the formulation of an individually tailored regimen. In its place, Cornaro advised sobriety in food and drink, a message that (he argued) was applicable to all, regardless of complexion or class.

In his widely translated *Hygiasticon*, Leys put some flesh on Cornaro's bare-bones account, as it were, providing a few details as to what simplicity and sobriety in diet, in order to live well and long, might mean. A mainstay of this was a dish called *panada* (also *panatella*): 'the Italian name of that kind of pap or gruel which is made of bread and water or some flesh-broth boyled together'. Indeed by eating just panada, 'and now and then an egge or two, a man may live very long and with great healthfulnesse', Leys wrote. The reason? Panada was very easily digested and similar to the chyle the stomach produced through the concoction of foods; it was temperate or balanced in its qualities; it was little subject to corruption or putrefaction in the body as other foods might be; and it bred an abundance of 'good blood'.[56] Panada was in fact Italian peasant food – a way of using precious but stale bread.

That said, in Leys's case, simplicity of diet was not to be confused with a vegetables-only diet. His warning against certain vegetables in particular followed the standard line of limiting consumption. 'When we say a man must warily abstain from these kinds of food', Leys wrote, 'it is not so to be understood as that a man may not (for example) eat a little colewort, onyons, cheese, beans, pease and the like … but that he ought not to eat them in any notable quantitie'. This warning aside, Leys's advice was remarkably similar to those advocating a 'Pythagorean' diet, and was a long way from the dietary pattern of his fellow Jesuits (as we saw in the previous chapter). Meat was to be avoided. Leys points to the 'many husbandmen [farmers] and others of mechanick trades [labourers], who ordinarily feed on bread, butter, pottage, pulse, herbs, cheese and the like, eating flesh very rarely; and yet they live long not onely with health but with strength'.[57]

The 'sober diet' as advocated by Leys had much going for it. By tempering the humours, it preserved man 'from almost all manner of diseases', whether generated from within the body or from without (like wounds), and it mitigated the effects of incurable diseases (like ulcers and urinary gravel).[58] It helped men to live long and to die without pain and made 'the bodie lightsome, agil, fresh and expedite' and the senses sound and vigorous.[59] It mitigated the passions and the affections, 'especially those of anger and melancholie', preserved memory, improved 'wit and understanding', the better to engage in 'prayer, meditation and contemplation', and assuaged lust.[60] There was a clear moralizing, not to say Christian element, to Leys's notion of sobriety and temperance, largely absent from Cornaro's manual. All of the people Leys mentions as long-lived because of their sober regimens are saints or holy men: 'I grant indeed that wicked men, and in particular homicides and blasphemers, do not for the most part live long, albeit they be temperate in their diets; for the divine vengeance persecuteth them'. And what better reason to aim for a long life than to be able to praise God with the wisdom of years?[61]

This moralizing ethos was shared by radical Protestants, for many of whom the total avoidance of meat took on the dimensions of a crusade. In England, sects like the Ranters advocated meat-avoidance for different reasons, from the notion that God was present in all living things to the desire to avoid the sensuality associated with meat and drink.[62] In 1655 a former 'haberdasher of hats', Roger Crab, sold his estate, gave the proceeds to the poor and took up a life of poverty on a rood of rented land (¼ acre or one-tenth of a hectare). Crab gave up meat, regarding it 'a sinne against his body and soul to eat flesh or to drinke any beer, ale or wine'. He ate only what he could grow, 'as corne, bread and bran, hearbs, roots, dock-leaves, mallowes and grasse', water his only drink. Crab declared himself 'neither for the Levellers, nor Quakers, nor Shakers, nor Ranters', but was in the radical tradition.[63] His dietary choices, like his 'hermeticall' lifestyle, were religious in nature rather than medical (as for Cornaro) or a combination of the two (as for Leys) (Figure 6.3).

Slightly more medical in tone was another hat-maker, Thomas Tryon, the most vociferous of this generation of English religious radicals. Tryon apprenticed as a hatter under an Anabaptist, and came to like the radical movement's ascetic lifestyle. At 18

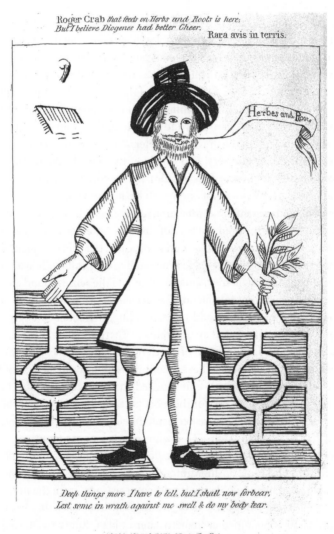

Roger Crab *that feeds on Herbs and Roots is here;*
But I believe Diogenes had better Cheer.
Rara avis in terris.

Herbes and Roots

Deep things more I have to tell, but I shall now forbear,
Lest some in wrath against me swell & do my body tear.

Figure 6.3 Roger Crab, frontispiece of *The English Hermite*, 1655 (Wellcome Library, London).

he moved to Barbados, to develop his hat trade and for the greater freedom of religion there; but, shocked by the cruelty of slavery, he returned to London. Here, Tryon heard what he called his 'inner voice' (1657). In numerous writings that followed, he sought to reconcile the teachings of the Bible, Pythagoras and Hinduism. For Tryon, spiritual progress meant a mixture of pacifism, non-violence to animals and temperance. He published a variety of books dealing with domestic matters, with an emphasis on health and diet.

Tryon's *Bill of Fare of Seventy-Five Noble Dishes of Excellent Food* (1691) is probably the first exercise in vegetables-only cookery advice. It included, in the author's words, 'several excellent dishes of food, easily procured without flesh and blood, or the dying groans of God's innocent and harmless creatures, which do as far exceed those made of flesh and fish as the light doth darkness or the day the night, and will satisfie all the wants of nature to the highest degree'.[64] These included 'bread and butter eaten with our thin gruel', 'eggs poached and some parsly boiled and cut small, and mixed with some bitter and vinegar melted', 'spinnage [spinach] boiled with the sound tops of mint and balm, seasoned with salt and butter, and eaten with bread', 'roasted or boiled potatoes eaten with butter, salt and vinegar', and a range of different pottages. In preparing these recipes Tryon insisted that simplicity was the key: 'therefore seek not many dishes, nor variety of foods, especially at one meal, for most diseases and distempers are contracted through excess and inordinate living'.[65]

Tryon himself lived a frugal life, including a vegetable-based diet (although he did not manage to persuade his wife to do so). A young Benjamin Franklin, then an apprentice printer, was a some-time convert after reading several of Tryon's books. Franklin was particularly struck by Tryon's notion of flesh-eating as murder, which complemented the more utilitarian motives of economy and clear-headedness that would result. Franklin's undoing was a combination of the aroma of freshly cooked cod, 'hot out of the frying pan', and a realization that if this fish could survive on eating other, smaller fish, 'I don't see why we may not eat you'. 'So I dined upon cod very heartily', Franklin relates in his *Autobiography* (1791), and 'return[ed] only now and then occasionally to a vegetable diet'.[66]

How did Pythagoras – he of the right-angled triangles – come into it? When early moderns wanted to refer to a diet lacking in the flesh of slaughtered animals they referred to a 'Pythagorean diet'. In addition to making numerous contributions to knowledge, including mathematics, Pythagoras was also the first Greek to promulgate a dogma for the existence of the soul. The soul was immortal and could be endlessly transformed into other living creatures. Therefore all life forms should be treated as kindred; ascetic practices were also necessary to ensure the soul's progress. Pythagoras argued that the more insubstantial the foods, the more the body was purified and the closer it could come to the gods. Apparently, Pythagoras practised what he preached: for breakfast he had honey, and for dinner millet or barley bread with raw or boiled vegetables. In the Christian West, his practices – via the early Church fathers, ascetics and the rule of St Benedict – influenced various orders of monks and nuns, like the Carthusians (discussed in the previous chapter).

Although Tryon styled himself a 'student of physic' and was certainly conversant on the subject,[67] he was not a doctor; and indeed many doctors remained as ambivalent about vegetable diets as they did about fasting. Few medical authors were willing to go so far as to recommend a vegetable-only diet, except for certain categories of sick people. It went against the best medical knowledge. Vegetables were certainly more welcomed now than two hundred years earlier; but physicians tended to pour scorn on the idea that 'one can substitute without risk a meagre (vegetable) diet for one of flesh ... that vegetables are more nourishing, fatten and fortify the body', to quote the regent of the Paris medical faculty Nicolas Andry.[68] And it went against orthodox Christianity. One had to be a religious radical indeed to reject God's bounty, as defined by the words of St Paul that 'every creature of God is good, and nothing [is] to be refused, if it be received with thanksgiving'.[69] The Catholic Church was loath to accept the advocacy of strict vegetarianism of the type affirmed by Andry's sparring partner Philippe Hecquet, on the grounds that it went against the notion of divine bounty (which included meat) and the Church's rejection of any sort of food taboo.[70] Monastic and saintly asceticism or periodic fasting were one thing, a dogmatic prohibition for all, whether on medical or religious grounds, was quite another. As a result, there was little of what we might call strict vegetarianism being advocated or followed by physicians; indeed the very term 'vegetarian' was not coined until 1847, when it was used by the newly founded Vegetarian Society in Britain.

At the same time there was an increasing reaction to the over-refinements of baroque cookery and a recommendation of increased simplicity and 'naturalness' in food. Both medical and cookery writers were in agreement on this, as we saw in Chapter 2. The English virtuoso and fellow of the Royal Society John Evelyn decried 'the generical difference of flesh, fish, fruit, &c. with other made dishes [prepared or complex dishes] and exotic sauces, which a wanton and expensive luxury has introduc'd, debauching the stomach and sharpening it to devour things of such difficult concoction, with those of more easie digestion and of contrary substances, more than it can well dispose of'.[71] These words come from Evelyn's *Acetaria* of 1699, written in praise of the 'wholesomness of the herby-diet'. Evelyn's enthusiasm for vegetable cultivation and consumption is evident in his translation of de Bonnefons's *The French Gardiner*, from which we have quoted. Evelyn was keen enough to prepare foods without meat that he collected recipes for them; and these, interspersed with delightful philosophic comments and some directions about gardening were assembled in the *Acetaria*. On the eve of a new century, the ancients continued to be a point of reference; but they were just as often disagreed with. Of vegetables, Evelyn notes that 'Galen indeed seems to exclude them all, unless well accompanied with their due correctives ... Nay, experience tells us, that they not only hurt not at all, but exceedingly benefit those who use them, indu'd [endowed] as they are with such admirable properties as they every day discover'.[72] Medical ideas change, as do tastes. 'The cucumber itself, now so universally eaten, being accounted little better than poyson, even within our memory', is but one example.[73]

The French physician and chemist Louis Lémery looked back to a golden age in his *Traité des aliments* (1702), extolling the value of the plant-based diet of primitive society, 'when men lived longer and were subject to less diseases than we'. 'The foods which plants afford us', Lémery went on, 'are in some measure to be preferr'd before all others, because they are lighter, easier of digestion and produce more temperate humours'.[74] The shift towards a chemical view of the digestive process, as seen in Lémery, meant that vegetables posed less of a threat to health than they had for Galenic physicians. Hecquet argued much the same thing, but from an iatromechanical perspective, a few years later (as we saw in the previous chapter). Rangoni would have been spinning in his grave! That said, Evelyn or Lémery might write enthusiastically about vegetables without ever abandoning meat. Hecquet, by contrast, kept to his ascetic and naturalistic principles, both in what he ate and in his medical practice.[75]

Much the same can be said of the Florentine Antonio Cocchi, who wrote in support of a vegetable diet thirty years after Hecquet. The iatromechanist and naturalist Cocchi was well known in English circles, having lived in England for three years (1723–1726) and being elected a fellow of the Royal Society (1736).[76] His *Del vitto pitagorico* was published in 1743, translated two years later into English as *The Pythagorean Diet*, and five years after that into French.[77] Cocchi's own clinical consultations from around this time, published after his death, suggest a practitioner dissatisfied with the drugs then available, who instead emphasizes the therapeutic role of diet (with meat broths, cooked vegetables and mineral waters most prominent) and hygiene (exercise or rest). On one occasion he writes favourably of the diet advocated by George Cheyne, one of the few other authorities he mentions by name.[78]

It provides evidence of how the Pythagorean attitude towards diet and health was taken up during the Enlightenment, in a spirit of rationalism and criticism of useless artifice. It accompanied a widespread promotion of natural foods and simple tastes. Cocchi turned to the ancient ascetic Pythagoras for his inspiration, and not the 'barbaric school' of ancient physicians, by whom he means Galen and his followers. Galen, as we know, had regarded fruits and vegetables as too watery and phlegmatic. Cocchi put his own gloss on the latest physiological understandings of the digestive process to explain how his dietary recommendations would benefit people. Optimal nutrition depended on what Cocchi called 'subtlety' – the lightness, clarity and mobility of the body's fluids. Fruits and plants provided a more readily abundant and usable form of fluid. How did this translate into actual recommendations? 'In' came fresh vegetables and herbs, milk and fresh cheese; 'out' went fermented beverages, bulbous roots (garlic, onion), legumes, dried fruits and nuts, and spices. It is important to note that this was not strict vegetarianism as some English radicals had known it or as we would term it today. Cocchi allowed for 'a mixture of some few and those chosen kinds of flesh, and especially flesh boiled with tender and fresh herbs', as apparently Pythagoras had done.[79] However, it came as close as doctors were generally willing to go.

In addition to pondering that great question – is marriage fit for literary men?[80] – and leading and active scholarly and professional life, Cocchi ate and lived modestly, limiting himself to one meal a day. True to his word, Cocchi's 'lunch consisted of several vegetable dishes, always of the freshest and best that could be got at the time of the year, in addition to the occasional chicken or other very good meat', while on fast days he had given up fish and vegetables to eat only 'milk, some good fruit and a little bread'.[81] (Given that Cocchi was a Mason, the decision to abstain must have been taken more for health than religious reasons.) He likewise eschewed the taking of medicines, practising on himself what he preached for others.[82]

Few of Cocchi's contemporaries were willing to go even as far as he did, as Ken Albala has pointed out.[83] The problem with vegetables, argued Cocchi's contemporary Giuseppe Antonio Pujati in his 'reflections on the Pythogorean diet', was precisely that they were too easy to digest. They were so easily expelled from the body that they provided little nutrition.[84] Pujati used the same theories about 'insensible transpiration' and the chemical content of foods as Cocchi had done to argue his point. But Pujati was against the whole premise of the health-giving nature of a vegetable diet, beginning with the very notion of a golden age when man lived long and healthily on vegetables. What were all those biblical shepherds doing with their sheep, then? He also criticized the specifics of Cocchi's recommendations, such as the validity of the milk cure for gout, which Cocchi favoured and which Pujati regarded as a matter of fashion and ineffective.[85] In general terms, Pujati argued that an exclusively vegetable diet, as in the case of the poor forced to subsist on wild plants, results, not in better health, as Cocchi alleged (with Tuscan peasants in mind); rather, it caused intestinal problems, vomiting and diarrhoea.[86] Pujati argued that vegetables should be considered as 'correctives' to meat dishes and certain physical conditions: 'the use of vegetables is a remedy, but not a food', he wrote.[87]

We can see the echoes of Galen in Pujati's criticism of Cocchi, reminding us that there was as much continuity as change in late eighteenth-century medicine. Who won the Cocchi-Pujati debate? If it can be decided in terms of prose style, then the clarity and elegance of Cocchi's vegetarian essay wins hands down over Pujati's turgid and overworked meaty counter-blast. But no one actually won; in fact the loser was the reader, none the wiser as a result, since both doctors were using the same medical theories to support their contrasting positions. What the debate does reveal is the revival of medical writing about diet, discussed in Chapter 2, consistent with the dominant medical philosophy of the late eighteenth century. Pujati returned to the age-old theme of offering medical advice to those living a sedentary lifestyle, such as scholars. However, unlike Galenic authors of the previous two centuries, such as Guglielmo Grataroli, he refrained from offering itemized dietary advice. His treatise on the subject, as indigestible as his *Riflessioni*, devotes twenty pages to 'cautions regarding diet'.[88] It contains hardly a reference to actual foods. This was no longer the point; more important was to ensure suitable quantitative intake and proper digestion, in the context of other factors like sleep and exercise. Pujati was more neo-Hippocratic, rather than strictly Galenic, in the way he placed diet back into the broader context of regimen or hygiene, which he then proposed as a way of staying healthy and treating disease.

A range of people, from cooks to doctors, were keen to contribute – or cash in – on the new 'herby' fashion. One of these was a Celestine Benedictine in Naples, Vincenzo Corrado, who turned a chapter on vegetable cookery, published in 1773, into a small treatise eight years later.[89] Corrado's stated motive in writing the book was to provide ways of preparing 'the simple Pythagorean food' that were not only 'pleasing to the palate' and able to 'meet standards of luxury in setting sumptuous tables', but that were also able 'to satisfy the delicate taste of noblemen and maintain the health of scholars'.[90] The Alsation doctor and botanist Pierre Buc'hoz likewise made his own modest contribution. His 1783 treatise dedicated to 'preparing the healthiest foods' contains a recipe for vegetable soup 'without butter and without any kind of fat', which he claims is 'better, healthier and cheaper' as a result.[91] At the same time, writers of regimens health manuals, like Andrew Harper, condemned the Englishman's fondness for meat while being equally suspicious of 'a thin, watery, vegetable diet', which 'rob[bed] the body of competent nourishment'. The result was to reduce the bodily 'system' to 'below the standard of health', predisposing it to diseases of 'debility and relaxation'.[92]

The majority opinion of most doctors at the end of our period can perhaps best be summed up by the great Scottish systematizer John Sinclair. Vegetables were a fundamental part of a healthy diet and more readily digested than meat, Sinclair noted, but had their limitations as the sole source of nourishment. First of all, 'it was evident from the structure of the human body, that it was calculated to be partly maintained on meat'. Moreover, 'the custom of eating animal food has become so general and is so deeply rooted in our habits of late that it could not now be given up'. And, finally, it was necessary for the people's nourishment 'in bleak and northern countries, where the finer and more useful sorts of vegetables are reared with difficulty'.[93]

Conclusion

In this chapter we have seen how a significant shift in foodways could catch physicians unawares. In less than two hundred years vegetable consumption went from being perceived as synonymous with ill health to being a source of good health; from being a sign of courtly licentious and disregard for the body it became an indicator of high morality and social consciousness. Against a backdrop of a rapidly spreading elite predilection for vegetables and fruits, physicians reacted by warning against overconsumption and 'abuse' and by providing suggestions on how to counter and temper their ill effects. Religious radicals took the debate to a new, moral level, forcing the 'Pythagorean diet' on to the agenda. Doctors eventually came round to the benefits of vegetables and fruits – as a result of their own direct observations and experiences, and because of the impact of chemical and mechanical ideas about the body, digestion and foods – even if most were reluctant to advocate a diet that excluded meat entirely.

CHAPTER 7
NEW WORLD FOOD: THE COLUMBIAN EXCHANGE AND ITS EUROPEAN IMPACT

Introduction

In 1560, almost seventy years after Columbus's first voyage in search of a westerly trade route to the Indies, it was still common to express a sense of wonder at the new worlds encountered. For the Lyonnais physician Jean Bruyérin-Champier nothing demonstrated 'the formidable power of Nature and the wonderful providence she offers man to nourish himself' than 'the regimen and foodstuffs of the new Indies or the New World', to which the author dedicates an entire chapter.[1] It was evidently still shocking that there existed places where 'the people know nothing of bread, wine and meat', the staples of Europe. And there was much more to marvel at. Bruyérin-Champier refers to beans (*phaseoli*) the size of a hazelnut as 'a curious trick of Nature', which seem 'chiselled, sculpted and polished by the hand of an artist or artisan'. Maize (*maïso*) is said by the natives of Hispaniola to be better for bread than wheat, although the people 'of our lands' who have gone 'down there' judge it to be 'hardly cultivable and of little dietary value'. Potatoes (*battatas*) are roots 'like large truffles or large turnips', white inside, which can be eaten raw but are best 'boiled in water or roasted in the fire'. Then there are birds with multicoloured plumage, like the exotic turkey (*gallinis indicis*), which merits its own entry in the section devoted to edible birds.[2] Of the foodstuffs Bruyérin-Champier discusses, only the turkey has made it back to France, on sale 'in the last few years', having been imported 'into our world' by the Portuguese and Spanish.

His curiosity towards the products of the New World was tempered by this warning: 'It should not shock us that new diseases are everyday declared, unheard of in the previous century, and spread from one country to another. In effect, we are adopting a new lifestyle [*ratio vivendi*] which we are importing from another world'. He concluded with the question, 'if we go looking for foods in the Indies, must we not expect to be contaminated by them?'[3] As an example, he referred to the arrival of venereal disease, the 'French pox', from the New World, which had quickly spread throughout Europe. By importing New World customs, including foods, we risked bringing in New World scourges, too.

Bruyérin-Champier's discussion of foods and places is a mixture of wonder, mistrust and hearsay, based largely on other authors, mainly the chroniclers of the discoveries. These texts expressed the 'newness' of this world, at least in their eyes: new civilizations, new landscapes, new riches, and new plants and animals. They were immensely successful as a literary genre well into the seventeenth century. By and large, our medical authors were less excited by the process, worried instead about the dangers these new foodstuffs might pose to the European population. Bruyérin-Champier was more curious than most contemporary medical authors when it came to the new exotic diets and foodstuffs, nor was he judgemental about them; but, then, he was making a conscious effort to be encyclopaedic. That said, he was more typical of his time in looking for classical antecedents in the foods and practices he relates, unconvinced that there could exist anything really new under the sun. Nor did he distinguish between east and west: both were still part of an undifferentiated and exotic 'Indies'. And yet, in his own small way, Bruyérin-Champier was a witness to the beginnings of what the environmental historian Allen Crosby has called 'the Columbian exchange'.[4] Columbus set in train the biological unification of the planet, bringing together two agricultural systems that had evolved separately hitherto. The result was an exchange of the fruits of the earth that continues to this day, an exchange not just of agricultural products, but of foodways too, which began between Europe and the Americas, but quickly extended to Africa and Asia.

Following the European 'discovery' of the New World, the European settlers brought with them European plants and animals. The plants included wheat, rye, barley, the olive, grapes, rice and sugar cane; as for the animals, they brought cattle, sheep, pigs and, of course, the horse. As for those they 'received', the experience of the arrival, reception and success of New World foodstuffs – maize, potatoes, tomatoes, chillies (not forgetting the turkey) – is unique. It was not just the novelty of these things in themselves that struck Europeans, but the different ways they were used. If many are now fundamental elements in the European diet, this was not a foregone conclusion. In a continent of pronounced regional differences, New World foodstuffs were not adopted equally throughout nor at the same time and pace. The assimilation of each has its own distinct trajectory, some finding acceptance in southern Europe, others in the north. Chilli pepper was assimilated within a few years but the potato took much longer to find its place as a staple; and while the tomato is today virtually synonymous with Mediterranean foods, given its perceived lack of nutritional or medicinal properties, it is a wonder it was adopted at all. And this is to say nothing of those foodstuffs which were not adopted at all in Europe, whether by choice or ignorance, such as cassava.[5]

How did early modern Europeans react to dietary novelty? This chapter will trace the trajectories of several New World products from what Stephen Greenblatt referred to as 'the ambiguous experience of wonder' to acceptance on European plates, alongside native ingredients.[6] The factors determining which plants were assimilated, when, where in Europe and in what ways, can tell us much about changing learned medical discourses during the period; but can also tell us about broader socio-cultural context for changing dietary practices.

Medical authors and New World plants

New World food plants and animals began to arrive in Europe at the same time as the first challenges to the elaborate and long-held Galenic schema of food qualities and their relation to the bodily humours. It is therefore logical to ask what role contemporary perceptions of these foods might have had in undermining the Galenic system. The second, larger question is the extent to which the attitudes of our medical authors to New World flora and fauna influenced or were shaped by changing dietary habits in the wider society.

The simple answer to the first question, concerning the impact of New World foods on Galenism, is very little, if not at all. This is because if medical authors examined the new foodstuffs in any detail, they had few difficulties in slotting them into their pre-existing categories. Determining whether these new food plants and animals were hot, dry, cold or moist, and to what degree, proved to be relatively straightforward. That is, when medical writers were interested in them at all. Although we might expect our medical dietary authors to be the first to mention the new plants, in actual fact they showed a distinct lack of enthusiasm and curiosity. With very few exceptions, their silence during the first hundred years following the first voyages of discovery is almost deafening. Instead, the first detailed descriptions of the new foods are to be found in narratives of the voyages of discovery and conquest, as mentioned.

There is no better illustration of this lack of early medical interest than the work of the Spanish physician Nicolás Monardes. In 1545 Monardes updated an old regimen, the *Sevillana medicina* by Juan de Aviñón. Despite reworking large parts of the fourteenth-century text, including its descriptions of the health benefits and risks of numerous foods, Monardes did not refer to any New World ingredients.[7] However, a quarter of a century later, when it came to how the new plants could provide financial gain, chiefly in the form of medicines, Monardes took the lead. He was the first person to write about them extensively from this point of view – but not in a dietary manual. Monardes, a native of Seville, came from a Genoese trading family. This cultural inheritance, combined with his own medical expertise, and the fact that he lived and worked in Seville, the official port of call for the fleets returning from New Spain, made it no accident that Monardes would write about the new products with such mercantile enthusiasm. His treatise was published in Seville in Spanish in 1569 and was soon widely translated. This included an English version of 1577, with the evocative title of *Joyfull Newes Out of the Newe Founde World*.[8] Monardes's 'keen ability to find utility in recently discovered things', noted by the literary historian Michael Solomon, manifested itself in ascertaining and promoting the pharmaceutical, rather than dietary, value of the new plants.[9]

As drugs, some of the plants Monardes described, such as guaiac bark and sarsaparilla, would quickly enter into European civic pharmacopoeias, the lists of medicinal ingredients sold by apothecaries. Botany would soon become 'big science and big business'.[10] But relatively few edible plants made the transition. Chilli pepper may have proved a worthwhile substitute for black pepper in the kitchen, as we shall see, and it even may have been sold in apothecaries' shops (at least in England), but it never replaced or even rivalled black pepper as a medical ingredient.[11] Apothecaries tended to stick to what they knew and were loathe to change.

This medical antipathy is strange. As Ken Albala has noted, earlier centuries had welcomed foreign foods and medicines and had worked them into their nutritional theories and pharmacopoeias.[12] Sugar and spices are the obvious very early examples of this process, as are ingredients like lemons and rhubarb, introduced into Europe in the Middle Ages. Rice arrived in the fourteenth century and was inserted into the dietary manuals of the day without difficulty and yet, as we shall see, the New World potato was rejected and treated with consternation. For every doctor who wrote enthusiastically of, say, chocolate, another wrote against it. This may have been down to timing: just as these New World products were coming to physicians' attentions, some dietary authors were learning to defend native food habits and native ingredients. In Chapter 4 we saw how the Paracelsians advocated the superiority of local medical ingredients over more expensive exotic ones. Likewise, when it came to diet, medical authors like Thomas Moffett were praising the foods of their own country, whatever Galen might have thought, and condemning imported foreign ones. Especially in northern Europe, foreignness was viewed as a sign of luxury, decay and moral weakness. The Parisian anatomist Charles Estienne (Carolus Stephanus), no great fan of seasonings at the best of times, wondered why people could not be content with native condiments, but had to go in search of rare and exotic aromatics overseas.[13] Bruyérin-Champier accused the Portuguese and Spanish of undertaking their explorations for no other reason than the pursuit of riches and luxury.[14] The Spaniard Francisco Nuñez de Oria felt pressed to address the criticism that far-flung voyages were being carried out, despite all dangers, merely to satisfy an 'insatiable appetite' for wealth and novelty.[15]

In addition to this feeling for the local, our sixteenth-century regimen authors wrote at a time of scepticism towards the potential of the New World, which had taken the place of the initial European expectations that the flora and fauna of the New World would yield up untold riches and health benefits. This scepticism would give way, in turn, to a curiosity and cautious appreciation of what the new plants might offer by way of foodstuffs. In this observation phase, regimens increasingly drew upon the accumulation of knowledge that accompanied the development of scientific botany and zoology, and sometimes contributed to it. This was followed by a naturalization phase, as the curiosity that had characterized the encounter with the new foods gave way to a feeling of normality, even commoness, as at least some of the plants and animals became naturalized in Europe – or 'noursed up', as John Parkinson put it (1629).[16] This was naturalization in the horticultural sense of acclimatization. Some plants, shipped as seeds or rootstocks, survived the transatlantic voyage back to Europe, prospered in botanic and pleasure gardens, and then made a smooth transition to farmers' fields. But it was also naturalization in a broader cultural sense, as they became perceived as 'natural' ingredients in local diets and were Europeanized in the process. The chronology of naturalization differs substantially from food to food and from place to place. The aim of the rest of this chapter is two fold: first of all, to examine the trajectories of the main New World food plants (and one animal), comparing the differing roles played by close analogy, negative analogy and no analogy in their take-up; and, secondly, to consider the extent to which medical opinion affected or simply reflected the trajectories of these new foods.

Close analogies

Imagine a world without strawberries: large, juicy and sweet. Before contact with the New World, Europeans knew only the small, wild strawberry. This was a popular fruit and by the beginning of our period plantsmen had developed three varieties for garden cultivation, with a range of medical uses (Figure. 7.1).[17] But it remained a tiny delicacy. Given this, Europeans not only welcomed larger, New World strawberries, but sought to hybridize them. From the discovery of the larger 'Virginia strawberry' in the early 1600s

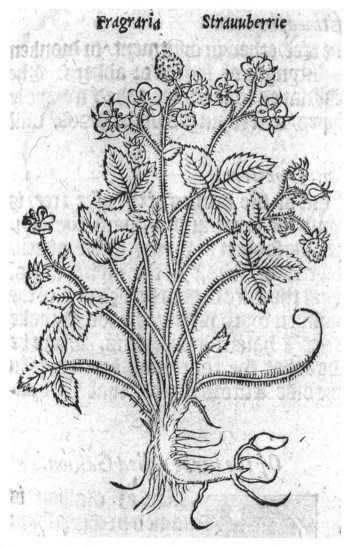

Figure 7.1 'Fragaria. Strawberrie', the wild strawberry. Woodcut from *The Seconde Parte of William Turner's Herball*, 1562 (Wellcome Library, London).

and the even larger Chilean strawberry, in 1714, the similarity of the fruits made these newcomers much in demand in Europe, until they were successfully crossed, in France, later in the century.[18] So popular was the resulting garden strawberry that its Latin name, *Fragaria ananassa*, associated it with another recent and equally chic New World import: the pineapple.

Different factors lay behind the pace at which New World foodstuffs were naturalized in Europe. First and foremost, as the example of the strawberry suggests, was that of analogy: their perceived resemblance to an existing plant or animal. The early naturalization of two New World foods, both in dietary theory and in dietary reality, confirms the role of analogy. The first are beans. Europeans knew only the broad bean and the black-eyed bean – all other beans originate from the New World. At first, new varieties had a cachet of curiosity and rarity that made them a must-have for the elites. Thus Parkinson considered broad beans a dish fit only for the poor, whereas the 'French or kidney beane' was 'a savory meate [food] to many mens palates ... a dish more oftentimes at rich mens tables than at the poore'.[19]

But this phase did not last long, so well did New World beans grow in Europe. In 1592 Gregorio de los Rios, chaplain and gardener to King Philip II of Spain, commented on the beans from the Indies 'of many colours'.[20] The New World varieties were accepted so quickly and without difficulty that medical authors tended to use the word 'bean' (*phaseolus* in Latin) to indicate them all.[21] Dietary writers classified New World beans exactly as they did the familiar species and indeed the New World beans only occasionally received separate mention or coverage. In his herbal of 1545, the German doctor and Lutheran pastor Hieronymus Bock referred to them as 'foreign beans' (*Welsch Bonen*), remarking on their tenderness, but grouped them together with European beans.[22] Louis Lémery made the distinction that the American bean was smaller than the European one. Although of the same form and colour, the American version generated more wind or, as Lémery's English translator put it, 'it very violently works both upwards and downwards'.[23] Writing in 1755, Jacques-Jean Bruhier envied the Americas, whose inhabitants were able to eat fresh beans all year round by sowing them regularly, thus sparing themselves what he delicately called the 'inconveniences' of dried beans.[24] The fact that these New World natives were called 'French beans' reminds us of the ongoing exchanges, linguistic and horticultural, between old and new worlds.

The same rapid and unproblematic acceptance was true of the chilli pepper, or capsicum.[25] Illustrated by Monardes in 1574, by 1590 the Jesuit José de Acosta wrote dismissively that 'this plante is well known, and therefore I will speake a little' (Figure 7.2). There may have been some lingering disagreement among physicians as to whether the chilli pepper was hot or cold in its workings in the body, but for Acosta the matter was already decided: it was 'a very mockery to say that it is not hote, seeing it is in the highest degree'.[26] In the chilli pepper's case the analogy lay with black pepper, as the semantic similarity of the two in many European languages suggests. This close analogy is responsible for the chilli's rapid acceptance both in Europe and, through the Portuguese port of Goa, into the Indian subcontinent and beyond.[27]

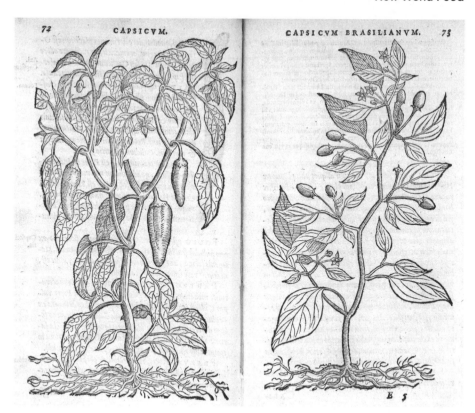

72   CAPSICVM.   CAPSICVM BRASILIANVM.   73

Figure 7.2 'Capsicum' (chilli pepper). Woodcut from Nicolás Monardes, *De simplicibus medicamentis ex Occidentali India delatis, quorum in medicina usus est*, 1574 (Wellcome Library, London).

In Europe, chilli peppers were at first regarded as a new variety of the spice; its seeds were even referred to as 'grains'. White, black and 'long' pepper, the three types as classified by early modern Europeans, had long been used in cooking. Pepper was a great favourite of our medical authors, when another, cold and moist ingredient needed to be heated and dried. It was also a useful medical ingredient, as it warmed the stomach, aiding concoction, without heating the rest of the body. European understanding of pepper and its origins was hazy and the New World 'variety' only complicated the picture. Indeed it was this confusion that hastened the spread of chilli, because it could so readily be associated with the spice. Moreover pepper was still fairly expensive, whereas chillies could be grown locally and cheaply, at least in southern Europe; and it is in southern Europe that the chilli was most used. In Italy, Spain and Portugal 'the graines are used for pepper all the yere, and are thought to commend meates condited with them, better than common pepper', wrote Walter Baley in a short essay of 1588.[28] Gianvettorio Soderini concurred, noting how chilli was 'used like black pepper ... on all dishes', with the added advantage of being 'stronger and more pungent and effective than the other'.[29] So effective was it that chilli was reportedly being used to 'falsify' black pepper.[30]

Chilli became a common condiment even in areas where the plant did not readily grow, such as England. When Baley wrote about it, he had only 'herbarians of our own time', like Mattioli, to go on. As regius professor of physic at Oxford and one of Queen Elizabeth I's physicians, Baley was certainly well informed, but he had never seen this new variety of pepper growing in England, which he called 'codded pepper', because the 'grains' grew in a cod or husk, which turned from green to red as it ripened. The dried 'cods' were then sold in London's apothecaries' shops. Just over a century later, by the time of John Evelyn's *Acetaria* (1699), the 'Indian capsicum' was well known enough in England to serve as substitute for 'vulgar pepper', even if the preparation needed to render it 'not only safe but very agreeable' was a little on the labour-intensive side.[31]

Chilli's diffusion as a spice then 'retreated' during the eighteenth century, declining throughout much of Europe, alongside other spices, while it remained prominent in areas like Spain. According to the Breton nobleman the marquis de Langle, writing at the end of the eighteenth century, the nobles of Aragon were inordinately fond of *pimiento*, a 'fruit as long as one's finger … which tastes like black pepper' and 'leaves your mouth burning and your breath on fire for the rest of the day'.[32] De Langle's travelogue is a work of pure fiction, but it is indicative of a prevailing stereotype. Another chilli stereotype closer to own time is the identification of Hungary with both its production and use, in the form of sweet and hot paprika, and the many dishes, especially stews, associated with it. But the Hungarian embrace of the chilli may well have occurred only in the ninetenth century, given that a Hungarian cookery book of 1826 still referred to it as a 'new spice'.[33]

Exoticism, or the Turco-Indian question

The integration of new food plants was not always so direct, as the issue of nomenclature reveals. Why should adjectives like 'Turkish' and 'Indian' crop up so often, even when contemporaries were aware of the New World origins of a plant or animal? In sixteenth-century Europe the Central American bird we call the turkey was known as *pavo de las Indias* in Spanish, *coq d'Inde* in French, *gallo d'India* in Italian and *indianischer Hahn* in German. The bird was thus 'Indian'; only in English was there a different association: 'Turkey cock/hen'. The same association befell maize, generally referred to as 'Indian' or 'Turkey' wheat/corn in the languages of Europe, as we shall see in this section.

To begin with 'Indian', the explanation is quite simple. 'The Indies' remained the common term for the Americas throughout the sixteenth and well into the seventeenth centuries. It also stood in for exoticism and abundance, regardless of a thing's origins: from ancient times, 'India' had represented a fantastical and vaguely understood land of oddities and hybrids. On to this was grafted, beginning in the sixteenth century, the connotation of anything originating from lands under Iberian control, whether American or Asian. When we add to this mix the lack, among Europeans, of accurate and detailed information about the native uses of things, we can begin to see why 'Indian' might refer to foods and objects from places as diverse as the Americas, Africa, Asia and the Levant.[34]

As for 'Turkey', when it comes to the bird, in English the adjective was applied to the peacock even before the European discovery of the Americas, just as it was used to interchangeably with the 'Guinea' in guinea fowl.[35] Here, 'Guinea' or 'Turkey' simply meant 'from over there'. As for 'Turkey corn' for maize, historians have really gone to town on this one: that the Ottoman Turks were the first to adopt the plant because they used it fatten up the women in their harems; or because the cob resembles a turban; or that it entered Venice by way of Bulgaria and Romania, then under Turkish rule; or that, in Italian *grano turco* is related to the name given to buckwheat – *grano saraceno* – because of a presumed non-Christian ancestry of that plant. In fact, this last suggestion is closest. 'Turkish' was used to indicate something foreign, exotic. For sixteenth-century Europeans, Turkey was then the source of many new flowering plants, such as the tulip and the crocus, and so applying it to a new food plant was not so far-fetched as might seem.

In the observation phase names helped render strange objects familiar, semantically linking the exotic to the native. This brings us back to analogy: if the new food could be viewed as a substitute for another food, then its chances of meeting with approbation were higher – especially if the medical advice was all in favour. Thus the turkey found quick favour in Europe because of its similarity to another, edible bird, the guinea fowl, originally from northern Africa (as its name suggests). Both were praised by doctors, who considered them one of the best of meats, light and easy to digest, suited to every age and constitution. So similar were the two birds in the minds of contemporaries that what we call the turkey was often conflated with the guinea fowl. Baldassare Pisanelli did this (referring to its origins in Numidia); so too did Konrad Heresbach (in his discussion of 'Ginny cocks and Turky cocks'), Joseph Du Chesne (commenting that they should really be called 'African') and Moffett (explaining that 'they were first brought from Numidia into Turky and thence to Europe, whereupon they were called turkies').[36] They might also be considered a North American variant of the North African bird, as Bruyérin-Champier and Lémery both did. Compared to the guinea fowl, Lémery describes the 'turkey-cock' as 'larger and better tasted'.[37] The confusion means that guinea fowls may lurk in some early descriptions of turkeys, and vice versa. Even Carl Linnaeus, in his late eighteenth-century binomial classification scheme that is still with us, did little to clear things up. He opted for *Meleagris gallopova*, which translated from the Latin means something like 'guinea fowl chicken-like peacock'. Meanwhile, in Turkey it was known as the *hindi* (Indian), while in India itself it was first called the *piru*, after the Portuguese name, since it entered the subcontinent via the Portuguese port of Goa. And to complicate an already complicated picture, the Portuguese *peru* reflects the (mistaken) belief that the bird originated from Peru.[38] Strangely, no one seems to have opted to call it the 'Mexican bird', which would at least have been accurate.

The documented European history of the turkey begins in 1511. In that year King Ferdinand of Spain ordered his chief-treasurer in the Indies to send ten turkeys – five cocks and five hens, for breeding purposes – with every ship sailing to the Casa de la Contratación de Indias in Seville (which had been established only eight years previously to foster and regulate trade with the New World).[39] The turkey quickly became a coveted item of courtly exchange. By the middle decades of the sixteenth century it was being reared and eaten throughout much of Europe, the first stage in its transition from curiosity to naturalized foodstuff. While it stood for New World abundance and novelty in the European mind, the bird itself remained a coveted rarity, and as such the object of conspicuous consumption.[40] In the sumptuary legislation discussed in Chapter 3, the Venetian authorities prohibited the eating of turkeys and partridges at the same meal: the inference being that one rare bird at a time ought to be enough. Similar legislation had been passed in England in 1541.[41] So valuable were her turkeys to the ten-year-old Jeanne d'Albret of Alençon, in Normandy, that when she left for Paris in 1538 she provided the chateau's gamekeeper with an annuity of thirty-four *livres*, eight *sols* and six *deniers* for the care of her six breeding pairs.[42] If the young Jeanne stipulated the payment in royal money of account rather than actual coins, it was because she was the king's niece (and later, queen of Navarre, better known to history as the spiritual force behind the French Huguenots).

Recipes penned by elite chefs also emerged. Bartolomeo Scappi, responsible for the papal kitchens from 1549, included instructions 'to roast an Indian cock and hen, which in some parts of Italy are known as Indian peacocks', in his *Opera* of 1570. The bird was still unusual enough to merit a full description by Scappi, but common enough for him to remark that 'in Rome they are eaten all year round'.[43] It remained an elite foodstuff for at least another century, 'very much appreciated on the tables of the great lords', in the words of the Bolognese cook to the Gonzaga of Mantua, Bartolomeo Stefani.[44] The turkey merited an enthusiastic chapter in Nicolas de Bonnefons' *Les délices de la campagne*, while Portugal's first cookery book, published in 1680, has a specific chapter devoted to the turkey, as well as recipes scattered in other sections – eighteen in all.[45]

The turkey had similar elite status in New England, although far from being eaten at the first Pilgrim thanksgiving in New England, in 1621, it seems that the first domesticated turkeys arrived some years later, imported from England, for the tables of the well-off.[46] In March 1661 'a great fatt turkey' was stolen from the household of magistrate and politician Simon Bradstreet in Andover, Massachusetts, which they were keeping for their daughter's wedding celebrations. Its theft warranted a criminal charge, which is why we know about the occurrence.[47]

For medical authors, the main risk posed by the turkey was to a nobleman's purse. The anatomist Estienne asserted, not without a touch of irony, that 'whoever he was that brought us these birdes from the island of India lately discovered by the Spanyards & Portingales ... hath more fitted and provided for the tooth then for any profit'. Turkeys were doubtless tasty, with 'fine and delicate flesh'; but they were not suitable for raising because of the vast quantities of feed needed to keep them.[48] All in all, the peacock was preferable, Estienne suggested.

His advice was ignored. The son of the book's German translator, Melchior Sebisch, even featured the turkey on the frontispiece of his own regimen (Figure 7.3).[49] And in France, according to cardinal Jacques Davy du Perron, the number of turkeys had 'increased wonderfully in a short time', such that they were being driven annually from Languedoc to Spain in flocks like sheep.[50] In the wake of this increasing rearing and

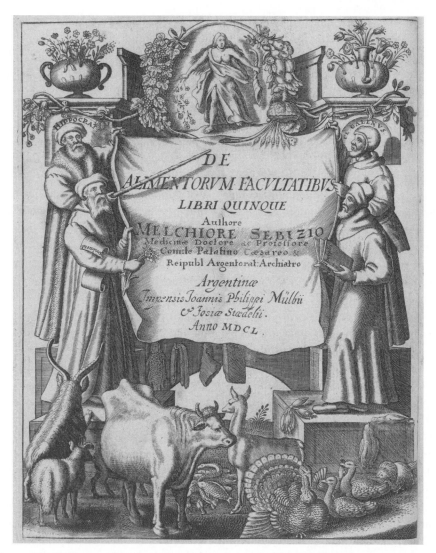

Figure 7.3 Title page of Melchior Sebisch's *De alimentorum facultatibis*, 1650, with turkey in evidence (Wellcome Library, London).

consumption, the seventeenth-century medical opinion was slightly more positive. The anonymous *Thrésor de santé* of 1607 noted that turkeys were 'commonly served at the tables of men of means'. One wealthy owner fed his prized bird entirely on anise seeds. 'The flesh was marvellously delicate, but the expense excessive', the author concludes. Turkeys might be hungry eaters, but given a normal diet the males especially repaid the investment by increasing greatly in size, providing a meat that was 'tender and delicate'.[51]

In the eighteenth century the turkey grew in medical favour, even if the reasoning changed. In his quest for 'lightness' in diet and 'ease of digestion', George Cheyne was a great fan. Because of the turkey's vegetable diet, because it was eaten fairly young and because of its light colouring, Cheyne argued, turkey was 'lighter' than either duck or goose.[52] In the same vein, the turkey suited the more 'natural', lighter and uncontrived style of cooks like François Marin in mid-eighteenth-century France.[53] By the end of the eighteenth century the turkey had become quite naturalized in parts of Europe. In the northern counties of England turkeys were raised in large numbers and driven to the London market in autumn.[54] And in Italy, the Naples-based Vincenzo Corrado devoted sixteen recipes to the bird, now quite at home among the 'domestic winged animals', like capons, hens and geese.[55] 'Turkey hen' became simply 'turkey', the French *coq d'Inde* became *dinde* (and *dindon*), and the Italian *gallo d'india* gave way to the now-familiar *tacchino*, perhaps in imitation of the bird's call.

If the European reception and assimilation of the turkey proved unproblematic to physicians and elite consumers alike, the path of 'Turkey wheat' was not so smooth. The problematic nature of the naturalization of maize is evident in three different aspects: trajectory, regionality and usage. Its trajectory was the opposit of the turkey's. If the turkey was popularized first among the elites, taking several centuries to achieve broader acceptance and accessibility, maize worked its way from the bottom up, progressing from animal fodder, to famine food, food for the poor and, eventually, for the well-off as well. Secondly, the success of maize in Europe took on a pronounced regional dimension. Finally, when it came to usage, the preparation and consumption patterns eventually adopted in Europe differed markedly from those customary in the New World.

Maize arrived soon enough, being one of the earliest New World arrivals to find a place in European art. When the painter Giovanni da Udine did the festoons for Raphael's frescoes in the Roman palace of the banker Agostino Chigi, in the years 1515–1517, he included ears of maize.[56] By the 1540s maize was widely cultivated as an object of curiosity in botanical and courtly pleasure gardens – which is not to say it was being eaten yet. Nuñez de Oria made the claim that bread made from maize was even lighter than wheat bread, while admitting that Spanish colonists did not always find it as tasty as their own bread.[57] We shall return to the colonial experience of maize later in this chapter; for their part, Europeans were reluctant to eat it. Few of the sixteenth-century regimens mention maize and when they do it regards the consumption of maize by Europeans and native inhabitants in the New World, not by Europeans in the Old World. None shared Nuñez de Oria's reserved praise; rather they universally decried maize bread as dry, poorly nourishing and hard to digest.

Their limited information came from the chroniclers of the Spanish conquest and from botanists like Leonhard Fuchs and Pietro Andrea Mattioli. In 1542 the German Fuchs had been the first to illustrate the entire plant, which he also noted was 'now growing in all gardens'.[58] But, as Mattioli points out, Fuchs was wrong about the plant's Turkish or Asian origin. (Mind you, Mattioli seems to have taken great pleasure in pointing out Fuchs's errors, to the point of including an entry to them in his book's index.) Mattioli regularly updated his commentary on Dioscorides, first published in 1544; the 1570 edition was the first to describe maize.[59] Mattioli tells his readers that maize bread is dry and hard, and so difficult to digest. He is fairly well informed about its American origins, native uses and types, but his view of maize as a foodstuff is typically negative. Mattioli compares it to millet, an inferior cereal, suitable for animals and only eaten by people in time of famine. Mattioli's description of maize shows that Europeans were still experimenting with the plant, still trying to see where and how to grow it and how to consume it, if at all. It was soon discovered that maize did not prosper as well in northern climes. John Gerard had managed to grow maize in his own garden, 'where it commeth to ripenes when the summer falleth out to be faire and hot'.[60]

Sixteenth-century husbandry manuals tend not to mention maize. The only one to describe it is the Florentine nobleman Soderini, exiled to his estate in the 1590s. Maize was good for 'fattening up any animal and they eat it with appetite', Soderini wrote in his manuscript, and its flour 'makes good bread during famines'.[61] In the middle of the following century, Vincenzo Tanara said much the same. The kernels it produces, 'in time of abundance are given to doves and hens, but in time of dearth are reduced to a flour and a sweet polenta made from it, and it is said by the peasants who eat it that it is very filling but gives little nourishment'.[62] This was in fact how maize began to make the transition from experimental plant to foodstuff: as desperation or famine food. This was also how European colonists in the New World first came to terms with it, as we saw in Chapter 4.

In the Americas, while European colonists and their descendants agonized over whether eating certain native foodstuffs compromised their European-ness, necessity played an important role in speeding the naturalization of maize. In the 1570s the colonists of the Spanish settlement of Santa Elena (Florida), had, in practice, already accepted it, planting maize in order 'to sustain our children', alongside a range of other New and Old World vegetables and fruits.[63] From the time of the first the conquistadors, as Fabio López Lázaro has put it, 'though dreaming of Aztec gold, most European immigrants starved for Mexican corn'.[64] To necessity we must add the role of Native American women. In this process of incorporation, they served as facilitators and vectors of European–Amerindian interaction.[65] Without them, maize – whose preparation was both labour intensive and the responsibility of women – would never have entered the diets of European settlers.

Grudging acceptance of maize became full-scale cultural assimilation in the following century, from south to north. This is evident in European attitudes to a similar way of preparing maize among the Amerindians, variously referred to as *atole*, samp and *sagamité*. The first to write in favour of it, in 1591, was the Spanish-born but Mexican-educated physician Juan de Cárdenas. He wrote for the educated Spanish and creole public of New Spain, missing no opportunity to criticize Old World authors when they misjudged or underrated New World foods and medicines.[66] His role as self-styled popularizer and translator of Amerindian knowledge and customs to the Spanish and creole population is evident in his discussion of *atole*: maize cooked with lime, then ground, mixed with water and baked. Cárdenas used Nahuatl terms to describe the maize plant, mentioning the different varieties of *atole* employed by Amerindians, including as a drink. Cárdenas appealed to direct experience – both his own and that of his readers – which enabled them to be sure of the temperate nature of maize, and therefore its suitability for European bodies. He was not afraid to take issue with one of the best known authorities of the day on materia medica, Mattioli, who had described maize as excessively hot and moist. Rather, Cárdenas praised maize as 'the most temperate sustenance that is known', possessing 'all the qualities one can wish for in a staple'. He concluded that had Hippocrates and Galen known of maize and *atole*, 'they would not have praised barley water so much'.[67]

In England and its colonies, Gerard's initial hostility to maize likewise gave way to the more favourable opinion of John Winthrop the younger, English Puritan and governor of the Connecticut Colony. Writing around 1662, Winthrop informed the fellows of the Royal Society in London, for whom his essay on 'Indian corne' was written, that 'it is now found by much experience, that it is wholesome and pleasant for food of which great variety may be made out of it'.[68] Winthrop even provided a recipe for 'the best sort of food which the English [in America] make of this corne', called 'sampe'.[69] Sampe or samp – the word comes from the Algonquin *nasamp* – required a careful processing of grains of maize, boiling, then adding butter or milk, with or without the addition of sugar, according to Winthrop. This Native American dish was evidently still a curiosity, but the addition of butter and sugar suggests that it had already undergone a degree of Europeanization. It was only in the middle of the eighteenth century, however, that well-off British Americans welcomed maize on to their plates. They did so in the form of hominy grits, as Trudy Eden has suggested. The dish may have resembled an English pottage, but it was prepared according to the lengthy and labour-intensive Native American technique of soaking, shelling and boiling the kernels first (as in samp). The dish was proclaimed wholesome, simple and easily digestible by the self-styled orator of the elite 'Tuesday Club', whose members met weekly to eat, drink and talk in Annapolis (Maryland) between 1745 and 1756.[70] No longer referred to as 'Indian corn', hominy could now be considered proper British-American fare. Moreover, its virtues were consistent with the latest iatromechanical ideas of digestion. The dish had not changed; the people, and their medical and dietary ideas, had.

Finally, further up the American continent, a similar transformation in European reactions occurred in New France. The French Jesuit Jérôme Lalement, active there during the middle of the seventeenth century, referred disparagingly to the 'bread of the land – if, however, that be bread: a mass of Indian corn meal soaked in water without leaven, which is not worth the bread which in France they make for the dogs'.[71] A century later, however, we learn from another French Jesuit that the French in New France were consuming maize in the form of *sagamité*: 'a sort of stew made of their Indian corn leached in ashes, ground by hand labour in wooden mortars, passed through grossly made sieves', 'which the Iroquois call *onnontara* in their language'.[72] Other than to say that 'pure *sagamité* is a light dish', so that it was usually eaten with meat or fish, the Jesuit Joseph-François Lafitau was not all critical about its consumption by French settlers. Lafitau was certainly more nuanced in his judgement of maize and its uses than many of his French predecessors (and contemporaries). Based on his nearly six years spent in New France, from 1711 to 1717, Lafitau noted how the Iroquois 'have especially a particular species [of maize] which they call *ogarita* and which we call *blé-fleuri* because the moment that it has felt the heat it bursts forth and blooms like a flower'. This was popcorn, and for Lafitau 'it surpasses all the others [uses of maize] in flavour'. He concludes, 'The French [in New France] like it very much'.[73]

If Europeans in the New World came to appreciate maize to the extent that they considered it their own, its reception in Europe remained more problematic.[74] As in the New World, necessity, in the form of famine, was the route by which maize made its way into Old World agriculture and diet. The fact that it was already being eaten by Europeans in the New World did not seem to make much of a difference. This was in clear contrast to the route for chocolate, where both the ingredient and the method of preparation were transported to Europe (as we shall see in the next chapter). The case of maize suggests how European acceptance and assimilation in the New World could follow quite a different trajectory from that of the Old: how Europeans in the Old World could adopt new ingredients while adapting them to traditional European foodways, transforming them in the process.

The first European doctor to refer to maize in a regimen was the Turinese Lodovico Bertaldi, in 1620. By then, maize bread and polenta was being eaten in the mountains of Piedmont and around Milan, 'during the winter by poor people'. Although maize bread was more 'crass and viscid' than wheat bread and could cause bodily 'obstructions', according to Bertaldi, when cooked in meat broth the flour was not an 'unagreeable food'.[75] Although it is unlikely that the 'poor peasants' to whom Bertaldi refers would have been able to prepare their polenta in this way, his suggestion is indicative of an incipient process of naturalization and an increasing acceptance of maize into the diet. By Bertaldi's time we find it in parts of northern Italy, Spain and France.

Grown initially in Europe as animal fodder, maize owed its spread to its use as famine food. Because of its growing cycle, a crop of maize could be planted and harvested after one of wheat, in the same year, so that if the wheat harvest failed, there might still be time to get a maize crop in. Maize was categorized alongside other 'famine foods', the other minor or inferior cereals, including millet, barley, buckwheat, oats and rye, but with the added benefit of extremely high yields. Considering it a cereal meant turning into flour or meal. If Europeans in the Americas assimilated maize in its Amerindian guise – soaking it in lime, grinding the kernels and variously boiling or baking it – in the Old World they dried and milled it, turning it either into bread or polenta.

At a time when only wheat bread was 'real' bread and everything else a substitute for it, French writers in particular were never enthusiastic towards maize bread, whether they encountered it in the New or Old World. For Lafitau, Iroquois maize bread 'is the heaviest and most insipid imaginable', very much like the maize bread 'sold in Italy to the common people', as well as in Gascony and Béarn. Describing the Italian version, Lafitau remarked that 'one must have a good stomach to digest it'.[76] In her travels in Spain, Madame d'Aulnoy found the maize bread remarkably sweet but heavy like a piece of lead in the stomach.[77] Their comments were consistent with contemporary medical advice thinking. For Louis Lémery (1705), maize bread was no substitute for wheat bread, being 'hard of digestion, heavy in the stomach, and does not agree with any but such as are of a robust and hale constitution'.[78]

More than as bread, maize tended to catch on in those places already accustomed to eating a kind of grain pottage, of the sort called by the ancient Romans *pulmentum*. For Tanara (1644) *polenta* was any grain pottage, customarily made with wheat.[79] But it could also be made from barley, millet, buckwheat or other 'inferior' or 'lesser' cereals. In northern Italy, Spain, parts of France and in Romania, all areas which had been Roman provinces, maize increasingly took the place of the other cereals in the making of polenta. Its growing importance is evident in a work of husbandry first published in 1569, Agostino Gallo's *Le venti giornate dell'agricoltura e de' piaceri della villa* (The twenty days of agriculture and the pleasures of the country estate), mentioned in the previous chapter. Originally, there was no entry on maize; however, when a publisher in Brescia (Giambattista Bossini) reprinted it in 1775, a twenty-five-page Appendix on maize was added.[80] Hitherto, it seems, people could read Gallo's treatise on agronomy and gardening in the Veneto without feeling the need for any reference to maize; but by the late eighteenth century, when maize had conquered many parts of Europe, this lacuna was no longer acceptable.

The Appendix reminds us that maize started at the bottom of the food chain and rose to the top. At first 'this very simple foodstuff' (maize) was eaten only by 'poor peasants'; more recently, 'artisans and town-dwellers' had started to eat it. Finally, 'the landowners themselves wanted to try this rustic foodstuff, rendered more civilised by their customary seasonings'. This reminds us that a foodstuff's assimilation is not only a factor of locale, but also one of class. In the process, maize's health warning changed. If the social elites were initially put off by medical 'scruples of the obstructions, bad humours and diseases it could cause', they now believed maize to be 'healthy, medicinal and beneficial for curing certain diseases and infirmities'.[81] Another case of medical opinion chasing evolving dietary practice.

If the elites were able to enrich polenta with cheese, meat sauces and other costly and refined additions, the poor had to make do with polenta on its own, with the addition of a little salt at most. By Bossini's time in the late eighteenth century, maize was having negative consequences that our medical authors, even those most critical of the new food plant, could not have foreseen. It had become a staple in some areas, to the point of excluding other foods, rendering the diet poorer rather than richer. And if this was not enough, doctors in Spain, France and Italy were beginning to associate maize with a new and terrible affliction, which first appeared and spread in areas of intensive maize farming and consumption. The first to do so was the Spaniard Gaspar Casal, a doctor in Oviedo (in the Asturias region of Spain), who labelled the disease 'Asturian leprosy', in 1735.[82] Later in the century, Italian doctors adopted the local peasant term for it, *pelle agra*, meaning 'rough skin'. But pellagra did not just affect the skin, causing it to peel off, as these two labels suggested; it also caused chronic diarrhoea, dizziness, extreme lethargy, before progressing to insanity and, often, death. Pellagra's association with a maize-based diet was increasingly hypothesized, but the exact link between maize and pellagra remained the subject of much, often heated, debate throughout the century (and, indeed, until the puzzle was conclusively solved in the 1930s).[83]

'Potatoes', from confusion to staple

If the trajectory of maize was problematic, in part due to the less than flattering analogy with inferior cereals, that of New World tubers – with little in the way of analogy – was remarkably varied. In 1629 the London apothecary and botanist John Parkinson noted the change in status of one such tuber, which he called 'Potato's of Canada'. Parkinson wrote that 'by reason of their great increasing, [they] have growne to be so common here with us at London, that even the most vulgar begin to despise them, whereas when they were first received among us, they were dainties for a Queene'.[84] The plant had gone from fashionable curiosity to dislike in less than a generation. The reason? 'Too frequent use, especially being so plentifull and cheape, hath rather bread a loathing then a liking of them', according to Parkinson.

The 'potato' he was writing about is what we call the Jerusalem artichoke (*Helianthus tuberosus*). The French explorer Samuel de Champlain had first tasted (and described) it while travelling along the coast of what is today New England, twenty-five years earlier. Champlain referred to them as 'roots … having the taste of artichoke', comparing the new tuber to what was then a very fashionable vegetable, as we saw in the previous chapter.[85] The comparison stuck: when it was grown as a curiosity in the gardens of Cardinal Farnese in Rome, it acquired the popular name of *girasole articiocco*, or 'sunflower artichoke', because of the similarity its flowers. This became 'Jersualem artichoke' in English. The name was first used in 1633 by John Goodyer, contributor to Thomas Johnson's greatly revised edition of John Gerard's *Herball*. The learned Goodyer distanced himself from the label, however, commenting that 'one may wel by the English name of this plant perceive that those that vulgarly impose names upon plants have little either judgement or knowledge of them'.[86] And confusion continued. When D. Hay translated Louis Lémery's *Traité des aliments* into English in 1745, over a century after Goodyer, Hay called them simply 'potatoes'.[87] Mind you, the tuber's name in French, *topinambour*, offers no clearer idea of its origins. It derives from a Brazilian tribe – for no other reason than that they both came to the attention of Parisians at the same time. In 1613 pedlars of what were known in France as 'truffes du Canada' capitalized on the sensation caused by a few members of the Tupinamba tribe then being exhibited in Paris, and the accompanying rage for all things Brazilian, by renaming their product to make it more enticing.[88]

A few decades after it had first come to the attention of Europeans, the Jerusalem artichoke had already ceased to be a rarity and a curiosity. Familiarity might breed contempt. On the plus side, Goodyer put a more positive take on the commonness of the tuber than his acquaintance Parkinson, referring to the many different ways the Jerusalem artichoke was being prepared and seasoned, by cooks 'led by their skill in cookerie'. But on the down side, two decades had been enough for Jersualem artichokes to acquire the characterization that they would never shed. 'Which way soever they be drest and eaten', Goodyer concluded, 'they stirre and cause a filthie loathsome stinking winde within the bodie, thereby causing the bellie to be pained and tormented'. As a result, they 'are meat more fit for swine, than men'.[89]

Did all this potato confusion assist the spread of another New World 'potato' in early modern Europe? If analogy could speed up naturalization of a foodstuff in Europe, its absence could slow it down. The potato so familiar to us today (*Solanum tuberosum*) had no analogous plant in Europe at the time, although comparisons to truffles or chestnuts were made by contemporaries. The closest analogues, Jerusalem artichokes and sweet potatoes, were themselves New World arrivals, with dubious reputations. As a result, the potato's 'observation phase', during which it lingered as a botanical curiosity, lasted for most of the early modern period, well into the eighteenth century – if we except its early naturalization in parts of the British Isles and the Low Countries. The European reaction to the potato, characterized by mistrust and suspicion, thus provides an evocative example of human 'food fears' throughout history, as explored by Madeleine Ferrières.[90]

Potatoes were not well regarded by European physicians, in part because they differed botanically from other known food plants and in part because of their association with root vegetables, best left for peasants. Their early association with the truffle provided a spark of excitement during the sixteenth century and a flurry of trading activity among the elites; but this soon subsided. If the name given the tuber by the Swiss physician-botanist Caspar Bauhin in 1596 predominated – *solanum tuberosum*, still what we call it today – so too did his view of its qualities: it caused wind, 'incited Venus' and provoked leprosy.[91] Over one hundred years after it had first come to the attention of Europeans, medical authors like Strasbourg physician Melchior Sebisch could still wonder whether it had been known to the likes of Dioscorides and Theophrastus. However Sebisch was in no doubt as to the potato's main characteristics, dismissing it as a cold and humid food that caused flatulence and harmful juices unless corrected by the use of aromatics.[92]

Only English authors were favourable. The potato caught on here more quickly than in the rest of Europe, and dietary writers approved of them and acknowledged them as a common food from a relatively early date. The acceptance of English medical authors may simply reflect the acceptance on the part of English farmers and consumers, accustomed as they were to root vegetables. It may also be that the English authors regarded potatoes as less 'foreign', and so less dangerous for English constitutions, because they were associated with the colony of Virginia, as John Gerard does in 1597 (Figure 7.4).[93] And it may be because medical writers agreed that English constitutions were well suited to digesting rough and heavy foods, so that there was no real reason to reject them. Whatever the reasons, English medical opinion was different from that of their continental colleagues. If Sebisch classified potatoes as cold and moist, for Thomas Moffett, writing in the 1590s, they were hot in the second degree. 'They nourish mightily, being either sodd [boiled], baked, or rosted', wrote Moffett. As a result, potatoes are 'now so common and known amongst us, that even the husbandman buyes them to please his wife'.[94]

Thirty years later the English naturalization of the potato was complete. In 1620 the physician Tobias Venner classified potatoes as temperate in quality, which made them 'very wholsome and good for every age and constitution, especially for them that be

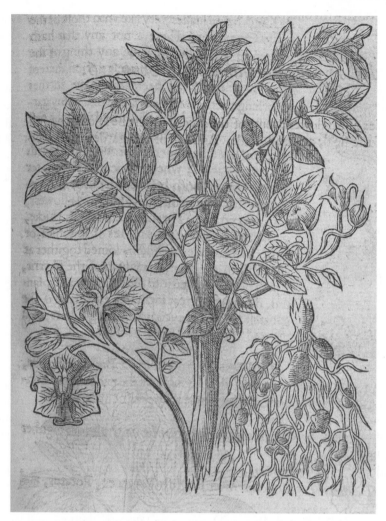

Figure 7.4 'Potato of Virginia'. Engraving from John Gerard, *The Herball or, Generall Historie of Plantes*, 1597 (Wellcome Library, London).

past their consistent age'. Furthermore, 'though somewhat windie', potatoes were 'verie substantiall, good and restorative, surpassing the nourishment of all other roots or fruits'. They did 'wonderfully comfort, nourish, and strengthen the bodie'. Equally important, 'they are very pleasant to the taste'. In Venner's own time potatoes were already widely accepted enough to be 'diversly dressed and prepared, according to every mans taste and liking'; 'sopped in wine' they were 'specially good'.[95] Across the North Sea, the Amsterdam apothecary Lambert Bidloo likewise noted how the once exotic 'Peruvian potato' was now 'grown in our own fields', completely naturalized with its own very Dutch name, *Aard-Appel* (earth-apple).[96]

But no one went as far as John Forster. If the English translator of Monardes could wax lyrical about 'joyfull newes out of the newe founde world', Forster was not to be outdone in proclaiming 'England's happiness increased' in 1664.[97] Forster has the honour of being the author of the first European work entirely devoted to the potato – even if the English government was little interested in his scheme to solve the hunger problem through potato cultivation. Nothing is known about Forster aside from what he reveals in this pamphlet: that he wrote from southern England but that his knowledge of potato cultivation and consumption came from Ireland. It was in Ireland, famously, that the potato was first adopted, towards the end of the sixteenth century (though whether due to contact with the English, the Spanish or the Basques is still much debated).[98] Potato cultivation took the place of oats when land became scarce due to the English conquest and land confiscation. Its dietary assimilation was easier where oat-based porridges and pottages, cooked in a cauldron over an open fire, were the norm, rather than bread. They made a welcome accompaniment to the milk 'whitmeates' and 'sower curds' which the traveller Fynes Moryson identified as a key element of the diet.[99] Seventeenth-century Irish peasants learned that the potato provided a family's subsistence on smaller area of land, in a way no other crop could in the Irish climate: a monotonous diet but an abundant one.[100] As a result, the potato advanced piecemeal through the island and was fully accepted by the 1730s.

What became the standard Irish combination of milk and potatoes turns out to be quite nutritious. The paradox is that, while the Irish peasantry was ridiculed as the most wretched of Europe, little different from the beasts they tended – witness Andrew Boorde's comments in Chapter 4 – they probably had the healthiest diet. This point was not lost on reform-minded thinkers elsewhere in Europe, who, during the late eighteenth century, advocated potato cultivation and consumption for their own peasantries (if rarely for themselves). The view found its way into the dietary recommendations of medical writers, such as William Buchan.[101] It seemed an obvious solution; there was no inkling of the risks a potato monoculture might pose if that crop should fail.

Forster's potato plea was based on the tuber's use as a means of combating poverty. Food shortages, wars and dire poverty help explain how the potato advanced, in fits and starts. As the *Annales* historian Michel Morineau observed, the English wars in Ireland, Louis XIV's war in Alsace and Lorraine, and the War of the Spanish Succession in Flanders all left the potato in their wake.[102] During the Thirty Years War (1618–1648) potato cultivation had first become common in Germanic countries; and this would happen again, through the vast plain of central Europe, during the War of the Austrian Succession (1740–1748) and the Seven Years War (1756–1763). Only potato cultivation, hidden underground, could survive marauding armies. And because of their climate, these were also parts of Europe most evidently conducive to the growing of potatoes. Add the crusading zeal of Frederick II of Prussia to the mix and the potato's continental success was assured (or so we are told).[103] But not so fast: in some areas it declined once the immediate food crisis had passed, only to return at a later date. And in most of Europe it remained associated with poverty, with crisis and with animals (since it was most customarily fed to livestock). The potato's really large-scale impact, both positive and negative, would not be felt until the middle of the nineteenth century, and this should not be read back into the early modern period, as surveys of the subject tend to do.[104]

Eighteenth-century medical authors remained divided on the potato's virtues. George Cheyne was keen. 'Nothing is so light and easy to the stomach, most certainly, as the farinaceous and mealy vegetables', Cheyne wrote, with the potato in mind.[105] This ought to have made it a blessing in the eyes of practitioners who advocated a vegetables-only diet, such as the Lyonnais surgeon Jean-Baptiste Pressavin. Potatoes might provide a 'rather abundant nutritive substance', admitted Pressavin, and this was fine during time of dearth. But that is as far as it went: one could not 'make a habitual and exclusive usage of them without harming one's constitution'.[106]

If the association with famine food, and indeed animal fodder, turned people away from eating potatoes, then distinguishing between different potato varieties could bring them back. In Haute-Alsace, from the mid-eighteenth century, a distinction was made from potatoes meant for animals, the *Erdapfel* ('earth apple', the same name given to the Jerusalem artichoke) and those favoured for humans, the *Grubieren*, or 'earth pears'. The preferred recipe was to eat them whole, baked in their jackets, with a bit of milk curd.[107] By around 1780 the chemist and doctor Antoine-Augustin Parmentier had several dozen varieties at his disposal, on which to conduct his analyses. Enlightenment reformers like Parmentier advocated cultivation and consumption of these two crops as a way of solving hunger crises and ongoing poverty. As a keen promoter of the potato, Parmentier even supplied recipes in his various treatises, to encourage people to eat them – although, strangely enough, the recipe today known as 'Parmentier potatoes' is not one of them.

Despite these reform-minded campaigns in favour of the potato, its acceptance as a staple food in areas of southern Europe, like France or Italy, would only come in the middle of the nineteenth century.[108] In the first stage of the potato's spread it had colonized areas of Europe with a strong dependence on root vegetables, particularly in northern Europe. In a second stage this began to take place among populations accustomed to chestnuts, this time in the mountains of Mediterranean Europe. From the mid-eighteenth century – but in particular during the nineteenth – baked or boiled potatoes took the place of bread in many parts of Europe to become the principal food of the poorer classes: easier to produce, cheaper to buy and just as nutritious.

The tomato's tale is similar. It likewise met with great suspicion on the part of medical authors and it likewise took many centuries before it became established and appreciated. There are several reasons for this suspicion on the part of our dietary authors. First of all, the analogies made between these two newcomers and similar European plants discouraged rather than encouraged their reception. Tomatoes were regarded as a variety of aubergine. Aubergines had only recently entered the diets of southern Europeans and were regarded by physicians as unhealthy, because of their cold and moist qualities. Their name of 'mad apples' (*mala insana*) tells you all you need to know. They were also widely associated with the Jews, as we saw in Chapter 5. If aubergines, according to Venetian Pietro Antonio Michiel, 'are harmful to the head, generating melancholic humours, cankers, leprosy, oppilations, long-lasting fevers and sickly colour', tomatoes 'are dangerous and harmful', their odour alone bringing about 'eye diseases and headaches'.[109] Sebisch also mentions tomatoes in his discussion of aubergines. The latter were regarded as harmful in Germany and were not generally cultivated or eaten. The tomato, likewise, 'although they grow easily and abundantly in gardens' is 'rejected by our cooks', although Sebisch admits to them being eaten elsewhere, seasoned with pepper, salt and oil.[110]

From a dietary point of view, physician-botanists and authors of regimens were asking basic questions of the new plants: what do you resemble? what do you taste like? what can you replace?[111] The potato was so unlike anything familiar to Europeans that is naturalization took place in fits and starts. Centuries had to pass before it entered all of Europe's food cultures and before medical authors outside of England and the Netherlands shed their reservations towards it. When it came to the tomato, the answer to the first question is clear: the aubergine. As to the second, taste, it is evident that the tomato was appreciated, if at all, for its tartness. The tomato had nothing much to offer, other than its bright colour. The naturalization of the tomato only came when southern Europeans (where the tomato grows best) began to experiment with it on its own terms, first as a condiment. This could only happen once they had shrugged off fears about its potential harmfulness. The tomato's moist and acidic qualities became valued when theories of how digestion worked, changed as a result of chemical and mechanical medicine.[112] As a result, from the middle of the seventeenth century the tomato was naturalized in parts of Italy, Spain and southern France; but it was only in the nineteenth century that it became a regular foodstuff and condiment.

Conclusion

Medical authors exercised little influence over what New World foods were eaten and when. They were slow to mention them; and when they did it was either with an underlying suspicion or to claim them as varieties of something they already knew. Indeed the regimens exhibited enthusiasm only with foodstuffs closely analogous to those found in the ancient authorities. In this case they tend to reflect broader dietary trends rather than bring them about. Once society at large had determined a use for something, there was little the medical authors could do to stop it.

In any case, we still know woefully little about the exact paths of exchange: the routes New World plants followed into Europe and back again – and, of course, on into Africa and Asia. Religious orders like the Jesuits (in the case of the drug guaiac into much of Europe) or the Carmelites (in the case of the potato into Italy) might be the agents of such exchange. So too were early botanists, herbalists and horticulturists, with their exchanges of plants, seeds and specimens, as well as botanical information. But plants did not always follow the most direct routes. In the sixteenth century the American plant *Magnolia grandiflora* made its way into Italy (Pisa, to be precise) not via Spain, but by way of Vienna, where the botanist Charles de l'Écluse had brought it.[113] The tomato made its way from Mexico to Argentina not by travelling south, but by crossing the ocean to Spain, making its way to Italy via Spanish contacts in the early sixteenth century, and then being brought to Argentina by Italian immigrants in the nineteenth century.[114] And the turkey arrived in Virginia and Massachusetts, not directly from Central America, but via Spain and then England, while its route to Brazil went via Portugal.[115]

More importantly, to what extent did New World foods alter the way Europeans ate during the early modern period? To answer this we must bear in mind both chronology and cultural practice. From today's standpoint it is easy to see how New World food plants transformed European foodways. So many of our 'traditional' dishes – from ratatouille to tomato pasta, from fish and chips to cassoulet, from gazpacho to polenta – would be unthinkable without them. And yet, on closer look, in their current guise many of these dishes turn out to be nineteenth-century affirmations. While some foods, like the turkey, chilli pepper and beans, were quickly assimilated into early modern Europe, the real impact of these foods was a long time in coming. The story is the same when viewed from an agricultural standpoint. The impact of these new crops on European farming is undeniable: in terms of acreage alone, crops like the potato came to dominate parts of northern Europe, and maize parts of southern Europe. But this impact was only felt towards the end of our period, and then even more throughout the nineteenth century.

If there are thus chronological limitations to impact in early modern Europe, there are also cultural ones, in terms of actual practices and uses. It has been said that Spain was less 'Mexicanized' than Mexico was 'Hispanicized' as a result of the Columbian exchange.[116] The statement could be extended to a comparison between the New World and the Old: the dietary impact of Europe on the Americas was greater than that of the Americas on Europe. Crops like the potato and maize only became widespread in Europe when they became necessary, due to the agricultural and economic crisis of the time. It was only this crisis that forced people to overcome their initial resistance to these two plants and allow them to enter the local food chain; the success of potatoes and maize was thus the *result* rather than the *cause* of this transformation in Europe's food system.

Moreover, rather than have their diets altered by New World plants, it was the Europeans who altered their uses. The process of assimilation into European diets witnessed profound change, with Europeans shaping these foods according to their own habits, preferences and needs. These were very different from those of the Native Americans who had first developed these plants. In Europe, maize was dried and milled and made into polenta, not macerated and shaped into tortillas. And Europeans from John Forster through to the Enlightenment reformers were desperate to turn potatoes into bread. So, although some of the New World plants acquired a massive place in European diets, they did not radically transform them; on the contrary, the plants were called upon to fortify, to bolster up and, eventually, to enrich these diets.

That said, three completely new arrivals did bring about a considerable transformation in the liquid food culture, as we shall see in the next chapter.

CHAPTER 8
LIQUID FOOD: DRINKING FOR HEALTH

Introduction

The previous chapters have all dealt with food: poor food, rich food, regional food, religious food, vegetable food and new food. What about drink? What did people wash all this food down with? How did early modern Europeans quench their thirst and stay healthy? According to Francesco Gallina, doctors viewed drinking as a necessity for two reasons. First, drinking 'moistens the inside of the body and fills those places which are dissolved and consumed with humid substance'. And, secondly, it 'takes nourishment to all the extremities and renders it sufficiently penetrative'.[1]

We distinguish between 'food' and 'drink', but in early modern Europe both were included under the same rubric, as those things ingested into the body that provided nourishment. Drinks like wine, beer and chocolate were considered foods because they fed the body – sometimes too much. (By contrast, milk was hardly considered at all in the regimens, aside from references to a Dutch fondness for it and, excepting breast milk, which was regarded as indispensable in the diet of infants.) In addition to this, beverages were taken dietetically, in the ongoing attempt to balance the humours in one's body, according to the Galenic model, or to provide that balance of salts, oils and spirits which stimulated appetite, facilitated digestion and fortified the nerves, according to the later iatrochemical model. More specifically, beverages, including alcoholic ones, were an important element in the medical pharmacopoeia. When the English cleric Ralph Josselin, aged 67, suffered shortness of breath and swollen limbs in 1683, his first recourse was to a well-known remedy of the day, Daffy's Elixir, whose principal ingredient was brandy. When 'it wrought much with mee', as he wrote in his diary, causing him to see double, he turned instead to a medicated beer to help him sleep.[2]

As this example suggests, the most notable difference between the early modern period and our own time is how much people drank, especially drinks containing alcohol. This included both regular and binge drinking. In terms of the former, people drank at all times of the day, day in day out, adults as well as children. The consumption of alcoholic beverages – wine or beer, and occasionally, cider, according to the region – reached extremely high levels during the early modern period. Alcohol was a necessary component of most people's diet; a crucial source of nourishment. It served as a social lubricant, a basic element in all festivities and business deals, as well as providing escape from the rigours and tribulations of life.

Binge drinking was also common, a basic element of many a celebration, from religious feasts to guild banquets. A monthly binge was even considered healthy, within a general regime of moderation. In the mid-1660s, a Bolognese priest travelling through France, Sebastiano Locatelli, remarked of one such binge: 'This debauch which, following the advice of cardinal Antonio Barberini's doctor, I needed at least once a month in order to cure my usual headaches, left me in perfect health.'[3] One can find doctors throughout the early modern period ready to affirm that the occasional spell of excess cleansed the stomach and restored the body, as Matthieu Lecoutre has observed.[4] However, habitual drunkenness was considered unhealthy, not just responsible for a long list of other afflictions but a disease in its own right: a point of view that survived changing medical theories well into the eighteenth century. To avoid inebriation, regimens advised a variety of ingredients which could be taken with one's wine, from the powder of different animal tusks to bitter almonds, or else consuming acidic or salty foods, as well as a range of 'antidotes' designed to counter the poison that too much drink was thought to form in the body. Towards the end of the seventeenth century, coffee would first be proposed as 'antidote to wine'.

Of course it is impossible to determine an 'average' quantity consumed that would be valid for all centuries, regions, social classes, sexes and ages, given the different ways and different conditions in which drinks were consumed. That said, when historians have attempted to calculate specific averages, these rarely go under a litre of wine per capita, and sometimes climb to two, three or even four litres per person, per day. When an 'Order of Temperance' was set up in Hesse in 1600, their idea of moderation was to limit consumption of wine by its members to seven glasses per meal, twice a day.[5] We know that grape cultivation increased throughout the period. In France, high cultivation increased further during the eighteenth century, testimony to increased demand and rising prices. If France was awash in plonk, the century also saw the development, refinement and marketing of some of France's more famous new premium wines, which accompanied the *nouvelle cuisine* of the period. The average consumption figures for beer are even higher than those of wine. In Sweden, during the sixteenth century, people drank forty times more, on average, than they do today. English families, during the seventeenth century, drank something like 350 litres per head – an average that includes children.[6]

At the start of our period, Europe was divided into an ale/beer-drinking north – stretching from the British Isles, across the North Sea to the Low Countries, Scandinavia and the Holy Roman Empire – and a largely wine-drinking south, from the Iberian peninsula in the west to Greece and the Balkans in the east. There was a broad swathe in the middle of the continent where the two cultures overlapped. This regional picture of food production and consumption, and the health notions that went with it, explored in Chapter 4, was complicated when it came to drink by factors of class and wealth. The elites throughout Europe generally preferred wine to beer and were willing to pay for the privilege. And just as there was a European geography of drinking preferences, so there was one of drunkenness. From the numerous references to drink in Fynes Moryson's *Itinerary* (1617), there emerges an approximate ranking of drunken drinkers, with the Saxons and Bohemians at the top, followed by the Dutch, then the Germans and Poles, Scots and Irish; at the moderate end of the ranking, the French and Italians edged out the English and Swiss (Figure 8.1).[7]

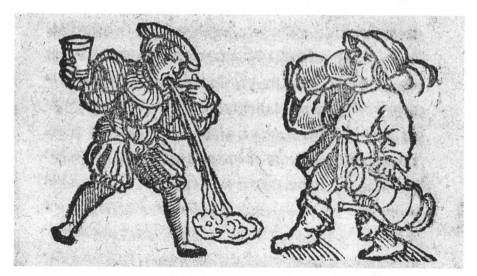

Figure 8.1 'De ebrietate' (drunkenness). Woodcut from Johann Brettschneider's *De tuenda bona valetudine*, 1550 (Wellcome Library, London).

Alvise Cornaro was so confident of the impact his sober treatise was having all over Europe, he boasted that 'Germany has begun to ban excessive drinking' as result of it.[8] Wishful thinking it might have been, but there was a co-relation to reactions against all this drink: not so much wine-against-beer parts of Europe, as wet-against-dry. Reactions to alcohol and drunkenness came first from northern Europe, at the end of the fifteenth century, partly in response to the spread of distilled spirits.[9] This call was taken up a few decades later by radical religious groups like the Anabaptists. While doctors and churchmen of all religious stripes advocated moderation, it was only certain Anabaptist reformers who pushed for total abstinence from their followers, gaining all Anabaptists the reputation as drinkers of water rather than of wine and beer, as Mack Holt has noted.[10] When worries about the dangers posed by habitual drunkenness increased during the eighteenth century, in tandem with the fashion for stronger wines and increasingly alcoholic beverages, it was northern European physicians who recommended a 'return' to water, the natural beverage of choice.

This chapter explores how the regimens responded to changing European habits in what and how people drank, and to what extent the former influenced the latter over the course of the early modern period. Opinions about the traditional liquids – water, wine, ale/beer – had to evolve to contend with the newer arrivals, like stronger spirits and the very different 'colonial beverages', chocolate, coffee and tea.

Water

As in all times and places, water was a necessity: at once ordinary and unremarkable, and a limited, precious good. It was crucial to the daily diet, for the daily soup or mixed with wine, if less often on its own. It tended not to be the drink of choice (for those able to choose what they drank) because it was not considered nourishing, unlike other beverages. To quote the Italian polymath Francesco Algarotti, writing in 1750, 'Water is indeed an excellent thing, and I drink plenty of it. Yet I do not fail to blend it with the divine drink of Homer' (meaning, wine).[11] It was also difficult to access water that met with the high standards demanded by medical writers: clear, clean and 'light'; tasteless and odourless; and sourced from fresh rainwater or swiftly flowing streams and springs.

The difficulty for the historian is water's very banality, making reference to it rather rare. That said, there is plenty of evidence denouncing putrid water entering urban fountains or in rural streams, resulting in dysenteries and fevers. Despite the words of caution from physicians, urban inhabitants regularly drank from city rivers, polluted by the many trades located along their banks. Poor water quality had consequences on the rest of diet as it is indispensable in the making of things like bread and beer. We know that towns went to great lengths to ensure a regular supply of water, whether through direct access to lakes, rivers or ponds, the channelling of springs, pumping from underground water sources, or the collection of rainwater in extensive underground cisterns. They also relied on water-sellers who brought in water from outside and peddled it in the streets (Figure 8.2). In eighteenth-century Paris there were some 20,000 water-sellers bringing water to the houses of Parisians.[12] This was just as well, given that the water of the River Seine, 'one of the best in the kingdom', in the view of physician Achille Le Bègue de Presle, 'acquires some very foul qualities as it passes through Paris, rendering it unhealthy'.[13]

During the early modern period, water became 'healthy', in the minds of (some) doctors and (some) consumers. To counter the widespread opinion that one had to drink wine in order to lead a healthy life, and to suggest that water-drinkers were actually healthier than wine-drinkers, the French physician Laurent Joubert gave the example of Ottoman Muslims. 'Do we not say, he is as strong as a Turk?', Joubert asked. He estimated that wine-drinkers constituted only a small minority of the world's population, around one per cent of human beings – probably an underestimate, but Joubert had made his point.[14] Water, especially water from fast flowing streams and fresh springs, was increasingly recommended as the beverage of choice. The most famous ode to wine, Francesco Redi's *Bacchus in Tuscany* (1685), which extols the qualities of the most famous wines of Redi's day, especially those of his native Tuscany, was written by a physician who drank very little of it, preferring water, a habit he also recommended for his patients.[15] George Cheyne (1724) took this advice still further in the strict regimen he favoured for his growing clientele. Cheyne considered water 'the primitive, original beverage', 'sufficient and effectual for all the purposes of human wants in drink'. Indeed, 'happy had it been for the race of mankind other mixt and artificial liquors had never been invented' – by which Cheyne means just about every other beverage we shall survey in this chapter.[16] For the Swiss physician Samuel-Auguste Tissot (1770), 'the water-drinker always relishes it', whereas 'he who drinks the most delicious wines will always desire new ones'. And it was the same with foods.[17] For doctors like Cheyne and Tissot, both advocates of a simpler and more 'natural' regimen, water was best.

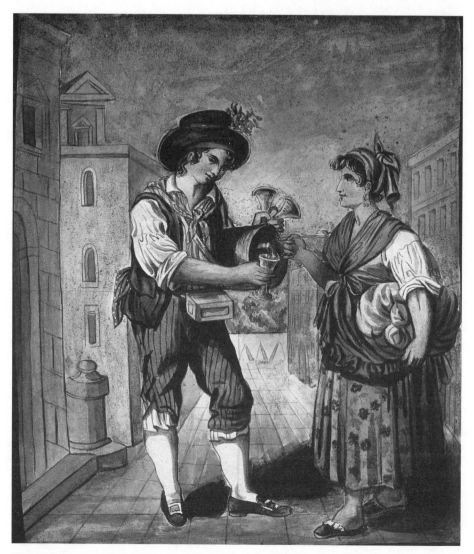

Figure 8.2 *Acquajolo di Napoli* (Neapolitan water seller). Watercolour, artist and date unknown (Wellcome Library, London).

Water was infinitely malleable. It might become a luxury good, as was increasingly the case over the course of the early modern period. The first fashion was the increasing popularity of named mineral waters, coming from specific springs. Redi's medical consultations, dating from the second half of the seventeenth century, are full of references to these, such as Tettuccio water (from Montecatini, in Tuscany) in treating diarrhoea and Nocera water (Umbria) drunk during meals to aid digestion.[18] Medical and social fashions went hand in hand. By 1762, the spa of Montecatini was already exporting 112 barrels of water a year. On the eve of the French Revolution, twenty-two types of water were available to elite Parisians, from places like Barèges, Plombières and Spa (over 300 kilometres away).[19]

Galenic advice had it that water should be neither too hot nor too cold, and so it was often drunk at room temperature. At the same time, water could also be adjusted to suit the individual drinker. For health reasons, French king Louis XIV had it served cold or hot according to the time, his desire or the advice of his doctors. And Madame Geoffrin, whose Paris salon was host to some of the leading figures of the Enlightenment during the 1750s and 1760s, was a great fan of glasses of hot water, taken morning, noon and night: part of a strict diet to which she ascribed her continuing good health.[20]

A second fashion was for chilled drinks, including wine, requiring the use of ice, and the consumption of 'snow' in the form of sherbets. Ice or compacted snow was a luxury good rather than a necessity like water, and its consumption went against Galenic medical advice. But the fashion spread from Italy from the sixteenth century and doctors soon adjusted their advice to suit the increasingly popular custom. (It helped that Galenic wisdom had it that what was pleasurable to us might also be good for us.) So, they argued, 'snow' was purifying, eliminating 'corrupt and evil humours' from the body.

If the use of ice to cool down drinks dates from ancient times, the use of snow to freeze liquids artificially in order to make iced desserts like *sorbetti* dates from the sixteenth century.[21] This was the result of new knowledge of the process by which a substance could be frozen in a vessel by surrounding it with a mixture of salt or saltpetre and snow or ice. Ice became a commodity and its provision an increasingly commercialized activity. In Rome, at the end of the seventeenth century, there were forty storehouses for ice and by 1809, 250,000 kg of ice were being distributed in the city.[22] And while iced desserts and drinks might still be a luxury in much of Europe, in their homeland, they had become something of a staple: Naples had thirty-five snow suppliers (*nevaioli*) in 1722 and forty-three in 1807.[23] The city's fifteen *sorbettieri* ran businesses, ice-cream shops, that ranked alongside the city's many coffee-houses in terms of social function and broad clientele. The Neapolitan physician Filippo Baldini even devoted a 'medico-physical essay' to *sorbetti* (1775). Baldini, who prided himself on being something of a medical experimenter and who was the author of a range of medical treatises, including one on the benefits of the potato, divided iced desserts into three types: subacid, aromatic and lactigenous. Each was purported to cure specific ailments. Thus, acid-based *sorbetti* (made from fruit) increased the fluidity of the humours in the body and helped against diarrhoea; aromatic ones (made from chocolate, cinnamon or coffee) encouraged animal vigour and propagation and helped with melancholy; while milk-based ones were also a remedy for diarrhoea.[24]

Wine

The consumption of water links us to the consumption of wine since the two were often drunk together. Water was purified by wine, but water also reduced the concentration of alcohol in the wine. Wine was considered an essential nutrient; a meal without it was a *caninum prandium*, or dog dinner (in Latin), so-called because only dogs had an aversion to wine.[25] It was the main beverage for most early modern Europeans: in southern Europe, of course, where the vine flourished, but also in the north, when and where people could afford it. Grapes were grown wherever climate permitted, but even in many peripheral areas where the vine could barely survive, and the finished product was invariably sour and weak.

Wine was much more than a common tipple, for three reasons. First of all, like bread, wine had fundamental religious associations. It was central to the Mass, from its being consumed at the Last Supper, as well as at many other occasions described in the Bible such as the wedding feast at Cana. It was thus indispensable for Christian worship, even though wine might not be offered to the whole congregation, a matter of controversy for Protestant reformers. Second, wine was widely regarded as the analogue of blood. Not only did its colour and substance suggest a close link, but also both blood and wine were believed to be made in the same way. Wine was made from harvested grapes the way blood was made from ingested food, both processes involving crushing, fermenting, separation from by-products and refining. The third reason for wine's importance followed from the second. Just as blood was essential for life, one of the body's four humours or fluids, so wine could regenerate the body. It was considered useful for all complexions, regions and ages, and especially for the aged, emaciated and convalescent. Because wine was the substance believed most easily converted into human blood and assimilated into the body, so it was the quickest to nourish. It was generally considered an indispensable nutrient, and for quenching the thirst or after strenuous labour, it was the beverage of choice for Renaissance doctors.

The perceived virtues of wine could fill a book – and sometimes did. The most famous was a treatise on the history and benefits of wine by Andrea Bacci. A native to Rome, Bacci was personal physician to pope Sixtus V and the author of several books on mineral springs and thermal waters before he turned his hand to wine. Bacci's 1595 treatise 'on the natural history of wines' is scholarly in tone, written in Latin and extending to 370 densely printed pages.[26] He describes the process of wine-making and the storage of wines; the benefits to health of different wines; the history of wine, with the focus on ancient Rome; and the characteristics of a wide range of different wines, Roman, Italian and foreign.

Bacci's treatise was a compendium, presenting the widely varying medical viewpoints on the virtues and vices of wine without attempting a synthesis. This reflected the fact that medical writers disagreed on many of the finer points, such as which wines were healthy and which harmful. It was also possible to disagree on which wine varieties suited which individual humoural temperaments, which wines best tempered the qualities of certain foods, at which point in the meal they were best drunk in order not to impede 'concoction' in the stomach, and at what temperature they were best drunk in order to benefit health. One thing the medical writers did manage to agree upon, as Lynn Martin has pointed out, was that the consumption of wine, and alcoholic beverages in general, was beneficial to the old.[27] This may be another instance of medical advice simply going along with what was regarded as widespread practice throughout Europe – namely, that old people drank more. Wine heated the cooling bodies of the aged, expelled their sadness and melancholy, brought on sleep and eased constipation. In the words of Thomas Elyot, 'God dyd ordeyn [wine] for mankynde, as a remedy againge the incommodities of age'.[28] Even that much-cited advocate and model of moderation, the famously long-lived Cornaro, drank fourteen ounces of wine a day, or around half a bottle, throughout his life.[29] On this basis, and citing wine's rejuvenating properties, the naval physician Thomas Trotter advised increasing doses according to age: two glasses of wine a day at forty, four at fifty and six at sixty.[30]

Early modern Europeans certainly drank plenty of wine, and the French most of all, if Locatelli is to be believed (which, coming from an Italian, you might think is the pot calling the kettle black). While in Lyon in 1664, Locatelli writes, 'Its three hundred thousand inhabitants drink more wine than is consumed in twelve cities in Italy'.[31] That said, most wine was drunk watered down, in Lyon as elsewhere. This was usually done by the drinkers themselves: a pitcher of water was placed beside the jug of wine, at table. The watering of wine was a custom that went back at least as far as the ancient Romans and during our period it was habitual to drink wine and water in Italy, Spain and France, but less so in northern Europe.

The rationale behind mixing wine and water had as much to do with health as with morality. In late-Renaissance art, watering wine was emblematic of the virtue of temperance, from the Latin *temperantia*, meaning moderation and self-control (but with an additional notion of what we might call time management) (Figure 8.3).[32] It was also axiomatic. The Spanish doctor Gerónimo Pardo used it as the title of a medical treatise, 'of watered wine and wined water', to illustrate how good health came from balancing these two opposites. For Pardo, 'watered wine is the mixing of wine and water, in proper proportion, to maintain human health, cure and prevent diseases'.[33] Renaissance physicians explained the benefits according to their notion of the 'subtlety' or lightness of wine, ready to evaporate in the air. Wine was watered so as to prevent it from fuming and rising into the head, causing dizziness and inebriation, and overly heating the body. And so it was in practice. In 1657, correspondence of the Spada-Veralli family in Rome reported that their wet-nurse 'is not eating foods which will heat her and she waters her wine very well'.[34]

Dietary authors differed on whether the water was intended to 'correct' the wine or whether the wine was tempering the water. Although there was general agreement that wine's hot and preservative qualities served to balance the putrescent and cold qualities of water, especially in cold, damp regions, there was little agreement over whether water or wine should predominate in the cup. But the Flemish physician Hugo Fridaevallis, certainly no fan of luxury, stated quite clearly: 'water should be added to wine, not wine to water'.[35]

While physicians debated the correct proportions, the wine that peasants and the urban poor could afford was already fairly watery, an accompaniment to the meagre diets discussed in Chapter 3. The peasant stand-by was a weaker drink made by adding

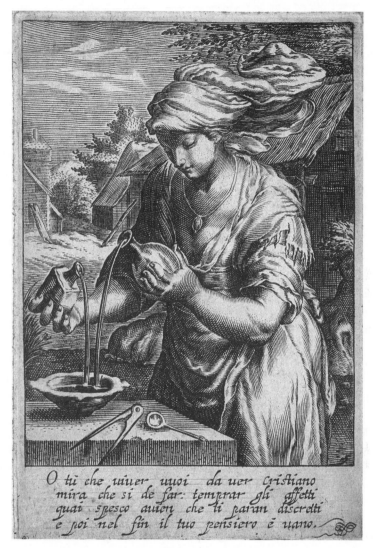

Figure 8.3 'Temperance', represented mixing water and wine into a drinking bowl. Engraving, artist unknown, late sixteenth century (Wellcome Library, London).

water to previously pressed grapes and allowed to ferment for two to three months, called *piquette* in France and *acquarello* in Italy (*acqua* being the word for water).[36] Most wine was consumed locally. And it was consumed young. Wine made from grapes harvested in September was considered 'old' by January, and by Easter, was well on its way to vinegar (in this age before sterilization, bottling and the addition of sulphites). If nothing else, the transitory nature of most wine helps to explain the prominence of vinegar as an ingredient in medieval and Renaissance cookery.

Higher-alcohol, sweet wines resisted better. As a result of this, there was a flourishing trade in the better-known wines, especially those sweet or strong enough to survive a long sea voyage and dubious storage conditions. By the seventeenth century, wine-making and retailing was becoming big business in some regions, and sweet wines such as Malmsey (Malvasia), Madeira and other varieties fetched high prices throughout Europe. Another solution was to fortify local wines with brandy, so they would survive export and transport. This is the origin of port and other fortified wines, which became favourites in England and elsewhere in northern Europe. For centuries, most of England's wine had been imported via France, but when war with France cut off wine supplies from Bordeaux, English trade with Portugal took off. When the English lowered tariffs with Portugal in 1703, the trade in port grew; henceforth, most wine drunk in England would come from either Portugal or Spain. (The Scots, by contrast, continued drinking French claret.[37]) Port was definitely not watered down by its English consumers, its high alcoholic content being one of its attractions – in 'an age when hard drinking was endemic among both sexes and in all ranks of society'.[38]

The growing English fondness for fortified wines during the eighteenth century would lead to a backlash against them, with a few physicians warning of the harm they caused. 'Wine is now become as common as water', according to Cheyne (which at least reminds us that water was common). For the many people who drank little besides wine, 'their blood becomes inflamed into gout, stone and rheumatism, raging fevers, pleurisies, small pox or measles; their passions are enraged into quarrels, murder, and blasphemy; their juices are dried up; and their solids [their flesh] scorch'd and shrivel'd'.[39] Cheyne was not alone. Of several thousand French medical consultations by letter for the period 1665–1789, 7 per cent of them recommended the avoidance of wine and strong liquors.[40] Then again, as Joseph Greene wrote to his brother following a medical consultation:

> The pleasantest advice they have given me, came at last: "that my solids being much relaxed, I must frequently mount my horse for exercise, and in my intermediate state, solace my self plentifully with good old Port". Peace to their Faculty-Wigs and Canes! Though they could not restore *my* health, have put me into a charitable method of drinking theirs.[41]

If medical writers at the start of our period had been generally favourable towards wines, while admittedly differing on the what, how and when, by the end of the early modern period there was much more ambivalence. This may explain why the Scottish aristocrat and systematizer John Sinclair concluded, in 1807, that 'there is no subject in which authors have differed more, than regarding the advantages and disadvantages of wine'.[42]

Cider, ale and beer

While the elites of northern Europe were able to afford wine, the majority of the population there regularly drank something else – either cider or ale and beer. If cider was generally regarded as a poor substitute for wine, along Galenic lines, there was at least one doctor who wrote enthusiastically about it – and did so several years before Bacci's treatise on wine. Julien Le Paulmier, a Protestant doctor from Normandy, was prompted to write on the virtues of the local tipple in response to its absence from ancient medical texts.[43] He thus fits into the category of medical authors who 'domesticated' Galen, examined in Chapter 4. In the best humanist tradition – Le Paulmier styled himself Palmarius – he explained that the ancients could not have known about cider as it was new to Normandy, going back no earlier than the start of the sixteenth century. Le Paulmier was the first author to take cider seriously, attentive to the different kinds and recommending that one should not mix different apple varieties. He was also the first to insert cider into a work of regimen, discoursing on its qualities – it is warm and moist like good wine, but moderately so – and its health-giving properties. Cider's advantage over wine was that it was less easily abused: less harmful than drinking wine without water. Cider was the preferred 'natural beverage': easy to digest and promptly assimilated by the body, it 'moistened and corrected the dryness of the [body's] solid parts' and quenched thirst.[44]

In England, where cider was reportedly 'the fifth kinde of drinke usuall heer', Thomas Cogan was much less enthusiastic. He judged cider to be cold in quality, only good for those with hot stomachs. For everyone else, 'it maketh even in youth the colour of the face pale and the skinne riveled [wrinkled]'. And as for pear cider, or perry, Cogan recalled that 'when I was a student at Oxforde, one mistresse G. sold perie in steede of Rhenish wine, and so beguiled manie a poore scholer'. *Caveat emptor*, he concluded.[45] Cogan was more positive about beer, especially small beer. Beer was not just for special occasions, but a regular food for most northern Europeans. It was also taken as medicine, with the addition of herbs and spices, like that consumed by Josselin. And, as our regimen writers often point out, it was a source of good old-fashioned drunkenness. The names given in England to local ales and beers leave this in little doubt: huffcap, mad dog, Father Whoreson, angels' food, dragon's milk, go-by-the-wall, stride wide and lift leg.[46]

Usually made from malted barley, ale and beer could also be made from wheat, rye and even oats. Beer and ale are similar, differing only in the method of fermentation and in the addition of hops (in the case of beer). Hopped beer – ale made with the addition of hops – was first introduced into England in 1520. As a rhyme penned in 1524 went, 'Greeke, heresie, turkey-cocks and beere/came into England all in a year'. (Mind you, the rhyme is inaccurate at least as far as the turkey is concerned, so should be taken with a pinch of salt.[47]) In England, the making of unhopped ale was traditionally part of the woman's domestic realm, and continued to be so until the age of urbanization and industrialization; hopped beer was made by men, in breweries, and would eventually predominate. As early as 1577, ale was described as 'sometime our only, but now taken with many for old and sick men's drink'.[48]

When it came to beer, the Milanese physician Girolamo Cardano was cautiously favourable, noting that 'although beer seems unpleasant at first taste, it grows on one with use'.[49] Renaissance physicians were normally less enthusiastic about ale and beer than they were about wine. Wine, because of its Mediterranean origins, was well known to ancient medical writers, but beer was not. Renaissance doctors associated beer with rustics and labourers and decided it was fit only for their robust constitutions. Guglielmo Grataroli mixed discussions of the virtues of wine with a Swiss Protestant zeal to ensure sobriety. As bad as getting drunk on wine might for one's health, getting drunk on beer was far worse. This was because, according to Grataroli, beer emits crass vapours that take a long time to dispel from the brain, so you actually stay drunk longer.[50] To make matters worse, for Cheyne, writing 150 years after Grataroli and operating under a new, mechanical model of digestion, ale was as difficult to digest as 'porke and pease-soup'. Cheyne's recommendation for Yorkshire or Nottingham ale? 'They make excellent bird lime [an adhesive applied to branches to trap birds], and when simmer'd some time over a gentle fire, make the most sticking and the best plaister for old strains that can be contriv'd'.[51] But then Cheyne did not really approve of alcohol of any kind.

Northern European physicians did sometimes make a virtue of necessity and write in praise of ale and beer. The English physician Andrew Boorde thought ale a 'naturall drinke' for Englishmen, as we saw in Chapter 4. In one of Johann Brettschneider's works on regimen, there is a whole treatise on the making and virtues of beer (1550).[52] Not unlike Bacci's later treatise on wine, the German Brettschneider surveys the history of beer and the art of brewing; compares dark and light beers; analyses the different flavours, brewing methods and storage for a range of different beers from German-speaking areas of Europe, including parts of what is now Poland and Lithuania; and concludes with a discussion of aromatic beers, flavoured variously with sage, hyssop, roses, ginger, cherries, prunes and so on. By the time he published his treatise, Brettschneider was drawing on a long tradition of beer-making. Some forty years earlier, the Bavarians had enacted their famous 'purity law' (*Reinheitsgebot*) of 1516. Rural households typically produced their own beer, while in towns it was brewed as a commercial enterprise, strictly regulated by government and guild regulations such as the Bavarian one.[53]

Throughout the seventeenth and eighteenth centuries, wine made inroads into previously beer-drinking areas. The greater use of bottles and the invention of the corkscrew made wine easier to transport, keep and drink. In some areas the price differential lessened, the result of increasing taxes on beer and ever-increasing wine production. That said, the first real threat to the production and consumption of beer, for example, in the Low Countries, came not from wine, but from brandy. In London the competition came from gin. Attracted to the higher alcoholic content of distilled drinks, the urban poor of northern Europe increasingly drank brandy and gin instead of beer. They were able to consume the same amount of alcohol at much less cost, but lost out on the nutrition that beer provided. The second threat to beer consumption came from coffee and tea, as we shall see below. That said, neither of these beverage types completely replaced beer. Indeed in some areas, such as London, Bavaria and some towns in the Low Countries, beer production actually went up in the eighteenth century. In part, brewers were keeping pace with a growing population; in part, they were developing new popular types of beer, like porter in England and pilsner in Bavaria.

Distillates of alcohol

By the start of the early modern period, new drinkable liquids were making their presence felt, beginning with distillates of alcohol. The distillation of alcohol was a by-product of alchemy: chemical research and exploration in pursuit of perfect substances. Practitioners of distillation were searching for a volatile spirit that they believed was analogous to the 'spirits' coursing through the human body, an artificial spirit that would thus prolong life. From this the name *aqua vitae*, or 'water of life'. At first, this *aqua vitae* was produced and used only for medicinal or chemical purposes, as a pain-reliever or solvent. But by the fifteenth and sixteenth centuries, it emerged from the confines of the apothecary's shop and entered houses and taverns. The expression also entered the vernacular languages of Europe: as *eau-de-vie* in French, *akvavit* in Scandinavian countries, *uisge beatha* in Gaelic (giving us 'whisky' in English). This was followed quickly by attempts to regulate its production, sale and consumption, made by the town councils of Nuremberg and Frankfurt, from the 1480s and 1490s. But in a satirical poem dedicated to revealing 'whether aqua vitae is healthy or harmful', the Nuremberg barber-surgeon and printer Hans Folz (1493) blamed the resulting social and health problems not on the drink but on its excessive consumption.[54] Early in the sixteenth century, the same councils intervened to stop the toasting ritual known as *Zutrinken*, made especially potent by the new beverage.[55]

By the seventeenth century it was competing with wine in consumption terms in certain areas of Europe. It could be distilled from a range of materials, distillation of wine being probably the oldest technique, borrowed from the Arabs and yielding a clear and fiery liquid. This is the origin of 'brandy', from the Dutch word *brandewijn*, or 'burnt wine'. Brandy gets it colour and nutty flavour from aging in wooden casks. Because it was more easily transported than wine, brandy became a staple on the long ocean voyages of the time. The trade was first encouraged by the Dutch, hence the origins of the English name, and later by the English – though in both cases the actual brandy was produced in France. Of course, *aqua vitae* could (and can) also be distilled from a wide range of other materials: the residual pits and skins left over from grape processing (grappa), various sweet fruits (kirsch), cereals like barley, wheat and rye (whisky and gin) and even potatoes (vodka and akvavit).

To this lengthening list of distillates, rum was added in the eighteenth century, during which time it became one of the most important and valuable commodities of the Atlantic trade. Distilled from molasses, rum was one of the principal uses for the sugarcane grown on plantations. For this reason, it was especially a New World drink, where it was the drink of choice in many a public house. So much so, in fact, that the reform-minded printer Timothy Green of Connecticut recommended tea as an alternative, despite his reservations regarding the latter. In his *Gazette* of 1772, Green published a piece by a certain 'Medicus', which noted that 'you will seldom see a thirst for rum and a thirst for tea in the same person' and concluded that 'for a single person whose life has been lost by tea, thousands have been slain by rum'.[56]

The final category of spirituous beverages consisted of liqueurs, a trade that originated in Italy in the seventeenth century and soon spread elsewhere. Concocted from a whole range of ingredients, from fruit blossoms to spices, these liqueurs had much vaunted health benefits. A treatise of 1783 by the doctor and botanist Pierre Buc'hoz abounds with recipes for them. For example, Buc'hoz claimed that his recipe for 'Peach liqueur à la Provençale', with the peaches preserved in alcohol, provided both a 'liqueur excellent to drink' and a 'fruit most agreable to eat', which also had medicinal properties: 'it is a specific for diseases of the lungs, it removes bad breath and is very good for bilious people'.[57]

When liqueurs became fashionable luxury goods in France during the eighteenth century, doctors were quick to express a medical opinion. Not surprisingly, perhaps, it was a divided one. For some, like Buc'hoz, liqueurs nourished the nervous system and enhanced mental abilities. For others, they were 'empty' foodstuffs, devoid of nourishment, whose only purpose was to provide pleasure by altering the body's mental state. Le Bègue warned that if drunk in any quantity, liqueurs 'weaken and destroy the body, madden the spirit, shorten life, accelerate the infirmities of old age, reduce the number of children, and harm those who are not thus prevented from being born'.[58] Sinclair believed them to be 'insidiously dangerous, as they are very palatable', 'fortunately more used on the Continent than in Great Britain'.[59]

Sellers of the liqueurs could appeal to iatrochemical models of mind and body in their sales pitches, as Emma Spary has noted.[60] Distillation itself, as a chemical process, found favour. The experienced distiller and retired café proprietor François-René-André Dubuisson published a treatise on the 'art of distillation' which met with the approval of Paris's Société Royale de Médecine. Dubuisson regarded his liqueurs as 'medicinal foodstuffs'. His experiments in distillation, he suggested, were directed towards improving the standards of liqueur production, the aim of which was to produce a more intense spirit, pure and of high quality. The end products may have been pleasurable, but they were also medicinal, in that they sought to isolate the medical components of plants for therapeutic uses. In any case, Dubuisson presented his rarefied luxury spirits as miles away from the cheap liqueurs made 'purely to satisfy the disordered appetite of the people'.[61]

In England at least, medical writers became increasingly critical of spirits during the eighteenth century. There was a widespread perception of increasing drunkenness, resulting in dependency and social disorder (Figure 8.4). John Moore, an English doctor who lived in Naples for a time, compared the Neapolitans' penchant for cold drinks with that of Londoners (1781):

Iced water and lemonade are among the luxuries of the lowest vulgar; they are carried about in little barrels, and sold in half-penny's worth. The half naked lazzarone is often tempted to spend the small pittance destined for the maintenance of his family, on this bewitching beverage, as the most dissolute of the low people in London spend their wages on gin and brandy; so that the same extravagance which cools the mob of one city, tends to inflame that of the other to acts of excess and brutality.[62]

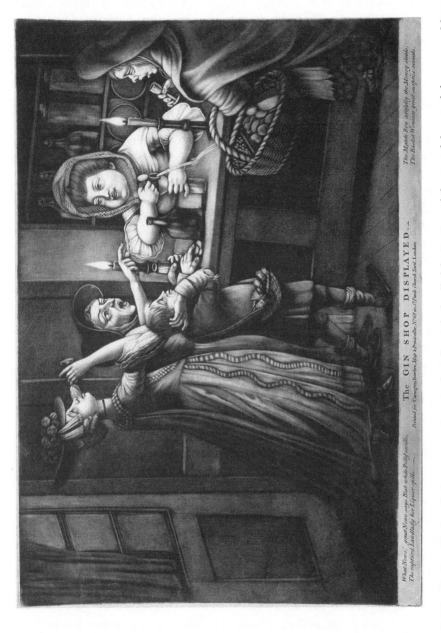

Figure 8.4 'The gin shop displayed': three women in a gin shop divert the landlady's attention while a match boy steals her money. Mezzotint by C. Bowles, 1765 (Wellcome Library, London).

Spirits like gin were viewed as overly heating, capable of generating fevers and inflammations. Cheyne argued that distilled liquors were never meant to be consumed as beverages. They were properly the stuff of apothecaries, an ingredient in certain medicines, not a drink.[63] They were full of high concentrations of salts and oils, which formed gluey particles in the body, clogging the circulation, heating the blood and burning the tissues. Moreover, the drunkenness that resulted was a moral threat to society.

Chocolate, coffee and tea

Cheyne did not think much of the new 'luxury' beverages either. They had come with European colonial expansion and, while not displacing either wine and beer or distilled drinks, they none the less transformed drinking habits. Although chocolate, coffee and tea had quite different geographical origins and would assume different trajectories in Europe, they were frequently grouped together in the minds of early modern Europeans. In the late seventeenth century, Samuel Pepys in London and Anthony Wood in Oxford were among England's earliest devotees of the new drinks, which in England arrived more or less at the same time. They consumed all three with equal zeal, often at a public coffee-house, although both men showed a preference for coffee.[64] And across the Channel, a merchant-grocer in the French city of Lyon, Philippe Sylvestre Dufour, wrote a three-part treatise on the three new beverages.[65] Dufour's methodology was the same in each section. He described the chemical properties and therapeutic uses of each, in the best Galenic regimen tradition; then he surveyed the ways to prepare and serve them; and finished with recipes for their preparation. Dufour's interests were more medical than recreational. If the reverend Locatelli had used binge drinking to treat his headaches two decades earlier, Dufour was now recommending coffee (Figure 8.5).

Chocolate was the first to have any real impact in Europe, and yet the initial reaction to it was anything but promising – in common with several other products of the New World, as we saw in the previous chapter. In the words of the Jesuit missionary José de Acosta, writing in 1590:

> The main use of cacao is a beverage called *chocolaté*, which is loathsome to such as are not acquainted with it, having a scum or froth that is very unpleasant to taste .... The Spaniards, both men and women, that are accustomed to the country, are very greedy of this *chocolaté*. They say they make diverse sorts of it, some hot, some cold, and some temperate, and put therein much of that *chili*; yea, they make paste thereof, the which they say is good for the stomach and against the catarrh.[66]

Spaniards in the Americas learned to like chocolate because of their proximity to and material dependence on the Indians, as Marcy Norton has shown.[67] It might happen like this: when the Spanish physician Antonio Colmenero de Ledesma, in the Indies, 'comming in a heat to visit a sicke person, and asking water to refresh me, they

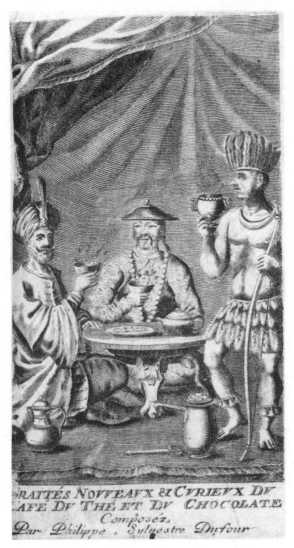

RAITÉS NOVVEAVX & CVRIEVX DV
AFE DV THÉ ET DV CHOCOLATE
Composéz.
Par Philippe . Sylvestre Dufour

Figure 8.5 Title page of Philippe Sylvestre Dufour's *Traitez nouveaux et curieux du cafe, du the et du chocolate*, 1688, showing three figures: Turkish, Chinese and Aztec (Wellcome Library, London).

perswaded me to take a draught of *chocolate*, which quencht my thirst'.[68] The aside comes from Colmenero's 1631 treatise on the virtues of chocolate, an indication of the positive impression the drink made on him.

As early as 1591, this New World drink was already being appropriated by Europeans as their own. In that year Juan de Cárdenas proclaimed it particularly good for the health of Spaniards and their Mexican-born descendants.[69] Even more than the Amerindians, it was the creoles of the Indies, in particular, its women, who had most realized the health potential of chocolate, he suggested. And Cárdenas provided them with the basic medical advice for its preparation and how, when and with what accompaniments to take it. As a drink favoured by women, by the early 1700s the sixty nuns of the convent of Santa Isabel in Mexico City were spending 2,916 pesos on chocolate for themselves, the sacristans and the priests, but only 390 pesos on poultry, eggs and wine.[70]

Already a valued trade good before the Spanish conquest, Spanish colonists developed the commerce in cacao in the Americas; but trade across the ocean took longer to become established. In Europe, its first consumers were the elites of Seville with connections to Spanish America. Shipments of cacao would be accompanied by the accoutrements necessary to prepare and drink the chocolate in domestic situations. Its reputation as a cheering and invigorating drink spread. From the 1620s cacao was on its way to becoming a commodity in Spain; by 1685 it was being 'adulterated' by shopkeepers – a sure sign of increasing demand; and by the early 1700s it was being consumed at all levels of Spanish society.[71]

It helped that the first European to conduct a serious investigation into cacao, and much else besides, the physician Francisco Hernández, praised the drink *cacahoatl* as neutral, which could be made hotter or colder according to the ingredients added, according to the humoural needs of the individual. Drinking chocolate increased vitality and alleviated melancholy and might be used in treating fevers and dysentery. But it also led to an increase in the libido, while excessive use 'obstructs the organs, drains colour, and induces cachexia and other incurable diseases'.[72] That said, generations of medical doctors after Hernández disagreed on its exact properties. Chocolate's astringent flavour suggested one set of humoural qualities (cold and dry), while its unctuousness and ability to nourish and fatten the body suggested another (hot and moist).[73] Despite (or because of) the physicians' competing claims about the medicinal virtues and vices of the beverage, chocolate largely owed its success in Europe to its consumption as a social beverage, not a medicine.

The thick, foamy drink was also favoured as something that could be consumed during periods of abstinence and fasting, referred to in Chapter 5. Liquids were allowed at such times and 'taking chocolate' had the advantage of providing nourishment. The issue was first put to papal consideration in 1577. In 1632, professors of theology representing the Benedictine, Franciscan, Dominican and Jesuit orders met in Salamanca to debate it, but the issue was never clearly resolved.[74] The most detailed Lenten dietary, Paolo Zacchia's 1636 *Vitto quaresimale*, makes no mention of chocolate: perhaps it had not yet become common in Rome. But forty years later the danger was that people might be tempted to consume chocolate to the exclusion of all else. During Lent of 1678, the wife of the Roman nobleman Orazio Spada begged him not to carry on having 'meals of just chocolate', for it made the stomach lazy and weakened the complexion. Orazio's doctor had advised him to reduce his chocolate consumption, 'especially not as thick as he drinks it' and his wife worried that 'by drinking too much chocolate he is making himself ill'.[75]

Chocolate's diffusion throughout Europe followed routes of Spanish political power and cultural influence. On a trip to Spain in 1668, the future grand-duke of Tuscany, Cosimo III, and King Carlos II enjoyed cups of chocolate while watching a bullfight. Back in Florence, the same grand-duke's 'foundry', a kind of experimental laboratory-cum-apothecary's shop under the directorship of Francesco Redi, would develop a secret and much sought-after jasmine-scented version.[76] For early modern Europeans, chocolate remained a beverage (eating chocolate as we know it today was only invented in the nineteenth century). It also retained its role and status as an object of commensality, an expression of hospitality and civility. By 1700 or so, drinking chocolate of the sugar-and-vanilla variety, accompanied by bread, brioche or other pastries, became the standard breakfast in aristocratic circles, in France and elsewhere. Chocolate maintained its elite connotations, becoming associated with aristocratic luxury and indolence. Its connotations with 'venery' and sensuality do not seem to have done it any harm.

Even so, drinking chocolate never became a phenomenon of mass consumption across Europe. Outside Spain – in Italy and France – chocolate remained limited to the social and religious elites. In Northern Europe, coffee, and later tea, were to have a much greater impact. If the first edition of Dufour's treatise, mentioned above, treated chocolate, coffee and tea at relatively equal length, the second edition of 1684 was emphatically about coffee. 'Amongst all the healthy things that [trade] has procured for us', Dufour wrote, 'the best and most universally good is in my opinion coffee'.[77] He especially appreciated the way coffee kept one sober and awake.

The medical angle proved effective as a marketing tool. At a time when coffee-drinking in England was still associated with the 'Turkey merchants' of the Levant Company, largely importing it for their own consumption, one trader, in the service of merchant Daniel Edwards, began to sell coffee in London. His name was Pasqua Rosee. In his handbill of 1652, Rosee boasted of the hot drink's abilities to 'prevent drowsiness and make one fit for business'.[78] No surprise there; more unusual to our ears were his claims that coffee was effective against headache, coughs, dropsy, gout, scurvy, miscarriage, 'hypocondriack winds' and any 'defluxion of rheums'. Coffee's growing success as a drink in Europe was due to its medical pretensions, with sellers like Rosee able to capitalize on widespread medical opinions about its virtues; a taste for the exotic, with its Arabic and Turkish associations; and its rising status as a social drink, consumed in public in the new coffee-houses. Coffee came with a health warning, however. The radical thinker Thomas Tryon – though here in agreement with medical opinion – warned that 'if a man be not wary, the use of it shall enslave him'.[79]

Native to eastern Africa (Abyssinia), coffee was adopted in Arab lands in the late Middle Ages, where it was viewed as a sober alternative to alcohol (the consumption of which was forbidden by Islamic law). Arab Sufi monks adopted coffee as a drink that would allow them to stay up for midnight prayers more easily. From religious aid, coffee passed into everyday usage, and coffee-houses soon spread throughout the Muslim Middle-East. European travel accounts first referred to this exotic beverage in the seventeenth century, by which time it was also being imported into Europe, mainly by Venetian merchants. Coffee and the coffee-house entered Europe as part of the same package and domestic consumption was rare at first. So exotic was it that when the merchant Pierre de la Roque returned to his native Marseille from his travels in the Levant, in 1644, he kept his coffee and coffee-making equipment in his cabinet of curiosities.[80] And yet, by 1696, both coffee and tea could be considered 'French' by at least one author.[81]

In 1686, the Sicilian Francesco Procopio Cutò opened the first café in Paris, 'Le Procope'. Cutò (Couteaux in French) had previously been shop assistant to an Armenian selling coffee, one of numerous 'Turks' to do so. The location of the 'Café Procope' across from Paris's main theatre, the Comédie Française, meant that actors, musicians, dramatists and other hangers-on congregated there. It started a trend, becoming the first literary coffee-house. So successful was Cutò that he was able to launch his eldest son, Michel, as a physician, while the younger son, Alexandre, inherited the business. The trend for *cafés*, coffee-houses, *Kaffeehäuser* and *botteghe di caffè* along the Parisian model spread throughout Europe. The first London coffee-house was Rosee's, established in 1652; eleven years later there were eighty-two in the City of London alone; and by 1734 London had 551 licensed coffee-houses, alongside numerous unlicensed ones.[82] What started in the mid-seventeenth century as a curiosity, quickly became a fashionable luxury, and ended the eighteenth century as an everyday good. Giuseppe Maria Galanti (1792) wrote how in Naples coffee-drinking had become widespread: 'even the vilest labourers want some in the morning; they regard it as a digestive'. 'Fortunately for their nerves', Galanti concluded, 'what is dispensed cheaply in the *botteghe* has but the colour of coffee'.[83]

Meanwhile, religious and medical men alike argued about its physiological properties. For Italian rabbi Moses Zacuto (1673) coffee was considered a medicinal drink and as such could be drunk before early morning prayers, where other 'liquid foods' like wine or beer were prohibited.[84] Others were less sure, concerned about the moral implications of a beverage which was at once sobering and exciting. If Zacuto's Mantua would have its own Jewish coffee-house in the mid-eighteenth century, for rabbis in London it was the coffee-house, and not the coffee, that constituted the problem (presumably risking contacts with non-Jews and the consumption of non-kosher foods). As pedlars and merchants, Jews were involved in the sale of coffee, like the exclusive rights granted to Flaminio Pesaro in the grand-duchy of Tuscany in 1665. Others ran coffee-houses, like Oxford's first, run from 1650 by a Jew named Jacob. And Jews were also enthusiastic consumers of coffee, like the population around them.[85]

As for the doctors, many were enthusiastic about coffee, even going so far as to consider it a universal remedy, a panacea, curing diseases of the heart, liver and stomach. Classed as hot and dry in the second degree in Galenic terms, coffee dried the body's own moisture. Result: far from increasing the libido like many other drinks, coffee actually reduced it. As Galenism gave way to iatrochemistry, coffee's qualities as mildly hot and drying were replaced by praise for its 'volatile salts'. But not everyone was convinced of its merits. Some Italian and French physicians feared that it would displace wine as the beverage of choice. Jean Gaulin, noting how coffee had become 'a fashion among women as well as among the common people', praised its former use as a medicine but was less certain of its use as a food.[86] The Heidelberg doctor Franz Anton Mai, sceptical of everything foreign, in particular, the French 'freedom and equality humbug', wrote disparagingly of the 'coffee epidemic'.[87] The historian August Ludwig Schlözer (1780) bemoaned the negative effects coffee was having on the German diet, which he argued did not suit the region's climate. Where once the Germans had been strong and healthy, drinking but small quantities of beer, the fashion was now for coffee, even though all warm drinks were harmful to the body, and coffee most of all.[88] And for Théodore Tronchin, most famous for being Voltaire's doctor, it was the fact that coffee was served hot that made it so harmful. If health was the balance between solids and fluids in the body, as it was for Tronchin, then hot beverages only served to dilute the body's strength. Mind you, this did little to dent Voltaire's penchant for coffee. On 23 January 1757, Voltaire wrote to Tronchin's cousin: 'I learn that a bale of coffee has arrived for me from Lorient, in spite of the doctor. He will not succeed in ridding us of our bad habits'.[89]

Convinced coffee-drinkers found they were able to play one doctor against another, in search of the medical advice that suited their predilections. In 1773 a Madame de la Ville Gille wrote to the Swiss physician Samuel-Auguste Tissot with this complaint: 'Every day I broke my fast with a cup of coffee with water and without sugar which usually made me go to stool. My physician has forbidden it, I admit that I have not yet had the courage to prevent myself'. In another, later letter to Tissot, she added, 'Pray tell me your feeling on the use of coffee. If it is absolutely contrary to me, I will renounce it. But if it is not harmful for me I would be very pleased not to deprive myself of it'.[90]

It was easy to parody the contradictory opinions of the medical community. A comedy performed by the Comédie Italienne in Paris, in 1730, had two poets disputing the purported benefits of coffee while seated in a coffee-house When the first poet claims that he can demonstrate that coffee is harmful on physical grounds, the second replies, 'And I, sir, shall prove the contrary, geometrically'. Poet One suggests, 'You see that [coffee] acts in a different manner and according to temperament. Let's draw a conclusion, now, whether it provokes sleep or troubles it, whether it stifles the senses or awakens them … makes the blood circulate too rapidly or else coagulates it'. But for Poet Two this was precisely the point: it was coffee's contrasting capacities which made it 'le véhicule universel'.[91]

From a social perspective, as Brian Cowan has written, coffee had all the attractions of the exotic but suited the new ethic of 'respectable' behaviour increasingly important to the middling and elite classes, with the emphasis on sobriety and civil conduct.[92] And because there was no associated fear of intoxication, coffee was well placed to become new social beverage: drunk in public settings but without the negative implications of wine or beer. Coffee-drinking and coffee-culture would be linked with the rationalistic culture of the eighteenth century. It went hand in hand with the idealized search for lucidity, clarity and freedom of thought. Unlike the tavern or inn, the café offered luxury ingredients, the respectability of its clientele and the pursuit of learning. The witty and spirited conversations held in the coffee-houses or in domestic salons were the sites for the expression of Enlightenment culture. The short-lived Milanese literary review *Il Caffè* (1764–1766) is emblematic of this environment. 'Born in a coffee shop', as it informed its readers, it was just the sort of periodical likely to be read and discussed in one.[93] But just as important in their own right were female gatherings like the *Kaffeekränzchen* or 'coffee circles' of eighteenth-century Germany, which contrast with the predominantly male spaces of Europe's seventeenth-century coffee-houses (Figure 8.6).[94] Indeed coffee-drinking suited the aims of northern Europe's rising bourgeoisie, where it was linked to the work ethic and increased productivity. Employers were told to welcome it among their workforce as an alternative to wine or beer. Wishful thinking perhaps, given that there is little evidence of workers' sobriety actually increasing.

As a stimulant, however, coffee exposed tensions in European society. This was especially so in German lands, where coffee was not accepted in the home until the

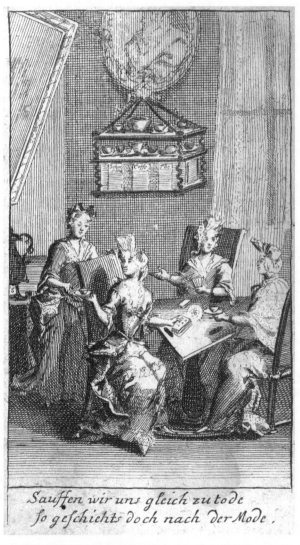

Sauffen wir uns gleich zu tode
so geschichts doch nach der Mode.

Figure 8.6 A group of women drinking coffee. Engaving from M. Duncan, *Von dem Missbrauch heisser und hitziger Speisen und Geträncke, sonderlich aber des Caffes, Schockolate, und Thees*, 1707 (Wellcome Library, London).

second half of the eighteenth century. This resistance was due to a mixture of three factors: a long-standing fondness for local beer; a general distrust of things considered 'un-German' and without overseas colonies to act as cultural mediators for exotic goods; and ongoing prohibition, taxes and criticisms especially directed against coffee.

The tensions are apparent in Johann Sebastian Bach's 'Coffee Cantata', a satirical operetta which provides a musical insight into some of the prevailing attitudes (*Schweigt stille, plaudert nicht*, or, 'Be quiet, stop chattering'). The work was first performed, fittingly enough, in Zimmerman's coffee-house in Leipzig, in 1734. It tells of the efforts of a stern father named Schlendrian – the name means 'stick-in-the-mud' – who attempts to check his daughter's propensity for coffee-drinking by threatening to make her choose between a husband and coffee. The father is perplexed that his dear daughter, Lieschen, drinks the hated coffee and he insists that she stop; she insists she needs the coffee buzz (or words to that effect). Lieschen sings an aria which begins, 'Ah, how sweet coffee tastes! Lovelier than a thousand kisses, sweeter far than muscatel wine!' And while dear dad goes searching for the beau, Lieschen makes it clear she will not marry any man that would deny her coffee. The gendering of the coffee compulsion was common in eighteenth-century representations of the subject.

The demand for coffee in Europe accompanied European expansion and empire-building. The Dutch planted it (in Java), as did the French (in the Caribbean), followed by the Spanish and Portuguese (in Central and South America). By the eighteenth century it was an international commodity. The story of tea is similar. In England and Holland, the suppliers of tea eventually overcame those of coffee. The first shipment of tea arrived around 1610 in Amsterdam, from India, where Europeans had encountered this ancient Chinese beverage. It was reported in 1635 in France, and then, courtesy of the Dutch, in England. In Amsterdam, tea replaced beer as the drink of choice by the 1680s and 1690s, and the same would happen in England during the eighteenth century, courtesy of the East India Company. Tea cost less than beer, and labourers came to prefer it, and it soon ousted coffee in popularity. John Sinclair put a medical gloss on this, explaining that the reason tea 'first came into general use' was due to the medical opinion that the most effectual means of improving health was by 'increasing the fluidity of the blood'.[95] Tea certainly met with Cheyne's approval. Cheyne considered green tea 'a very proper diluent, when softened with a little milk, to cleanse the alimentary passages and wash off the scorbutick and urinous salts, for breakfast'.[96] Tea was favoured as a digestive, which 'quenches thirst and exhilarates the spirit', in Andrew Harper's words.[97] But Harper was fighting a losing battle in considering tea as a medical rather than dietary drink, and the quantities of tea imbibed soon far exceeded Cheyne's moderate recommendations. From 1760 to 1795, English tea imports went from 5 million pounds to 20 million: this means something like 2 pounds per inhabitant (a year), to say nothing of contraband tea (given that it was taxed).

Chocolate, coffee and tea were grouped together as 'colonial beverages' because of their association with empire-building and overseas trade. Despite pronounced regional differences throughout Europe, some which persist to this day, their history is closely intertwined. All three drinks were served hot, usually with the addition of sugar; they made use of new implements, which might become luxury goods; they generated or accompanied new forms of social behaviour; and they were all stimulants in a way beverages had not been in the past. Whereas wine, beer and spirits numbed the mind with lesser or greater amounts of alcohol, chocolate, coffee and tea provided liquid refreshment that imparted a sense of energy and alertness. This was combined with the somewhat louche connotations of chocolate and coffee to embody a cultural contradiction, as Piero Camporesi pointed out: of a society 'highly-strung yet lazy, keen yet listless, industrious yet hedonistic, a late-sleeper yet an early riser'.[98]

It would be a mistake to posit alcoholic and stimulating beverages as polar opposites, with the former edged out by the latter. In Parisian cafés like the Café Suédois, some customers ordered coffee alone, but most ordered spirits (brandy, liqueurs, fortified wine, beer) with coffee on the side.[99] Alcohol remained the social beverage par excellence in Europe, regardless – or because of – the ensuing drunkenness and disorder. As important as coffee-houses were for the spread of knowledge and social reform, they were rarely the places openly accessible to all groups and ranks that was sometimes claimed. Different classes had their own coffee-houses or met in the same coffee-house at different times of the day. In many European cities, Jews had their own, even after ghetto walls came down. And just as chocolate, coffee and tea did not replace, but came to exist alongside previous beverages, so the coffee-house did not marginalize or displace other sorts of drinking establishments. Taverns remained central to European sociability, in particular for the labouring and artisanal classes. During the eighteenth century new kinds of drinking places added to this provision. The London elites had their private clubs, the site of all-male conviviality and heavy drinking. In Paris the *guinguettes* opened by wine merchants on the outskirts of the city provided entertainment and larger indoor and outdoor spaces than the traditional, neighbourhood taverns. *Guinguettes* offered a different kind of sociality and a different kind of leisure, where the cheaper wine on offer was only part of the story.[100]

Conclusion

By the seventeenth century the old liquid standbys of wine and beer were witnessing the spread of new drinks spread throughout Europe, drinks which came to exist either alongside wine and beer or else gradually replaced them, depending on the context. The result was a radical transformation in drinking habits. On the one hand, we have the distilled drinks, notably stronger in terms of their alcoholic content, such as brandy, gin and a range of liqueurs. On the other hand, we have the arrival of quite different drinks, in the form of chocolate, coffee and tea. Medical writers did not generally consider chocolate, coffee and tea as foods, in the way that wine and beer had been. Rather, they regarded them more as drugs: in both senses of the word, medicinal as well as euphoria- or escape-inducing. Throughout, medical writers sought to come to terms with the new arrivals, sometimes reflecting changing fashions, sometimes seeking to reign them in. Although keen observers, investigators and commentators, they appear as bystanders rarely able to shape events and behaviours.

CONCLUSION

There ought to be nothing simpler, nothing more natural, than eating and drinking. In reality, nothing is more complex and less spontaneous. Choosing what to eat and how to nourish our bodies is as much a natural act as a constructed one, involving cultural, social, moral and political forces.[1] In early modern Europe, to what extent was it shaped by medical forces, too? Or, to put it another way, how did medical authors attempt to shape what Europeans ate and drank as part of a healthy regimen? To that end, one of the aims of this book has been to problematize the relationship between diet and dietetics in early modern Europe.

The field of regimen lay at the intersection of more or less informed consumers, medical authority and food habits. The early modern regimen was not only a successful literary genre, it was a varied one. Printed advice on eating for health was subject to a range of conditioning factors, such as rank and occupation, nation and region, religion and morality, and the reaction to novelty. And, as this suggests, the genre was also a changing one. Regimens underwent the ups and downs of shifting medical philosophies and adapted to changing foodways in society at large. The whole field of preventive medicine underwent something of a revival during the Renaissance, with Galen as the key ancient authority and with a focus on foods and their nature. The ascendancy of Paracelsian and chemical medicine in the seventeenth century witnessed a shift to predominantly medicinal solutions to health problems and the consequential marginalization of regimen. In turn, a criticism of these often harsh medicines came in the eighteenth century, with the revival of preventive medicine, in a more Hippocratic guise, with a more generalized interest in food as one element in the broader context of regimen.

Despite these changes in medical thinking, the regimens themselves exhibit an underlying conservatism. This is evident both in their structure and approach, as well as in the actual advice. In Chapter 3 we observed how notions of what fare was suited to the elites and what to the rest of society remained little changed over the period, regardless of changing medical ideologies. And yet regimens were far from static. Even limiting ourselves to the early part of our period, that of the Galenic revival, it is evident that Galenism was flexible as a doctrine. So flexible, in fact, that it allowed medical writers to disagree over the 'qualities' of different foodstuffs and their effects on the body. When Renaissance doctors were confronted with changing or local preferences that went against the best Galenic advice, they 'domesticated' it. They argued that, had Galen known of our beef (in England), our maize (in New Spain) and our cider (in Normandy), he would no doubt have approved them. They did so on the basis of their own observation and their own experience on the ground. This observation and experience was also Galenism's undoing, because it seemed much more consonant with iatrochemical and iatromechanical approaches. But they too debated the nature of individual foodstuffs. Only authors writing as part of the regimen revival of the eighteenth century seemed much more in agreement with one another, but then it may also have been due to the fact that they were less concerned with itemizing the nature and effects of different foods, and more interested in general principles.

At times, we see regimens and society evolving along the same lines, in parallel. This is the case with elite cookery, which jettisoned its attachment to Galenic 'checks and balances' in favour of lighter, more 'natural' tastes and dishes, at the same time as medicine opted for a lighter touch, as we saw in Chapter 2. Labelled 'modern' by its proponents, to set it apart from the traditional cookery of the Renaissance, it developed first in France and soon became fashionable throughout much of Europe. The trend ran parallel to medical theories advising restraint, moderation and simplicity, as much at the table as at the sick bed.

Likewise, ideas about the relationship between nation and diet followed the course of changing experiences, both in Europe and overseas, and changing understandings of physiology, climate and race. As we observed in Chapter 4, the link between food, nature and nation was tightest in Galenic regimens: what you were determined what you ate and what you ate determined what you were. That was the surest way to health; any change in this custom was bound to cause serious health problems. This belief also fostered a fear of difference, for what was foreign became, at the very least, a source of ridicule, or much more likely, a threat. The shift in medical philosophies towards the chemical and the mechanical in the seventeenth century rendered what one ate much less problematic. It severed the direct link between nature and nation, turning foodways into a matter of taste and fashion in the eighteenth-century regimens.

A similar pattern of society and regimens evolving in tandem is evident in the religious dieting examined in Chapter 5. When it came to religious dietary habits, in particular fasting, Renaissance doctors found themselves in a quandary. Moderate fasting might be a good thing, but anything too extreme – too 'religious' – was harmful to the body. Christian abstinence was made worse by the fact that the main alternative to meat was fish, about which Galenic physicians were rarely enthusiastic. With the Reformation, Protestant doctors were able to voice their reservations quite openly; meanwhile Catholic doctors sought to point out the health advantages of fasting. The more flexible approach of the Catholic Church towards abstinence and Lenten observance during the eighteenth century reflected a changing attitude towards the consumption of food which was a closer fit to medical ideas, although it would be wrong to see this as an unequivocal sign of secularization.

If the regimen genre was thus far from static, it is also true that fashions in food were quicker to change than medical opinions. When it came to the consumption of vegetables and fruits, Renaissance doctors fought a losing battle against changing dietary habits which spread from Italy to France and across Europe. Rather than attempt outright prohibition, regimen writers generally reacted by suggesting ways vegetables and fruits could be tempered to render them less unhealthy (if not actually healthy). By the eighteenth century, however, doctors considered them very healthy indeed, even to the point of advocating (if not always practising) a vegetables-only diet. Salads went from being the epitome of courtly depravity to a source of lightness and virtue. The decline of Galenism, replaced by iatrochemical and iatromechanical philosophies, was partly responsible for this shift in opinion, as was the role of observation and experience. Or were doctors simply adjusting their views to suit actual food habits?

New World foodstuffs offer another test case for the capability of our medical authors to cope with change. They did not cope very well. Not only were they slow to mention the plants and animals of the Americas, they invariably condemned them as well. Only when they were perceived as analogous to foods already present on European tables did they welcome them. Even when their American cousins made a meal of maize, and when European peasants transformed it into polenta, our medical authors were still reluctant. After decades of confusion over the potato, it continued to divide medical opinion long after it had become a staple in much of northern Europe.

Given all of these variables, it is easy to understand why medical authors so often disagreed with one another. Thus, as a body of knowledge, regimens were contradictory, eminently adaptable, open-ended, just as their underlying framework and principles remained quite conservative. But is it useful to regard health manuals as a body of knowledge at all? Perhaps not, given that they were meant to be consulted and used by their readers. And these readers were just as likely to adapt (or indeed disregard) the advice as they saw fit, appropriating the information as their own.

In this sense the regimens were less a body of knowledge than a tool for problem-solving, based around a series of fixed points and rules through which readers might negotiate themselves in their quest for health. Medical writers sought to respond to this, adapting and modelling their regimens around evolving behaviour, just as they sought to shape this behaviour. Regimens thus provide an example of how knowledge circulated in the early modern period. First and foremost, we have seen how doctors and other medical writers reacted to changing food habits and preferences as these occurred on the macro level of whole social groups and geographical regions. We have only secondarily been able to touch on how this advice was variously received, appropriated and, often, ignored on an individual or micro level; and this merits much further, detailed, archival study.

NOTES

Introduction

1 Pressavin, J. B. (1786), *L'art de prolonger la vie et de conserver la santé, ou traité d'hygiene*. Lyon: J. S. Grabit, ii, xxv. All translations are my own unless noted otherwise.

2 Álvarez de Miraval, B. (1601), *De la conservación de la salud del cuerpo y del alma*. Salamanca: Andres Renaut, p. 76.

3 Joubert, L. (1995 [1578]), *The Second Part of the Popular Errors*. Trans. G. D. De Rocher. Tuscaloosa: University of Alabama Press, p. 113.

4 Guptill, A., Copelton, D. and Lucal, B. (2013), *Food and Society: Principles and Paradoxes*. Cambridge: Polity Press, 2013, p. 61.

5 Nestle, M. (2007), *Food Politics: How the Food Industry Influences Nutrition and Health*. Berkeley, CA: University of California Press.

6 Proctor, R. (2008), 'Agnotology: a missing term to describe the cultural production of ignorance (and its study)', in R. Proctor and L. Schiebinger (eds), *Agnotology: The Making and Unmaking of Ignorance*. Stanford, CA: Stanford University Press, pp. 1–33.

7 As an example of the social construction of healthy eating today, we need go no further than 'five-a-day': the campaign to encourage us all to eat more fruit and vegetables and the social response to it. From the 1990s, armed with plenty of good intentions but without much in the way of hard scientific data, governments in the global north have promoted this advice, shaped by food and health lobbies of various kinds, and presented in a bewildering array of configurations, from food 'pyramids' and 'plates' to 'wheels' and 'compasses', and permutations, from percentage of daily intake to portion size or portion numbers (ranging from five to nine, depending on the country in which you live). For the differing recommendations within Europe alone, see: http://www.eufic.org/article/en/page/RARCHIVE/expid/food-based-dietary-guidelines-in-europe/.

8 Céard, J. (1982), 'La diététique dans la médecine de la Renaissance', in J.-C. Margolin and R. Sauzet (eds), *Pratiques et discours alimentaires à la Renaissance: actes du colloque de Tours 1979*. Paris: Maisonneuve et Larose, p. 31.

9 Chen, N. (2009), *Food, Medicine, and the Quest for Good Health: Nutrition, Medicine, and Culture*. New York, NY: Columbia University Press, xi.

10 Claflin, K. (2012), 'Food among the historians: early modern Europe', in K. Claflin and P. Scholliers (eds), *Writing Food History: A Global Perspective*. London and New York: Berg, p. 38.

11 Jordanova, L. (1995), 'The social construction of medical knowledge'. *Social History of Medicine*, 8, 361–81.

12 Wear, A. (1992), 'Editor's introduction', in A. Wear (ed), *Medicine in Society: Historical Essays*. Cambridge: Cambridge University Press; Jordanova, L. (1993), 'Has the social history of medicine come of age?'. *The Historical Journal*, 36, 437–49.

13 The history of the discipline, and its changing approaches and methodologies, is surveyed in: Meyzie, P. (2010), *L'alimentation en Europe à l'époque moderne: manger et boire, XIVe siècle–XIXe siècle*. Paris: Armand Colin, pp. 7–27; Claflin, 'Food among the historians'.

14 On the 'cultural turn', see Burke, P. (2012), 'Cultural history and its neighbours'. *Culture & History: Digital Journal*, 1, 1, online at: http://dx.doi.org/10.3989/chdj.2012.006.

15 The past ten years of research in food history are critically discussed in: *Food & History*, 10:2 (2012): 'Studia alimentorum 2003–2013. Une décennie de recherche/A Decade of Research'.

16 Turner, B. (1982), 'The government of the body: medical regimens and the rationalization of diet'. *The British Journal of Sociology*, 33:2, 254–69; Turner, B. (1982), 'The discourse of diet'. *Theory, Culture and Society*, 1:1, 23–32.

17 Wear, A. (2000), *Knowledge and Practice in English Medicine, 1550–1680*. Cambridge: Cambridge University Press, pp. 154–209.

18 Slack, P. (1979), 'Mirrors of health and treasures of poor men: the uses of the vernacular medical literature of Tudor England', in C. Webster (ed), *Health, Medicine and Mortality in the Sixteenth Century*. Cambridge: Cambridge University Press, pp. 237–73.

19 Ackerknecht, E. (1973), *Therapeutics: From the Primitives to the Twentieth Century, with an Appendix History of Dietetics*. London: Collier-Macmillan.

20 Mikkeli, H. (1999), *Hygiene in the Early Modern Medical Tradition*. Helsinki: Academia Scientiarum Fennica; Albala, K. (2002), *Eating Right in the Renaissance*. Berkeley, CA: University of California Press; Bergdolt, K. (2008), *Wellbeing: A Cultural History of Healthy Living*. Trans. J. Dewhurst. Cambridge: Polity; Nicoud, M. (2007), *Les régimes de santé au moyen âge*. Rome: École Française de Rome, two vols.; Shapin, S. (2003), 'How to eat like a gentleman: dietetics and ethics in early modern England', in C. Rosenberg (ed), *Right Living: An Anglo-American Tradition of Self-Help Medicine and Hygiene*. Baltimore, MD: Johns Hopkins University Press, pp. 21–58, and (2003), 'Trusting George Cheyne: scientific expertise, common sense, and moral authority in early eighteenth-century dietetic medicine'. *Bulletin of the History of Medicine*, 77, 263–97.

21 Mikkeli, *Hygiene*, pp. 176–7.

22 Sinclair, J. (1807–08), *The Code of Health and Longevity: Or, a Concise View of the Principles Calculated for the Preservation of Health and the Attainment of Long Life*. Edinburgh: Arch. Constable, vol. 1, p. 170.

23 Tacitus, *Annals*, VI, xlvi, in G. Apperson (2006), *The Wordsworth Dictionary of Proverbs*. Ware: Wordsworth, p. 210.

24 Cavallo, S. and Storey, T. (2013), *Healthy Living in Late Renaissance Italy*. Oxford: Oxford University Press.

25 Rankin, A. (2013), *Panaceia's Daughter: Noblewomen as Healers in Early Modern Germany*. Chicago: University of Chicago Press, pp. 168–203.

26 Bacon, F. (1831 [1638]), 'History of life and death', in *The Works of Francis Bacon*. London: William Pickering, vol. XIV, p. 357.

27 Sinclair, *Code of Health*, vol. 2, pp. 185–301; also discussed in Palmer, R. (1991), 'Health, hygiene and longevity in Medieval and Renaissance Europe', in Y. Kawakita, S. Sakai and Y. Otsuka (eds), *History of Hygiene*. Tokyo: Ishiyaku, pp. 77–98.

28 Siraisi, N. (1997), *The Clock and the Mirror: Girolamo Cardano and Renaissance Medicine*. Princeton, NJ: Princeton University Press, p. 70.

29 Slack, 'Mirrors of health', pp. 237, 247.

30 Durante, C. (1586), *Tesoro della sanità, nel quale si dà il modo di conservar la sanità et prolungar la vita*. Rome: F. Zanetti; Rhodes, D. (1968), *La vita e le opere di Castore Durante e della sua famiglia*. Viterbo: Agnesotti, pp. 42–4.

31 Durante, C. (1686), *A Family-Herbal or the Treasure of Health*. Trans. J. Chamberlayne. London: W. Crooke; Fissell, M. (2007), 'The marketplace of print', in M. Jenner and P. Wallis (eds), *Medicine and the Market in England and Its Colonies, c. 1450–c. 1850*. Houndmills: Palgrave Macmillan, p. 114.

32 Smith, G. (1985), 'Prescribing the rules of health: self-help and advice in the late eighteenth century', in R. Porter (ed), *Patients and Practitioners: Lay Perceptions of Medicine in Pre-Industrial Society*. Cambridge: Cambridge University Press, p. 256.

33 Cornaro, A. (2014), *Writings on the Sober Life: The Art and Grace of Living Long*. Trans. H. Fudemoto (ed). Toronto: University of Toronto Press, p. xxii, 199, 207.

34 Reyher, J. G. (1790), *Anleitung zur Erhaltung der Gesundheit für den Landmann*. Schwerin: cit. in Bergdolt, *Wellbeing*, p. 244.

35 On ideas about children and the elderly as separate categories, see Newton, H. (2012), *The Sick Child in Early Modern England, 1580–1720*. Oxford: Oxford University Press, pp. 67–78, and Schäfer, D. (2011), *Old Age and Disease in Early Modern Medicine*. Trans. P. Baker. London: Pickering & Chatto.

Chapter 1

1 Venette, N. (1683), *L'art de tailler des arbres fruitiers, avec … un traité de l'usage des fruits des arbres pour se conserver en santé ou pour se guérir lorsqu'on est malade*. Paris: Charles de Sercy, part II, p. 2.

2 De Montaigne, M. (1811 [1580]), 'Of experience', in *The Essays of Michel de Montaigne*. Trans. P. Coste. London: W. Miller, vol. 3, pp. 357–431.

3 De Cervantes, M. (1885 [1615]), *Don Quixote of La Mancha*. Trans. J. Ormsby. London: Smith, Elder and Co., book II, chapter 47. Available online at: http://ebooks.adelaide.edu.au/c/cervantes/c41d/index.html.

4 Albala, *Eating Right in the Renaissance*, p. 4.

5 Ackerknecht, *Therapeutics: From the Primitives to the Twentieth Century, with an Appendix History of Dietetics*, p. 168.

6 Mikkeli, H. (1999), *Hygiene in the Early Modern Medical Tradition*. Helsinki: Finnish Academy of Science and Letters, pp. 10–11.

7 Nicoud, M. (2013), 'I *regimina sanitatis*: un genere medico tra salute, prevenzione e terapia', in M. Conforti, A. Carlino and A. Clericuzio (eds), *Interpretare e curare. Medicine e salute nel Rinascimento*. Rome: Carocci, p. 44.

8 Capone, P. (2005), *L'arte del vivere sano. Il 'Regimen Sanitatis Salernitanum' e l'età moderna*. Milan: Guerini e Associati.

9 Anon. (1608), *The Englishmans Doctor: Or the Schoole of Salerne, or Physicall Observations for the Perfect Preserving of the Body of Man in Continuall Health*. Trans. J. Harington. London: J. Helme, available online at: http://user.icx.net/~richmond/rsr/ajax/harington.html. The leek is the national emblem of Wales, and was formerly worn on St David's Day (1 March). Harrington would have approved of the modern-day preference for wearing a daffodil flower instead.

10 Sigerist, H. (1956), *Landmarks in the History of Hygiene*. Oxford: Oxford University Press, pp. 1–19; Green, R. (1951), *A Translation of Galen's 'Hygiene' (De sanitate tuenda)*. Springfield, IL: C. Thomas; Galen (2003), *On the Properties of Foodstuffs*. Trans. O. Powell (ed). Cambridge: Cambridge University Press.

11   Savonarola, M. (1991 [1515]), *Libreto di tutte le cose che se manzano*. Padua: Programma; Pisanelli, B. (2000 [1583]), *Trattato de' cibi et del bere*. Carmagnola: Arktos.

12   Albala, *Eating Right*, pp. 7–8, 26–37.

13   Mikkeli, *Hygiene*, p. 70.

14   Baley, W. (1588), *A Short Discourse of the Three Kinds of Peppers in Common Use*. London: Eliot's Court Press.

15   Mattioli, P. A. (1544), *Di Pedacio Dioscoride Anazarbeo libri cinque. Della historia et materia medicinale tradotti in lingua volgare …* Venice: N. De Bascarini. For discussions of the evolution of the work, see Stannard, J. (1969), 'P. A. Mattioli: sixteenth century commentator on Dioscorides'. *Bibliographical Contributions*, 1, 59–81, and Sboarina, F. (2000), *Il lessico medico nel* Dioscoride *di Pietro Antonio Mattioli*. Frankfurt: Peter Lang, pp. 53–62.

16   García-Ballester, L. (1993), 'On the origin of the six non-natural things in Galen', in J. Kollesch and D. Nickel (eds), *Galen und das hellenistische Erbe*. Stuttgart: Steiner, p. 115.

17   Jarcho, S. (1970), 'Galen's six non-naturals'. *Bulletin of the History of Medicine*, 44, 372–77, and Niebyl, P. H. (1971), 'The non-naturals'. *Bulletin of the History of Medicine*, 45, 486–92.

18   Anon. (1561), *Régime de vivre*. Paris: V. Sertenas, 16v.–17r., cit. in Céard, 'Diététique', p. 26.

19   We may yet return to this ancient notion. Following the mapping of the human genome sequence, modern genomics has laid out the promise of a more individualized medicine, including personalized nutrition. Thus the new field of 'nutrigenomics' aims to provide dietary recommendations based on a person's genetic profile. We shall see! Walsh, M. and Kuhn, S. (2012), 'Developments in personalised nutrition', *Nutrition Bulletin*, 37:4, 380–3.

20   Coleman, W. (1974), 'Health and hygiene in the *Encyclopédie*: a medical doctrine for the bourgeosie'. *Journal of the History of Medicine and Allied Sciences*, 29, 406.

21   Guarinoni, I. [Guarinonius] (1610), *Die Greuel des Verwüstung menschlichen Geschlechts*. Ingolstadt, cit. in Bergdolt, *Wellbeing*, pp. 199–200.

22   Albala, *Eating Right*, pp. 49–51.

23   Venner, T. (1620), *Via Recta ad Vitam Longam, or A Plaine Philosophical Discourse of the Nature, Faculties, and Effects, of All Such Things, as by Way of Nourishments, and Dieticall Obseruations, Make for the Preservation of Health*. London: Edward Griffin, pp. 33–4.

24   Albala, *Eating right*, pp. 176–7.

25   Howell, J. (1642), *Instructions for Forreine Travel*. London: Humphrey Mosley, p. 43.

26   Anon. (1607), *Le thresor de santé ou, mesnage de la vie humaine*. Lyon: Jean Ant. Huguetan, preface, p. 4.

27   Grataroli, G. [Gratarolus] (1574), *A Direction for the Health of Magistrates and Studentes*. Trans. T. Newton. London: William How; Dubois, J. [Sylvius] (1574), *De studiosorum et eorum qui corporis exercitationibus addicti non sunt*. Douai: Joannes Bogardi.

28   Petronio, A. (1592), *Del vivere delli Romani et del conservare la sanità*: Rome: Domenico Basa; Da Fonseca, F. (1626), *Regimento pera conservar a saude e vida … de qualidades do ar, de sitios e mantimentos do termo da cidade de Lisboa*. Lisbon: Geraldo da Vinha.

29   Abraham, N. (1600), *Gouvernement nécessaire à chacun pour vivre longuement en santé*. Paris: Michel Sonnius; Leys, L. [Lessius] (1634), *Hygiasticon: Or the Right Course of Preserving Life and Health unto Extream Old Age*. Trans. G. Herbert. Cambridge: Roger Daniel, 1634.

30   Grataroli, *Direction*.

31   Zuccolin, G. (2011), 'Nascere in latino e in volgare. Tra la *Practica maior* e il *De regimine pregnantium*', in C. Crisciani and G. Zuccolin (eds), *Michele Savonarola. Medicina e cultura di corte*. Florence: SISMEL-Galluzzo, pp. 137–209.

32 Prosperi, L. (2007), 'Le pouvoir de la nourriture sur la reproduction humaine: discours diététique et différences de genre d'après l'ouvrage de Giovanni Marinello (Italie-France, XVIe et XVIIe siècles)', in F. Audoin-Rouzeau and F. Sabban (eds), *Un aliment sain dans un corps sain: perspectives historiques.* Tours: Presses Universitaires François Rabelais, pp. 291–307.

33 Green, M. (2009), 'The sources of Eucharius Rösslin's "Rosegarden for Pregnant Women and Midwives" (1513)', *Medical History*, 53:2, pp. 167–92.

34 Valverda, J. (1552), *De animi et corporis sanitate tuenda libellus.* Paris: Carolus Stephanus, p. 41, cit. in Albala, *Eating Right*, p. 129.

35 Gentilcore, D. (2010), 'The *Levitico*, or how to feed a hundred Jesuits'. *Food & History*, 8:1, 87–120.

36 Boorde, A. (1542), *A Compendyous Regyment or Dyetary of Helth.* London: William Copland, ch. xviii; Cogan, T. (1584), *The Haven of Health Chiefly Gathered for the Comfort of Students, and Consequently of All Those That Have a Care of Their Health.* London: Henrie Midleton, p. 98.

37 Albala, *Eating Right*, pp. 48–77, 78–114.

38 Moffett, T. (1655), *Health's Improvement: Or, Rules Comprizing and Discovering the Nature, Method, and Manner of Preparing All Sorts of Food Used in This Nation.* London: Thomas Newcomb, p. 235.

39 Moffett, *Health's Improvement*, p. 31.

40 Grieco, A. (1991), 'The social politics of pre-Linnaean botanical classification', *I Tatti Studies*, 4, pp. 131–49.

41 Della Porta, G. B. (1658 [1558]), *Natural Magick.* London: Young and Speed, p. 254.

42 Savonarola, *Libreto*, p. 2r. The theme is discussed in Past, E. (2011), 'Una ricetta per *longo e iocundo* vivere: il *Libreto di tutte le cosse che se magnano*', in C. Crisciani and G. Zuccolin (eds), *Michele Savonarola. Medicina e cultura di corte.* Florence: SISMEL-Galluzzo, pp. 113–25.

43 Joubert, *The Second Part of the Popular Errors*, p. 113.

44 Archer, J. (1673), *Every Man His Own Doctor.* London: Printed for the author, p. 18.

45 Cornaro *Writings on the Sober Life*, p. 102.

46 Suhr, C. (2010), 'Regimens and health guides', in I. Taavitsainen and P. Pahta (eds), *Early Modern English Medical Texts: Corpus Description and Studies.* Amsterdam and Philadelphia: John Benjamins, pp. 111–18.

47 Méndez, G. (1562), *Regimiento de salud.* Salamanca: Pedro de Castro, fol. 2r., cit. in Solomon, M. (2010), *Fictions of Well-Being: Sickly Readers and Vernacular Medical Writing in Late Medieval and Early Modern Spain.* Philadelphia, PA: University of Pennsylvania Press, p. 24.

48 Álvarez de Miraval, B. (1601), *La conservación de la salud del cuerpo y del alma.* Salamanca: Andres Renaut.

49 Slack, P. (1979), 'Mirrors of health and treasures of poor men: the uses of the vernacular medical literature of Tudor England', in C. Webster (ed), *Health, Medicine and Mortality in the Sixteenth Century.* Cambridge: Cambridge University Press, p. 248.

50 Elyot, T. (1539), *The Castel of Helthe … Whereby Every Man May Knowe the State of His Owne Body, the Preservation of Helthe, and How to Instruct Well His Phisition in Sicknes, That He Be Not Deceyved.* London: Thomae Bertheleti, p. 83.

51 Paschetti, B. (1602), *Del conservare la sanità et del vivere de' Genovesi.* Genoa: Giuseppe Pavoni, pp. 4–6.

52 Rangoni, T. [Philologus] (1533), *De vita hominis ultra cxx annos potrahenda*. Venice: Nicolinus Sabiensis. Available online at: http://reader.digitale-sammlungen.de/resolve/display/bsb10166407.html.

53 Du Chesne, J. (1620 [1606]), *Le pourtraict de la santé, où est au vif représentée la reigle universelle et particulière de bien sainement et longuement vivre*. Paris: Claude Morel, p. 359.

54 Rodriguez Cardoso, F. (1620), *Tractatus absolutissimus … de sex rebus non naturalibus*. Frankfurt: Paul Jacobi, pp. 2r., 4r.–v.

55 Cardano, G. (1580), *Opus novum cunctis de sanitate tuenda*. Rome: Francesco Zanetti, p. 118.

56 Dubois, J. [Sylvius] (1544), *Régime de santé pour les povres, facile à tenir*. Paris: Jacques Gazeau, cit. in Dupèbe, J. (1982), 'La diététique et l'alimentation des pauvres selon Sylvius', in J.-C. Margolin and R. Sauzet (eds), *Pratiques et discours alimentaires à la Renaissance: actes du colloque de Tours 1979*. Paris: Maisonneuve et Larose, p. 42.

57 Dubois, *Régime de santé*, p. 41r., cit. in Dupèbe, 'Diététique', p. 50.

58 Cavallo, S. and Storey, T. (2013), *Healthy Living in Late Renaissance Italy*. Oxford: Oxford University Press, pp. 7, 270.

59 Ibid., p. 210.

60 Pardo-Tomás, J. and Martínez-Vidal, A. (2008), 'Stories of disease written by patients and lay mediators in the Spanish republic of letters (1680–1720)'. *Journal of Medieval and Early Modern Studies*, 38:3, 478.

61 Ponsonby, A. (1923), *English Diaries: A Review of English Diaries from the Sixteenth to the Twentieth Century*. London: Methuen, p. 144, cit. in Lane, J. (1985), ' "The doctor scolds me": the diaries and correspondence of patients in eighteenth century England', in R. Porter (ed), *Patients and Practitioners: Lay Perceptions of Medicine in Pre-Industrial Society*. Cambridge: Cambridge University Press, p. 244.

62 Le Roy Ladurie, E. (1987), *The French Peasantry, 1450–1660*. Trans. A. Sheridan. Aldershot: Scolar, pp. 219–20.

63 Joubert, *Popular Errors*, pp. 127–72.

64 Rankin, A. (2013), *Panaceia's Daughter: Noblewomen as Healers in Early Modern Germany*. Chicago: University of Chicago Press, pp. 168–203.

65 Ibid., p. 195, note 122.

66 Ibid., p. 196, note 124.

67 Pahta, P. and Ratia, M. 'Treatises on specific topics', in *Early Modern English Medical Texts*, pp. 84–5.

68 Albala, *Eating Right*, pp. 46–7.

69 Cavallo and Storey, *Healthy Living*, pp. 272–3.

Chapter 2

1 Baker, G. (1772), 'The case of Mr Thomas wood, a miller, of Billericay, in the county of Essex … read at the College on September 9, 1767'. *Medical Transactions*, 2, 259–74.

2 Cheyne, G. (1725 [1724]), *An Essay of Health and Long Life*. Dublin: George Ewing, xviii–xix. Italics in the original.

3   Dacome, L. (2005), 'Useless and pernicious matter: corpulence in eighteenth-century England', in C. Forth and A. Carden-Coyne (eds), *Cultures of the Abdomen: Diet, Digestion and Fat in the Modern World*. Houndmills: Palgrave Macmillan, 185–204.

4   Coleman, Health and hygiene in the *Encyclopédie* 419–20; Smith, Prescribing the rules of health, p. 281.

5   Ferrières, M. (2006), *Sacred Cow, Mad Cow: A History of Food Fears*. Trans. J. Gladding. New York, NY: Columbia University Press, p. 255; Porter, R. (1985), 'Laymen, doctors and medical knowledge in the eighteenth century: the evidence of the *Gentlemen's Magazine*', *Patients and Practitioners*, 283–314.

6   Le Bègue de Presle, A. (1763), *Le conservateur de la santé, ou avis sur les dangers qu'il importe à chacun d'éviter, pour se conserver en bonne santé et prolonger sa vie*. Paris: P. Didot, iii.

7   Ibid., xiii.

8   Mikkeli, *Hygiene in the Early Modern Medical Tradition*, pp. 109–10.

9   Paracelsus, T. (1993 [c.1520]), *The Herbarius of Theophrastus [Paracelsus], Concerning the Powers of the Herbs, Roots, Seeds, etc. of the Native Land and Realm of Germany*. Trans. B. Moran, in 'The *Herbarius* of Paracelsus'. *Pharmacy in History*, 35:3, 104.

10 Willard, T. (2011), 'Living the long life: physical and spiritual health in two early Paracelsian tracts', in A. Classen (ed), *Religion und Gesundheit: der heilkundliche Diskurs im 16. Jahrhundert*. Berlin: de Gruyter, 347–80.

11 Van Helmont, J. B. (1662), *Oriatrike, or, Physick Refined*. Trans. J. Chandler. London: Lodowick Loyd, p. 455.

12 Wear, *Knowledge and Practice in English Medicine, 1550–1680*, p. 405.

13 Thomson, G. (1675), *Orthomethodos Iatro Chimiche, or the Direct Method of Curing Chymically*. London: B. Billingsley, pp. 29, 33, cit. in Wear, *Knowledge and Practice*, pp. 403–5.

14 Ibid., p. 489.

15 Du Chesne, *Le pourtraict de la santé, où est au vif reprsentée la reigle universelle et particulière de bien sainement et longuement vivre*, pp. 203–15.

16 Santorio, S. (1676 [1614]), *Medicina Statica, or Rules of Health, in Eight Sections of Aphorisms*. Trans. J. D. London: John Starkey, p. 177.

17 Brockliss, L. (1989), 'The medico-religious universe of an early eighteenth-century Parisian doctor: the case of Philippe Hacquet', in R. French and A. Wear (eds), *The Medical Revolution of the Seventeenth Century*. Cambridge: Cambridge University Press, p. 202.

18 Hoffmann, F. (1971 [1695]), *Fundamenta Medicinae*. Trans. L. King. London: Macdonald, p. 104, cit. in Estes, J. W. (1996), 'The medical properties of food in the eighteenth century'. *Journal of the History of Medicine and Allied Sciences*, 51, 130.

19 Lémery, L. (1706 [1702]), *A Treatise of Foods in General*. London: Andrew Bell.

20 Ibid., viii.

21 Ibid., pp. 29–30.

22 Tyrkkö, J. (2010), 'Sign terms in specific medical genres in early modern medical texts', in I. Taavitsainen and P. Pahta (eds), *Early Modern English Medical Texts: Corpus Description and Studies*. Amsterdam and Philadelphia: John Benjamins, pp. 176–7, 186.

23 Pinsonnat, F. [Sieur de la Cour] (1690 [1686]), *Régime de santé pour se procurer une longue vie et une vieillesse heureuse*. Paris: Maurice Villery, p. 127.

24 Ibid., p. 65.

25 Crignon-De Oliveira, C. (2011), 'Peut-on vieillir sans médecins? La réponse des auteurs de régimes de santé ou «conseils pour vivre longtemps» aux xviiᵉ et xviiiᵉ siècles'. *Astérion*, online at: http://asterion.revues.org/2018.

26 Stolberg, M. (2011), *Experiencing Illness and the Sick Body in Early Modern Europe*. Trans. L. Unglaub and L. Kennedy. London: Palgrave Macmillan, p. 41.

27 Pardo-Tomás and Martínez-Vidal (2008), 'Stories of disease written by patients and lay mediators in the Spanish republic of letters (1680–1720)'.

28 Ibid., p. 477.

29 Conlin, J. (1977), 'Another side to William Byrd of Westover: an explanation of the food in his secret diaries'. *Virginia Cavalcade*, 26:3, 124–33; Eden, T. (2008), *The Early American Table: Food and Society in the New World*. DeKalb, IL: Northern Illinois University Press, pp. 124–32.

30 Pilloud, S. (2013), *Les mots du corps. Expérience de la maladie dans les lettres de patients à un médecin du 18ᵉ siècle: Samuel Auguste Tissot*. Lausanne: BHMS, pp. 208–12.

31 Spary, E. M. (2012), *Eating the Enlightenment: Food and the Sciences in Paris, 1670–1760*. Chicago: University of Chicago Press, p. 276.

32 Ackerknecht, *Therapeutics*, p. 179.

33 Weston, R. (2013), *Medical Consulting by Letter in France, 1665–1789*. Farnham: Ashgate, p. 179.

34 Stolberg, *Experiencing Illness*, p. 44.

35 Lémery, L. (1755), *Traité des alimens … augmenté … par Jacques Jean Bruhier*. Paris: Durand, xlviii–xlix.

36 Flandrin, J.-L. (1999), 'From dietetics to gastronomy, the liberation of the gourmet', in J.-L. Flandrin and M. Montanari (eds), *Food: A Culinary History*. New York, NY: Columbia University Press, p. 427.

37 Forster, W. (1746), *A Treatise on the Causes of Most Diseases*. London: J. Clarke, G. Hawkins and W. Reeve, pp. 212–16, cit. in Estes, 'Medical properties', pp. 135–6.

38 Smith, W. (1776), *A Sure Guide in Sickness and Health, in the Choice of Food, and Use of Medicine*. London: J. Bew and J. Walter, pp. 59, 66–7.

39 Cheyne, *Essay of Health*, pp. 11, 12.

40 Ibid., p. 15.

41 Guerrini, A. (2000), *Obesity and Depression in the Enlightenment: The Life and Times of George Cheyne*. Norman, OK: University of Oklahoma Press, pp. 89–117.

42 George Cheyne to Samuel Richardson, 9 March 1742, cit. in ibid., p. 177.

43 John Wesley to Edmund Gibson, 11 June 1747, cit. in ibid., p. 160.

44 Wesley, J. (1880 [1747]), *Primitive Physic*. Chicago, IL: O.W. Gordon, preface, pp. 9–10, 14–15, cit. in ibid., p. 184. See also, Wallace, C. (2003), 'Eating and drinking with John Wesley: the logic of his practice'. *Bulletin of the John Rylands University Library of Manchester*, 85:2, 137–55.

45 John Wesley, journal entry for 28 June 1770, in *The Works of John Wesley* (1975–). Oxford: Clarendon Press, vol. 22, pp. 236–7, cit. in Grumett, D. and Muers, R. (2010), *Theology on the Menu: Asceticism, Meat and Christian Diet*. London: Routledge, p. 61.

46 Guerrini, *Obesity and Depression*, p. 163.

47 Anon. (1702), *L'anti-Cornaro ou remarques critiques sur le traité de la vie sobre de Louis Cornaro venitien*. Paris: Claude Barré, pp. 6–7.

48 Falconer, W. (1778), *Observations on Some of the Articles of Diet and Regimen Usually Recommended to Valetudinarians*. London: Edward and Charles Dilly, pp. 1–2, cit. in Estes, 'Medical properties', p. 148.

49 Graham, J. (1790), *The Guardian of Health, Long-Life and Happiness*. Newcastle upon Tyne: S. Hodgson, p. 1.

50 Triller, D. W. (1783), *Diätetische Lebensregelen oder Belehrung, wie es anzufangen ein hohes Alter zu erlangen*. Frankfurt. Discussed in Bergdolt, *Wellbeing: A Cultural History of Healthy Living*, p. 243.

51 Knoeff, R. (1997), 'Practicing chemistry "after the Hippocratical manner": Hippocrates and the importance of chemistry in Boerhaave's medicine', in L. Principe (ed), *New Narratives in Eighteenth-Century Chemistry*. Dordrecht: Springer, 63–76.

52 Buchan, W. (1774 [1769]), *Domestic Medicine: Or, a Treatise on the Prevention and Cure of Diseases by Regimen and Simple Medicines*. London: W. Strahan, ix.

53 Black, W. (1782), *An Historical Sketch of Medicine and Surgery*. London: J. Johnson, p. 225.

54 Buchan, W. (1797), 'Observations concerning the diet of the common people, recommending a method of living less expensive, and more conducive to health, than the present', in *Domestic Medicine*. London: A. Strahan, ch. 56, pp. 647–79.

55 Archer, J. (1671), *Every Man His Own Doctor… Shewing How Every One May Know His Own Constitution, the Nature of All Food, What Is Good or Hurtful to Any*. London: Peter Lillicrap for the author, in Fissell, 'The marketplace of print', p. 122. In fact, Archer's short work is more an advertisement for his own remedies than a regimen.

56 Harper, A. (1785), *The Oeconomy of Health: Or, a Medical Essay Containing New and Familiar Instructions for the Attainment of Health, Happiness and Longevity*. London: C. Stalker, p. 38.

57 Tissot, S. A. (1765 [1761]), *Advice to the People in General, with Regard to Their Health*. Trans. J. Kirkpatrick. London: T. Becket, pp. 52–4.

58 Ibid., p. 61.

59 Emch-Dériaz, A. (1992), 'The non-naturals made easy', in R. Porter (ed), *The Popularization of Medicine, 1650–1850*. London: Routledge, pp. 142–3.

60 Tissot, S. A. (1772 [1768]), *A Treatise on the Diseases Incident to Literary and Sedentary Persons*. Edinburgh: Donaldson.

61 Ibid., p. 105.

62 Mikkeli, *Hygiene*, pp. 156–7.

63 Neves Abreu, J. L. (2010), 'Higiene e conservação da saúde no pensamento médico luso-brasileiro do século XVIII'. *Asclepio: Revista de Historia de la Medicina y de la Ciencia*, 62, 225–50.

64 Goulin, J. (1771), *Le médecin des dames, ou l'art de les conserver en santé*. Paris: Vincent. A companion volume on men's health was published the following year: [Goulin, J.] (1772), *Le médecin des hommes, depuis la puberté jusqu'à l'extrême vieillesse*. Paris: Vincent.

65 'Supplément en faveur des jeunes dames, ou extrait de la toilette de Vénus', in Goulin, *Médecin de dames*, pp. 409–65; see also, Martin, M. (2005), 'Doctoring beauty: the control of women's *toilettes* in France, 1750–1820'. *Medical History*, 49, 353–68.

66 Findlen, P. (1995), 'Translating the New Science: women and the circulation of knowledge in Enlightenment Italy'. *Configurations*, 3:2, 167–206.

67 Fara, P. (2004), *Pandora's Breeches: Women, Science and Power in the Enlightenment*. London: Pimlico.

68 Da Fonseca Henriques, F. (1731 [1721]), *Âncora medicinal para conservar a vida com saúde*. Lisbon: Miguel Rodrigues.

69 István, M. (1762–64), *Diaetetica, az az, a' jó egészség' meg tartásának modját fundamentomoson elö-ado könyv*. Kolozsvár: István Páldi. Available online at: http://mek .oszk.hu/08500/08581/; briefly discussed in Szlatky, M. (1992), 'Tissot as part of the medical Enlightenment in Hungary', in Porter, *Popularization of Medicine*, p. 206.

70 Pujati, G. (1768), *Della preservazione della salute de' letterati e della gente applicata e sedentaria*. Venice: Antonio Zatta, pp. 203–36.

71 Smith, *Sure Guide*, pp. 69–77.

72 Buc'hoz, P. (1783), *L'art alimentaire ou methode pour préparer les aliments les plus sains pour l'homme*. Paris: chez l'auteur.

73 Flandrin, 'From dietetics', p. 418.

74 Pinkard, S. (2009), *A Revolution in Taste: The Rise of French Cuisine*. Cambridge: Cambridge University Press, pp. 165–71.

75 Spary, *Eating the Enlightenment*, pp. 280–1.

76 [Menon] (1749), *La science du maître d'hôtel cuisinier, avec des observations sur la conoissance et proprietés des alimens*, Paris: Paulus du Mesnil, p. xxv, cit. in von Hoffmann, V. (2013), *Goûter le monde. Une histoire culturelle du goût à l'époque moderne*. Bruxelles: Peter Lang, p. 210.

77 [Menon] (1758), *Cuisine et office de santé, propre à ceux qui vivent avec œconomie et régime*. Paris: Le Clerc, Prault, Babuty.

78 Spallanzani, L. (1776), *Opuscoli di fisica animale e vegetabile*. Modena: Società Tipografica; Corrado, V. (1786), *Il cuoco galante: opera meccanica*. Naples: Stamperia Raimondiana, p. 9.

79 Hunter, A. (1810 [1804]), *Culina Famulatrix Medicinæ: Or, Receipts in Modern Cookery, with a Medical Commentary*. York: Wilson and Son, p. 7.

80 Ibid., p. 7.

81 Ibid., pp. 179–80, 244–5. Hunter's book is notable for its numerous recipes for 'macaroni', as well as for 'tomata sauce', so it is a shame Hunter did not think to combine the two, as he would have been one of the first! On the origins of *pasta al pomodoro*, see Gentilcore, D. (2010), *Pomodoro! A History of the Tomato in Italy*. New York, NY: Columbia University Press, pp. 69–98.

Chapter 3

1 Bruyérin-Champier, J. (1560), *De re cibaria, libri xxii. Omnium ciborum genera, omium gentium moribus et usu probata complectentes*. Lyon: Sebast. Honoratum, p. 188. Available online at: http://reader.digitale-sammlungen.de/resolve/display/bsb10191089.html. Available in French translation by Amundsen, S. (1998), *L'Alimentation de tous les peuples et de tous les temps jusqu'au XVIe siècle*. Paris: Dumas.

2 Moyer, J. (2013), '"The food police": sumptuary prohibitions on food in the Reformation', in K. Albala and T. Eden (eds), *Food and Faith in Christian Culture*. New York, NY: Columbia University Press, pp. 59–81.

3 *Provysion Made by the Kynges Hyghness and His Counsayll for the Puttynge a Parte the Excessive Fare and Redusynge the Same* (1518). London: Richard Pynson.

4   'The Regulation of Banquets', Senate decree, Republic of Venice, 8 October 1562; from Chambers, D., Fletcher, J. and Pullan, B. (eds) (1992), *Venice: A Documentary History, 1450–1630*. Oxford: Blackwell, pp. 178–9.

5   Moyer, J. (1997), *Sumptuary Law in Ancient Regime France, 1229–1806*, unpublished PhD dissertation, University of Syracuse, 1997; Killerby, C. (2002), *Sumptuary Law in Italy, 1200–1500*. Oxford: Oxford University Press.

6   De Montaigne, M. (1811 [1580]), 'Of sumptuary laws', in *The Essays of Michel de Montaigne*. Trans. P. Coste. London: W. Miller, 3 vols., vol. 1, p. 353.

7   Carbonelli, G. (ed) (1906), *Il 'De sanitatis custodia' di maestro Giacomo Albini di Moncalieri: con altri documenti sulla storia della medicina negli stati sabaudi nei secoli XIV e XV*. Pinerolo: Tip. Sociale.

8   Braudel, F. (1981), *The Structures of Everyday Life: The Limits of the Possible*. Trans. S. Reynolds. London: William Collins, pp. 190–4.

9   Bruyérin-Champier, *De re cibaria*, p. 239.

10 Cholmley, H. (1652), *Some Passages from a History of the Cholmley Family*. York and London, pp. 388–9, cit. in Hurren, E. (2013), 'Cultures of the body, medical regimen, and physic at the Tudor court', in T. Betteridge and S. Lipscomb (eds), *Henry VIII and the Court: Art, Politics and Performance*. Farnham: Ashgate, pp. 75–6.

11 Albala, K. (2007), *The Banquet: Dining in the Great Courts of Late Renaissance Europe*. Urbana, IL: University of Illinois Press, pp. 1–26.

12 Montanari, M. (2008), *L'Europa a tavola. Storia dell'alimentazione dal Medioevo a oggi*. Rome: Laterza, pp. 96–7.

13 Meyzie, *L'alimentation en Europe à l'époque moderne*, pp. 77–8.

14 Savonarola, *Libreto di tutte le cose che se manzano*.

15 Hurren, 'Cultures of the body', pp. 66–8.

16 Moyer, 'Food police', p. 69.

17 Albala, *Eating Right*, p. 205.

18 Grataroli, G. (1574 [1555]), *A Direction for the Health of Magistrates and Studentes*. London: William How.

19 Muffett, T. (1655), *Health's Improvement: Or, Rules Comprizing and Discovering the Nature, Method, and Manner of Preparing All Sorts of Food Used in This Nation*. London: Thomas Newcomb, pp. 80, 229, 294.

20 Archivio di Stato, Rome, *Fondo Spada Veralli*, B.463, cap. xxxii, cit. in Cavallo, S. and Storey, T. (2013), *Healthy Living in Late Renaissance Italy*. Oxford: Oxford University Press, p. 213.

21 O'Reilly, W. (2009), 'Last chances of the House of Hapsburg'. *Austrian History Yearbook*, 40, 70 note 102.

22 Muffett, *Health's Improvement*, p. 80.

23 Cardano, G. (1654 [1576]), *De vita propria liber*. Amsterdam: Johannem Ravesteinium, p. 25.

24 Muffett, *Health's Improvement*, pp. 231, 154, 94. The latter can be found in Pisanelli, B. (1589), *Trattato de' cibi et del bere, con molte dotte et belle annotazioni di Francesco Gallina*. Carmagnola: Marc'Antonio Bellone, p. 31.

25 Braudel, F. (1972), *The Mediterranean and the Mediterranean World in the Age of Philip II*. Trans. S. Reynolds. London: William Collins, vol. 1, p. 404.

26 Livi-Bacci, M. (1991), *Population and Nutrition: An Essay on European Demographic History*. Trans. T. Croft-Murray. Cambridge: Cambridge University Press, p. 92.

27 Braudel, *Structures of Everyday Life*, p. 196.

28 Ibid., pp. 194–5.

29 Thomas, D. (1996), *Henri IV: images d'un roi entre réalité et mythe*. Pau: Heracles, p. 378.

30 Bruyérin-Champier, *De re cibaria*, p. 238.

31 Bruegel, M., J.-M. Chevet and S. Lecocq (2014), 'Animal protein and rational choice: diet in the eighteenth century', *Journal of Interdisciplinary History*, 44:4, 427–52.

32 Meyzie, *Alimentation*, pp. 39–40.

33 Johnson, S. (1755), *Dictionary of the English Language*. London: W. Strahan, *sub voce*, no pagination.

34 Nuñez de Oria, F. (1586), *Regimiento y aviso de sanidad*. Medina del Campo: Francisco del Canto, p. 40v.

35 De Azara, F. (1846), *Viajes por la América del Sur desde 1789 hasta 1801*. Montevideo: Comercio del Plata, pp. 8–9.

36 Estienne, C. and Liébault, J. (1600 [1572]), *Maison rustique, or the countrie farme*. Trans. R. Surflet. London: E. Bollifant, pp. 717–18.

37 Hoffmann, F. (1695), *De pane grossiori Westphalorum, vulgo Bonpournickel*. Halle, cit. in Bergdolt, K. (2008), *Wellbeing: A Cultural History of Healthy Living*. Trans. J. Dewhurst. Cambridge: Polity Press, p. 227; Hoffmann, F. (1761), *A Treatise on the Nature of Aliments, or Foods in General*. London: L. Davis and C. Reymer, pp. 8–9.

38 Le Roy Ladurie, E. (1976), *The Peasants of Languedoc*. Trans. J. Day. Urbana, IL: University of Illinois Press, pp. 51–83.

39 Livi-Bacci, *Population and Nutrition*, p. 91.

40 Scheurer, R. (1985), 'Passage, accueil et intégration des réfugiés huguenots en Suisse', in M. Magdelaine and R. van Thadden (eds), *Le refuge huguenot*. Paris: Armand Colin, pp. 45–62.

41 Croce, G. C. (1617), *Contrasto del pane di formento e quello di fava per la precedenza*. Bologna: Bartolomeo Cochi. Available online at: http://www.giuliocesarecroce.it/trascrizioni.html.

42 Camporesi, P. (1989), *Bread of Dreams: Food and Fantasy in Early Modern Europe*. Trans. D. Gentilcore. Cambridge: Polity Press, pp. 120–30.

43 Cogan, *Haven of Health*, pp. 27–8.

44 Bruyérin-Champier, *De re cibaria*, pp. 367–8. Bruyérin-Champier's use of 'recently' with regard to shelled oats here is relative, since the preparation and consumption of *avenatus* was already described in the *Rosa Anglica*, a dietary written in 1314 by John of Gaddesden, court physician to Edward II (available online at: http://www.ucc.ie/celt/).

45 Lémery, L. (1745), *A Treatise of All Sorts of Foods, Both Animal and Vegetable: Also of Drinkables*. Trans. D. Hay. London: T. Osborne, p. 91.

46 Buchan, W. (1797), 'Observations concerning the diet of the common people, recommending a method of living less expensive, and more conducive to health, than the present', added to the 1797 edition of his *Domestic Medicine*. London: A. Strahan, pp. 647–79, at p. 652.

47 Ibid., p. 652.

48 Lémery, *Traité des alimens … augmenté … par Jacques Jean Bruhier*, p. 358. The opinion is Bruhier's.

49 Buchan, 'Observations', p. 656.

50 Ibid., p. 653. Italics in the original.

51 Ibid., p. 655.

52 Buchan, 'Observations', p. 671.

53 Where 'meate' stands for food in general, 'meete' for suitable, and 'grosse' for coarse (in both senses). Cogan, *Haven of Health*, p. 58, where he gives the expression in Latin: *crassa enim (ut aiunt) crassis conveniunt*. The English rendering can be found in the 1596 edition of the same book (London: Richard Field), p. 57. The Dutch humanist Rudolph Agricola quoted the saying, identifying it as proverbial, in his influential 1479 study of the role of invention and commonplace in logic, *De inventione dialectica libri tres* (s.l., 1528), p. 3.

54 Pisanelli, *Trattato de' cibi*, pp. 118, 122, 132, 138, 139. Pisanelli had a higher opinion of lentils, chickpeas and chestnuts, provided they were eaten at the right time of year and properly prepared.

55 Albala, K. (2007), *Beans: A History*. Oxford: Berg, pp. 135–46.

56 Pisanelli, *Trattato de' cibi*, p. 137; Castelvetro, G. (1989 [1614]), *The Fruit, Herbs and Vegetables of Italy*. Trans. and ed. G. Riley. London: Viking/Penguin, p. 60. Italian original available online at: http://www.liberliber.it/mediateca/libri/c/castelvetro/brieve_racconto _di_tutte_le_radici_etc/pdf/brieve_p.pdf.

57 Cogan, *Haven of Health*, p. 31.

58 Cardano, G. (1663), *Opera omnia*. Lyon: Huguetan and Ravaut, vol. 7, p. 56, cit. in Albala, K. (2003), *Food in Early Modern Europe*. Westport, CT: Greenwood Press, pp. 27–8.

59 Audiger. (1692), *La maison reglée et l'art de deriger une maison d'un grand seigneur*. Paris: Nicolas Le Gras, pp. 168–9.

60 Lémery, *Treatise of All Sorts of Foods*, pp. 77, 84, 92, 133, 135.

61 Ibid., p. 118.

62 Ibid., p. 85.

63 Ibid., pp. 225, 242.

64 Quellier, F. (2013), *La table des Français: une histoire culturelle (XVe–XIXe siècle)*. Rennes and Tours: Presses Universitaires de Rennes and Presses Universitaires François Rabelais, pp. 38–44.

65 Quellier, F. (2008), 'Le repas de funéilles de Bonhomme Jacques. Faut-il reconsidér le dossier de l'alimentation paysanne des temps modernes?'. *Food & History*, 6:1, 9–30.

66 Paulet, J.-J. (1793), *Traité des champignons*. Paris: Imprimerie nationale exécutive du Louvre, p. 21. Available online at: http://www.biodiversitylibrary.org/bibliography/5417#/summary.

67 Pisanelli, *Trattato de' cibi*, p. 181.

68 Schaechter, E. (1997), *In the Company of Mushrooms: A Biologist's Tale*. Cambridge MA: Harvard University Press, pp. 7–13.

69 Paulet, *Champignons*, p. 22.

70 Guyon, L. (1596), *Remonstrance au peuple champestre du haut et bas pays de Lymosin, pour les oster de l'erreur qu'ilz hont de ne point payer de tailles*. Limoges, cit. in Meyzie, *Alimentation*, p. 127.

71 Pleij, H. (2001), *Dreaming of Cockaigne: Medieval Fantasies of the Perfect Life*. Trans. D. Webb. New York, NY: Columbia University Press, p. 91.

72 Van Bavel, B. and Gelderblom, O. (2009), 'Land of milk and butter: the economic origins of cleanliness in the Dutch golden age'. *Past and Present*, 205, 41–69.

73 Malvasia, C. C. (1678), *Felsina pittrice. Vite de pittori bolognesi*. Bologna: Barbieri, vol. 2, p. 69, cit. in Natale, A. (2011), 'Formaggi', in G. M. Anselmi and G. Ruozzi (eds), *Banchetti letterari: cibi, pietanze e ricette nella letteratura italiana da Dante a Camilleri*. Rome: Carocci, p. 185.

74 Lotichius, J. P. (1643), *De casei nequitia, tractatus medico-philologicus novus*. Frankfurt am Main: Johannis Friderici Weissii.

75 Schoock, M. [Schoockius] (1664), *Tractatus de butyro. Accessit ejusdem diatriba de adversatione casei*. Groningen: Johannis Cöllen.

76 Moffett, *Health's Improvement*, p. 131.

77 Mattioli, P. A. (1595), *I discorsi ... di Pedacio Dioscoride anazarbeo della materia medicinale*. Venice: Felice Valgrisio, p. 288.

78 Heresbach, K. (1578 [1568]), *Foure Bookes of Husbandry*. Trans. B. George. London: John Wight, pp. 54r.–63v.

79 Fioravanti, L. (1570), *Il tesoro della vita humana*. Venice: Eredi di Melchior Sessa, p. 64v., cit. in Camporesi, P. (1995), *La terra e la luna: alimentazione, folklore, società* (Milan: Garzanti, 1995), p. 82.

80 Moffett, *Health's Improvement*, p. 131.

81 Lémery, *Treatise of All Sorts of Foods*, pp. 221–4.

82 Meyzie, *Alimentation*, p. 128.

83 Lemasson, J.-P. (2011), *L'incroyable odyssée de la tourtière*. Montréal: Del Busso, pp. 32–3.

84 Pennell, S. (1998), 'Pots and pans history: the material culture of the kitchen in early modern England'. *Journal of Design History*, 11: 3, p. 209.

85 Radeff, A. (1996), *Du café dans le chaudron. Économie globale d'ancien régime: Suisse Occidentale, Franche-Compté et Savoie*. Lausanne: Société d'Histoire de la Suisse Romande.

86 Ferrières, M. (2007), *Nourritures canailles*. Paris: Seuil, p. 10.

87 Meyzie, *Alimentation*, p. 132.

88 Montenach, A. (2011), 'Formal and informal economy in an urban context: the case of food trade in seventeenth-century Lyon', in T. Buchner and P. R. Hoffmann-Rehnitz (eds), *Shadow Economies and Irregular Work in Urban Europe, 16th to Early 20th Centuries*. Vienna: Verlag, p. 91–106.

89 Pinkard, S. (2009), *A Revolution in Taste: The Rise of French Cuisine, 1650–1800*. Cambridge: Cambridge University Press, pp. 85–91.

90 De Bonnefons, N. (1655), *Les délices de la campagne suitte du Jardinier françois*. Amsterdam: Raphael Smith, p. 253.

91 Du Chesne, *Le pourtraict de la santé, où est au vif reprsentée la reigle universelle et particulière de bien sainement et longuement vivre*, pp. 211–13.

92 Du Chesne, *Pourtraict de la santé*, p. 479.

93 Lémery, L. (1705), *Traité des aliments*. Paris: Pierre Witte, p. 282.

94 Ibid., xx–xxi.

95 Lémery, *Traité des alimens ... augmenté ... par Jacques Jean Bruhier*, lii.

96 De Bonnefons, *Les délices de la campagne suitte du Jardinier françois*, 'Aux maistres d'hotels. Epistre', pp. 108–16.

97 May, R. (1660), *The Accomplish't Cook, or the Art and Mystery of Cookery*. London: Nathaniel Brooke.

98 D'Hauteville, G. (1686), *Relation historique de la Pologne*. Paris, in Flandrin, J.-L. (1999), 'Dietary choices and culinary technique, 1500–1800', in J.-L. Flandrin and M. Montanari (eds), *Food: A Culinary History*. New York, NY: Columbia University Press, p. 411.

99 D'Aulnoy, Marie-Catherine. (1705), *Rélation du voyage d'Espagne*. La Haye: Henri van Bulderen, pp. 24, 113.

100 Meyzie, *Alimentation*, pp. 88–90.

101 Caraccioli, L.-A. (1776), *L'Europe française par l'auteur de la gaité*. Paris, cit. in Meyzie, *Alimentation*, p. 89.

102 Harper, *The Oeconomy of Health: Or, a Medical Essay Containing New and Familiar Instructions for the Attainment of Health, Happiness and Longevity*, pp. 32–3.

Chapter 4

1 Smith, J. B. (1986), *The Complete Works of Captain John Smith*, P. Barbour (ed). Chapel Hill, NC: University of North Carolina Press, vol. 1, pp. 264–5, cit. in Eden, T. (2008), *The Early American Table: Food and Society in the New World*. DeKalb, IL: Northern Illinois University Press, p. 59. The event is also discussed in LaCombe, M. (2012), *Political Gastronomy: Food and Authority in the English Atlantic World*. Philadelphia, PA: University of Pennsylvania Press, pp. 51–3.

2 Brown, A. (1890), *The Genesis of the United States: A Narrative of the Movement in England, 1605–1616, Which Resulted in the Plantation of North America by Englishmen*. Boston: Houghton, Mifflin and Co., vol. 2, p. 660.

3 Hammond, J. (1656), *Leah and Rachel: Or, the Two Fruitfull Sisters Virginia and Maryland: Their Present Condition, Impartially Stated and Related*. London: T. Mabb, pp. 10, 12. Available online at: http://etext.lib.virginia.edu/etcbin/jamestown-browse?id=J1026.

4 Gerard, J. (1597), *The Herball, or Generall Historie of Plantes*. London: John Norton, p. 77.

5 Wood, W. (1634), *New England's Prospect*. London, p. 63, cit. in LaCombe, *Political Gastronomy*, p. 61.

6 Columbus, C. (1971), *Los cuatro viajes del almirante y su testamento*, I. Anzoátegui (ed). Madrid: Espasa, p. 158, cit. in Earle, R. (2012), *The Body of the Conquistador: Food, Race and the Colonial Experience in Spanish America, 1492–1700*. Cambridge: Cambridge University Press, p. 1.

7 'Description of a voyage from Lisbon to the island of São Thomé' (1942 [c.1540]), in Blake, J. (ed), *Europeans in West Africa, 1450–1560*. London: The Hakluyt Society, vol. 1, p. 157.

8 Langton, C. (1547), *A Very Brefe Treatise, Ordrely Declaring the Pri[n]cipal Partes of Phisick*. London: Edward Whitchurch, book 1, ch. x.

9 Anon. (1561), *Régime de vivre et conservation du corps humain*. Paris: Vincent Sertenas, p. 17v.

10 Huarte, J. (1594), *Examen de Ingenios, or The Examination of Mens Wits*. Trans. R[ichard] C[arew]. London: Adam Islip, p. 22.

11 It is referred to in Joubert, *Popular Errors*, p. 113.

12 Albala, *Eating Right*, pp. 217–40.

13 Nuñez de Oria, *Regimiento*, ch. 3, pp. 8r.–30r.

14 Ibid., p. 33v.

15 Rangoni, T. (1577 [1558]), *Come il serenissimo doge di Vinegia... e li Venetiani possano vivere sempre sani*. Venice: Marco Bindoni, pp. 7v, 1r.

16 Paschetti, *Del conservare la sanità et del vivere de' Genovesi*, p. 114.

17 Petronio, *Del vivere delli Romani et del conservare la sanità*, p. 1.

18 Ibid., p. 197.

19 Ibid., p. 253.

20 Albala, *Eating Right*, p. 225.

21 von Hutten, U. (1521), 'Die Anschawenien', in *Gesprächbüchlin herr Vlrichs von Hutten*. Strassburg: Johann Schott, fol. 12, cit. in Johnson, C. (2008), *The German Discovery of the World: Renaissance Encounters with the Strange and Marvelous*. Charlottesville, VA: University of Virginia Press, p. 143.

22 van Beverwyck, J. (1644), *Autarkeia Bataviae, sive introductio ad medicinam indigenam*. Leiden: Joh. Maire, p. 5, cit. in Cooper, A. (2007), *Inventing the Indigenous: Local Knowledge and Natural History in Early Modern Europe*. Cambridge: Cambridge University Press, p. 44.

23 Cook, H. (2007), *Matters of Exchange: Commerce, Medicine and Science in the Dutch Golden Age*. New Haven, CT: Yale University Press, pp. 317–25.

24 van Beverwyck, *Autarkeia Bataviae*, pp. 76–7.

25 Bruyérin-Champier, J. (1560), *De re cibaria, libri xxii. Omnium ciborum genera, omium gentium moribus et usu probata complectentes*. Lyon: Sebast. Honoratum, p. 91.

26 Ibid., pp. 95–6.

27 Boorde, A. (1555), *The Fyrst Boke of the Introduction of Knowledge. The whych Dothe Teache a Man to Speake Parte of all Maner of Languages, and to Knowe the Usage and Fashion of al Maner of Countreys*. London: William Copland.

28 Bright, T. (1580), *Treatise: Wherein Is Declared the Sufficiencie of English Medicines, for Cure of All Diseases*. London: Henry Midleton, pp. 16, 12–13.

29 Aignan, F. M. (1696), *Le prestre medecin, ou discours physique sur l'établissement de la medecine. Avec un traité du caffé e du thé de France*. Paris: Laurent D'Houry, p. 215. Curiously, Aignan's localism sits alongside discussions of the uses of tea and coffee, as well as New World drugs like cinchona and ipepacuana, now regarded as safely 'French' by Aignan.

30 Monardes, N. (1577), *Ioyfull Newes Out of the Newe Founde Worlde: Wherein Is Declared the Rare and Singuler Vertues of Diverse and Sundrie Hearbes, Trees, Oyles, Plantes, and Stones, with Their Aplications, as Well for Phisicke as Chirurgerie*. Trans. J. Frampton. London: William Norton.

31 Du Chesne, *Le pourtraict de la santé, où est au vif representée la reigle universelle et particulière de bien sainement et longuement vivre*, p. 199.

32 Ibid., pp. 183–242 in section II and all of section III.

33 Giacomotto-Charra, V. (2012), 'Un médecin géographe: voyages, chorographie et médecine pratique dans *Le pourtraict de la santé* de Joseph Du Chesne'. *Camenæ*, 14, online at: http://www.paris-sorbonne.fr/article/camenae-14.

34 Turler, J. (1575), *The Traveiler*. London: William How, pp. 101–2.

35 Cogan, T. (1584), *The Haven of Health Chiefely Gathered for the Comfort of Students, and Consequently of All Those That Have a Care of Their Health*. London: Henrie Midleton, p. 4r.

36 Thomas, W. (1549), *The Historie of Italy*. London: Thomas Berthelet, p. 2v.

37 Letter from Ignatius Loyola to Adrian Adriaenssens, 12 May 1556, in M. Gioia (ed) (1977), *Gli scritti di Ignazio di Loyola*. Turin: UTET, pp. 758–9.

38 Coe, S. (1994), *America's First Cuisines*. Austin, TX: University of Texas Press, pp. 27–8.

39 Thwaites, R. (ed) (1896–1901), *The Jesuit Relations and Allied Documents*. Cleveland, Ohio: Burrows Brothers, vol. 39, p. 48, cit. in Millones Figueroa, L. (2010), 'The staff of life: wheat and "Indian bread" in the New World'. *Colonial Latin American Review*, 19:2, pp. 304–5.

40 Earle, *Body of the Conquistador*, pp. 150–1.

41 Relation of Reverend Paul Lejeune (1972 [1634]), *Relations des Jésuites, 1611–1636*. Montreal: Éditions du jour, vol. 1, p. 90, cit. in Guillaume Plunian (forthcoming), 'L'alimentation du "Sauvage" dans les récits de voyage français. Perceptions et évolutions du regard sur la Nouvelle-France (1603–1704)', *Food & History*.

42 Nuñez de Oria, *Regimiento*, p. 7v.

43 Cisneros, D. (1618), *Sitio, naturaleza y propriedades de la ciudad de México*. Mexico City, p. 114v., cit. in Earle, *Body of the Conquistador*, p. 87.

44 'Relación de Querétaro' (1986 [1582]), in R. Acuña (ed), *Relaciones geográficas del siglo XVI: Michoacán*. Mexico City, p. 243, cit. in Earle, *Body of the Conquistador*, p. 127.

45 Norton, M. (2006), 'Tasting empire: chocolate and the European internalization of Mesoamerican aesthetics'. *The American Historical Review*, 111, 688.

46 De Cárdenas, J. (1591), *Problemas y secretos maravillosos de las Indias*. Mexico: Pedro Ocharte, p. 176v.

47 Eden, *Early American Table*, pp. 100, 104.

48 Gerard, *Herball*, p. 274

49 Olsen, T. (2003), 'Poisoned figs and Italian sallets: nation, diet and the early modern English traveler'. *Annali d'Italianistica*, 21, 233–53.

50 Nuñez de Oria, *Regimiento*, pp. 195v.–196r.

51 Gratarolo, G. (1574), *A Direction for the Health of Magistrates and Studentes*. Trans. T.N. London: William How, p. 2v.

52 Albala, *Eating Right*, p. 229.

53 Du Chesne, *Pourtraict de la santé*, pp. 378–9.

54 Boorde, A. (1542), *A Compendyous Regyment or Dyetary of Helth*. London: William Copland, ch. x.

55 Thomas, W. (1861 [1546]), *The Pilgrim*. J. A. Froude (ed). London: Parker, Son, and Bourne, pp. 5–6.

56 Cogan, *Haven of Health*, pp. 113–14. As we saw in Chapter 3, Cogan says the same thing about oats, contrasting Galen's judgement that it was a food for beasts of burden to widespread consumption in northern England, where it keept the people healthy and strong (ibid., p. 28).

57 Muffet, *Healths Improvement*, p. 59.

58 Ibid., p. 58.

59 Olsen, 'Poisoned figs'; Lloyd, P. (2012), 'Dietary advice and fruit-eating in late Tudor and early Stuart England'. *Journal of the History of Medicine and Allied Sciences*, 67:4, 553–86.

60 Flandrin, 'Dietary choices and culinary technique, 1500–1800', p. 414.

61 Calderón de la Barca, P. (1983), *Los Guisados (mojiganga)*, in E. Rodríguez and A. Tordera (eds), *Entremeses, jácaras y mojigangas*. Madrid: Castalia, pp. 404–14. Available online at: http://www.cervantesvirtual.com/obra/los-guisados-mojiganga.

62 Nadeau, C. (2005), 'Spanish culinary history in Cervantes' "Bodas de Camacho"'. *Revista Canadiense de Estudios Hispánicos*, 29:2, 347–61.

63 Mercurio, S. (1645 [1603]), *De gli errori popolari d'Italia*. Verona: Francesco Rossi, p. 511.

64 Pujati, *Della preservazione della salute de' letterati e della gente applicata e sedentaria*, p. 208.

65 Sebisch, M. [Sebizius] (1650), *De alimentorum facultatibus*. Strasbourg: Johannis Philippi Mülbii et Josiae Stedelii, cit. in Albala, *Eating Right*, pp. 280–1.

66 *XV Bücher von dem Feldbaw* (1588). Strasbourg: Jobin, cit. in Fleischer, M. (1981), 'The first German agricultural manuals'. *Agricultural History*, 55:1, p. 1 note 3.

67 Meyzie, *Alimentation*, p. 49.

68 Nuñez de Oria, *Regimiento*, p. 41v.

69 Gage, T. (1648), *The English-American, His Travail by Sea and Land: Or, A New Survey of the West-India's*. London: R. Cotes, p. 79.

70 Ibid., p. 200.

71 Howell, *Instructions for Forreine Travell*, p. 166.

72 Ibid., p. 75.

73 Ibid., p. 64. Italics in the original.

74 Ibid., pp. 69–70, 78, 80, 85.

75 Ibid., pp. 92, 93.

76 Ibid., pp. 8–9.

77 Ibid., pp. 175–6.

78 Locatelli, S. (1905), *Voyage de France: moeurs et coutumes françaises (1664–1665)*. Trans. and ed. A. Vautier. Paris: Alphonse Picard, p. 91.

79 Ibid., pp. 51, 53, 54.

80 Dapper, O. (1717), *Exoticus Curiosus*. Frankfurt and Leipzig: Michel Rohrlachs, fol. 3r.–v., cit. in Cooper, *Inventing the Indigenous*, p. 40. In a series of books published in the 1670s and 80s, Dapper wrote about much of the known world, though he never left his native Netherlands.

81 Lémery, L. (1706), *A Treatise of Foods*. London: Andrew Bell, p. 143.

82 Ibid., pp. 152–3.

83 Ibid., pp. 306–9.

84 Pinsonnat, *Régime de santé pour se procurer une longue vie et une vieillesse heureuse*, pp. 102–3.

85 Anon. (1702), *L'anti-Cornaro ou remarques critiques sur le traité de la vie sobre de Louis Cornaro venitien*. Paris: Claude Barré, pp. 33–4.

86 Harper, *The Oeconomy of Health: Or, a Medical Essay Containing New and Familiar Instructions for the Attainment of Health, Happiness and Longevity*, pp. 35–6.

87 Buchan, W. (1797 [1769]), *Domestic Medicine: Or, a Treatise on the Prevention and Cure of Diseases by Regimen and Simple Medicines*. London: A. Strahan, pp. 61, 74.

88 Ibid., p. 63.

89 Buchan, W. (1797), 'Observations concerning the diet of the common people, recommending a method of living less expensive, and more conducive to health, than the present', new appendix to 1797 edition of *Domestic Medicine*, pp. 647–79, at p. 648.

90 Ibid., p. 649.

91 Ibid., p. 650.

92 Ibid., p. 675.

93 Jefferson, T. (1787), *Notes on the State of Virginia*. London: John Stockdale. See also, Eden, *Early American Table*, pp. 157–60.

94 Jefferson, *Notes*, pp. 71–2.

95 Ibid., p. 107.

96 Ibid., p. 230.

97 Meyzie, *Alimentation*, p. 252.

Chapter 5

1 Grumett and Muers, *Theology on the Menu*, viii.

2 *The Rule of St Benedict* (1989), Trans. J. McCann. London: Sheed and Ward, pp. 39, 44, 46, discussed in Grumett and Muers, *Theology on the Menu*, ix, 18.

3 Van den Berghe, A. [Montanus] (1662), *Diatriba de esu carnium et quadragesima pontificiorum*. Amsterdam: Aegidius Valkenier.

4 Zacchia, P. (1636), *Il vitto quaresimale… ove insegnasi come senza offender la sanità si possa viver nella Quaresima*. Rome: Pietro Antonio Facciotti.

5 Quellier, *La table des Français: une histoire culturelle (XVe–XIXe siècle)*, pp. 137–9.

6 Meyzie, *L'alimentation en Europe à l'époque moderne*, p. 38. On trade and consumption of salt-cod in Spain, see Grafe, R. (2012), *Distant Tyranny: Markets, Power and Backwardness in Spain, 1650–1800*. Princeton, NJ: Princeton University Press, pp. 52–79.

7 Huldrich Zwingli, 'Liberty respecting food in Lent' [1522], cit. in Grummet and Muers, *Theology on the Menu*, p. 54.

8 Luther, M. (1961 [1520]), Address to the nobility of the German nation, in J. Dillenberger (ed), *Martin Luther: Selections from His Writings*. Garden City, NY: Anchor, p. 456. Discussed in Albala, *Food in Early Modern Europe*, p. 200.

9 Flandrin, J.-L. (2007), *Arranging the Meal: A History of Table Service in France*. Trans. J. Jonshon. Berkeley, CA: University of California Press, p. 33.

10 Erasmus, D. (1522), *De interdicto esu carnium ad Christophorum episcopum Basilien. epistola apologetica*.

11 Erasmus, D. (1964 [1526]), Concerning the Eating of Fish, in J. Dolan (ed), *The Essential Erasmus*. New York and London: Mentor, pp. 276–326.

12 Martin Luther, *Treatise on Good Works*, cit. in Grumett and Muer, *Theology on the Menu*, p. 55.

13 Moyer, "The food police", p. 75.

14 De Sales, F. (1770 [1619]), *Philothea, or an Introduction to a Devout Life*. London: J. P. Coghlan, part III, chapter 39, 'On the honourableness of the marriage bed'.

15 Bell, R. (1987), *Holy Anorexia*. Chicago, IL: University of Chicago Press; but see also, Walker Bynum, C. (1987), *Holy Feast and Holy Fast: The Religious Significance of Food to Medieval Women*. Berkeley, CA: University of California Press, esp. pp. 194–207.

16 Revel, J. (1975), 'Les privilèges d'une capitale: l'approvisionnement de Rome à l'époque moderne'. *Mélanges de l'École française de Rome. Moyen-Age, Temps modernes*, 87: 2, 492.

17 Gentilcore, 'The *Levitico*, or how to feed a hundred Jesuits'.

18 Cepari, V. (1762), *Vita di S. Luigi Gonzaga della Compagnia di Gesu*. Rome: Gioacchino Puccinelli, pp. 39–40.

19 Ercolani, G. L. (2001), *Il pane dei santi. Storia e curiosità sull'alimentazione dei santi*. Lugano: Todaro, p. 143.

20 Bernini, D. (1786), *Vita di S. Giuseppe da Copertino sacerdote professo dell'Ordine de' Minori Conventuali di S. Francesco*. Florence: stamperia Bonducciana, pp. 22–3.

21 de La Salle, J. B. (1956 [1703]), *Règles de la bienséance et de la civilité chrétienne*. Paris: Ligel, pp. 330–1, cit. in von Hoffmann, *Goûter le monde*, pp. 64–5.

22 Strupp (Struppius), J. (1573), *Nützliche Reformation zu guter Gesundheit und christlicher Ordnung*. Frankfurt, cit. in Bergdolt, *Wellbeing*, p. 170.

23 Durante, C. (1643 [1586]), *Il tesoro della sanità*, Venice: Domenico Imberti, p. 50.

24 Albala, *Eating Right in the Renaissance*, p. 105.

25 Rangoni, *Come il serenissimo doge di Vinegia … e li Venetiani possano vivere sempre sani*, p. 13v.

26 Boorde, *A Compendyous Regyment or Dyetary of Helth*, ch. ix.

27 Mason, H. (1627), *Christian Humiliation, or, the Christian's Fast*. London: John Clarke, 'The conclusion, touching the physicall use of fasting', pp. 186–92, quoting verbatim Fernel's *Therapeutica universalis*.

28 Ibid.

29 Moffett, *Health's Improvement*, p. 278.

30 Sebisch, M. [Sebizius] (1650), *De alimentorum facultatibis*. Strasbourg: Joannis Philippi Mülbii et Josiae Stedelii, p. 1431, cit. in Albala, *Eating Right*, p. 202.

31 Cardano, *Opus novum cunctis de sanitate tuenda*, discussed in Siraisi *The Clock and the Mirror*, p. 85.

32 Nonnius, L. (1645 [1627]), *Diaeteticon, sive re cibaria*. Antwerp: Petri Belleri, pp. 304–10, discussed in Albala, *Eating Right*, p. 44.

33 De Bonnefons, *Les délices de la campagne suitte du Jardinier françois*, pp. 373–80.

34 Da Fonseca Henriques, *Âncora medicinal para conservar a vida com saúde*, pp. 186–253.

35 Archivio di Stato, Rome, *Fondo Spada Veralli*, B.618, correspondence of February–April, 1678, cit. in Cavallo and Storey, *Healthy Living in Late Renaissance Italy*, p. 217.

36 Montenach, A. (2001), 'Esquisse d'une économie de l'illicite. Le marché parallèle de la viande à Lyon pendant le Carème (1658–1714)'. *Crime, histoire et société/Crime, History and Societies*, 5:1, 7–25.

37 Zacchia, *Vitto quaresimale*, pp. 2–8.

38 The dietary alone is over one hundred pages long. Zacchia, *Vitto quaresimale*, pp. 66–180.

39 Nuñez de Oria, *Regimiento y aviso de sanidad*, p. 94.

40 No reference; discussed in Williams, J. (2013), *Flesh and Faith: Meat-Eating and Religious Identities in Late Medieval and Early Modern Valencia*, unpublished PhD thesis, Department of Historical Studies, University of Bristol, p. 193.

41 Ibid., pp. 202–3, 207.

42 De Castro, T. (2002), 'L'émergence d'une identité alimentaire. Musulmans et chrétiens dans le royaume de Granade', in M. Bruegel and B. Laurioux (eds), *Histoire et identités alimentaires en Europe*. Paris: Hachette, pp. 199–215.

43 Pisanelli, B. (1589), *Trattato della natura de' cibi et del bere*. Carmagnola: Marc'Antonio Belloni, p. 29.

44 Ioly Zorattini, P. C. (1980), *Processi del S. Uffizio di Venezia contro ebrei e giudaizzanti*. Florence, vol. 1, p. 271, cit. in Toaff, A. (2000), *Mangiare alla giudia: la cucina ebraica in Italia dal Rinascimento all'età moderna*. Bologna: il Mulino, p. 59.

45 Toaff, *Mangiare alla giudia*, p. 61.

46 Zorattini, *Processi*, vol. 3, p. 190, cit. in Toaff, *Mangiare alla giudia*, p. 65.

47 For instance, in Anon. (1607), *Le thrésor de santé, ou mesnage de la via humaine*. Lyon: Jean Huguetan, pp. 210–13.

48 Laguna, A. (1566), *Pedacio Dioscorides Anazarbeo, acerca de la materia medicinal y de los venenos mortiferos*. Salamanca: Mathias Gast, p. 425.

49 Nuñez de Oria, *Regimiento*, pp. 245–6.

50 Gil, J. (2009), 'Berenjeneros: the aubergine-eaters', in K. Ingram (ed), *The Conversos and Moriscos in Late Medieval Spain and Beyond*, vol. 1, *Departures and Change*. Leiden: Brill, p. 129.

51 Laguna, *Dioscorides*, p. 425.

52 Delicado, F. [Delgado] (1528), *Retrato de la Lozana andaluza*. Venice, cit. in Gil, 'Berenjeneros', p. 128. *Boronía* is a savoury pudding made with aubergines, cheese, breadcrumbs and honey.

53 Tanara, V. (1651 [1644]), *L'economia del cittadino in villa*. Rome: Gio. Battista e Giuseppe Corvo, p. 241.

54 *Spiritual Exercises*, week three, in Gioia, *Gli scritti di Ignazio di Loyola*, pp. 144–6.

55 Such permissions were granted reluctantly and rarely – on only eighteen occasions between 1670 and 1754 in France – so were not necessarily part of a new ecclesiastical scepticism. Watts, S. (2013), 'Enlightened fasting: religious conviction, scientific inquiry, and medical knowledge in early modern France', in Albala and Eden, *Food and Faith*, p. 108.

56 De Acosta, J. (1604), *The Naturall and Morall History of the East and West Indies*. Trans. E[dward] G[rimstone]. London: Val. Sims, p. 164.

57 Interestingly, the same did not happen in other Protestant countries like Scotland, the Netherlands and Norway, where fish consumption was evidently important enough economically, and a generally welcomed element of local diet, that the end of enforced fasting did not have much effect. Meyzie, *Alimentation*, p. 179.

58 Young, A. (1792), *Travels, During the Years 1787, 1788, and 1789, Undertaken More Particularly with a View of Ascertaining the Cultivation, Wealth, Resources, and National Prosperity, of the Kingdom of France*. London: W. Richardson, p. 49.

59 Galinier-Pallerola, J.-F. (2005), 'La gourmandise: péché capitale ou vertu mondaine? Le discours sur le goût en France au XVIIIe siècle', in A.-M. Cocula and J. Pontet (eds), *Au contact des Lumières. Mélanges offerts à Philippe Loupès*. Bordeaux: Presses Universitaires de Bordeaux, pp. 132–3.

60 Ibid., p. 135.

61 Watts, 'Enlightened fasting', p. 111.

62 Hecquet, P. (1710 [1709]), *Traité des dispenses du Carême*. Paris: Francois Fournier. The debate is discussed in Abad, R. (1999), 'Un indice de déchristianisation? L'évolution de la consommation de viande à Paris en carême sous l'Ancien Régime. *Revue historique*, CCCI:2, esp. pp. 249–54; Renan, L. (2009), 'Les bienfaits controversés du régime maigre: le *Traité des*

dispenses du carême de Philippe Hecquet et sa réception (1709–1714)'. *Dix-huitième siècle*, 41:1, 409–30; and Watts, 'Enlightened fasting', esp. pp. 114–20.

63   Brockliss, 'The medico-religious universe of an early eighteenth-century Parisian doctor: the case of Philippe Hecquet', pp. 191–221.

64   Andry, N. (1713), *Traité des aliments de Caresme*. Paris: Jean-Baptiste Coignard, p. 6.

65   Turrini, M. (2006), *Il 'giovin signore' in Collegio. I Gesuiti e l'educazione della nobiltà nelle consuetudini del Collegio ducale di Parma*. Bologna: CLUEB, p. 120.

66   Abad, 'Indice', pp. 254–9.

67   Mercier, L.-S. (1994 [1781–88]), *Tableau de Paris*. Paris: Jean-Claude Bonnet, p. 1178, cit. in Abad, 'Indice', p. 266.

68   Redman, B. (ed) (1977), *The Portable Voltaire*. Harmondsworth: Penguin, p. 147.

69   Grafe, *Distant Tyranny*, pp. 72–8.

70   Kitowicz, J. (1985), *Opis obyczjów za panowania Augusta III*. Warsaw: Panstwowny Instytut Wydawniczy, p. 106, cit. in Topolski, J. (1997), 'Religious fasting as a kind of the food taboo in Poland in the 16th–17th centuries', in S. Cavaciocchi (ed), *Alimentazione e nutrizione, secc. XIII–XVIII*. Prato: Istituto Datini, p. 560.

71   Kitowicz, *Opis*, pp. 229–30, cit. in Topolski, 'Religious fasting', p. 567.

72   Kowecka, E. (1991), *Dwór 'Najrzadniejszego w Polszcze magnata'*. Warsaw: Instytut Historii Kultury Materialnej Polskiej Akademii Nauk, pp. 179–80, cit. in Topolski, 'Religious fasting', pp. 558–9.

73   John Wesley, 'Upon our Lord's sermon on the Mount' (1741), in Grumett and Muers, *Theology on the Menu*, p. 62.

74   John Wesley, 'The more excellent way', cit. in Wallace, Eating and drinking with John Wesley, 145–6.

75   Hoffmann, F. (1740), *Gründliche Anweisung wie ein Mensch vor dem frühzeitigen Tod und allerhand Arten Kranckheiten*. Halle. Discussed in Bergdolt, *Wellbeing*, p. 228.

76   Marmontel, J.-F. (1804), *Œuvres posthumes… Mémoires*. Paris: Xhrouet.

77   Spary, *Eating the Enlightenment*, p. 261.

Chapter 6

1   Rangoni, *De vita hominis ultra cxx annos potrahenda*

2   Palmer, 'Health, hygiene and longevity in Medieval and Renaissance Europe', p. 93; Carrington, J. (2000), 'Rangoni, Tommaso, Italian physician, philologist and patron', in *Encyclopedia of Italian Renaissance and Mannerist Art*. London and New York: Macmillan, Grove's Dictionaries, vol. 2, pp. 1315–16.

3   Rangoni, *De vita*, especially pp. 48r.–57r.

4   Sorapán de Rieros, J. (1616), *Medicina española contenida en proverbios vulgares de nuestra lingua*. Madrid: Martin Fernandez Zambrano, p. 234.

5   Gentilcore, *Pomodoro! A History of the Tomato in Italy*, pp. 27–44; Giannetti, L. (2010), 'Italian food-fashioning, or the triumph of greens'. *California Italian Studies Journal*, 1:2, 1–16, available online at: http://escholarship.org/uc/item/1n97s00d.

6   Bruyérin-Champier, *De re cibaria*, p. 468.

7 Pisanelli, *Trattato de' cibi et del bere*, pp. 118–19.

8 Ibid., pp. 126, 132.

9 Ibid., p. 128.

10 Ibid., p. 105.

11 Lloyd, 'Dietary advice and fruit-eating in late Tudor and early Stuart England'.

12 Harrington, J. (1607), *The Englishmans Doctor: Or the Schoole of Salerne*. London: John Busby, p. 11.

13 Dallington, R. (1605), *A Survey of the Great Dukes State of Tuscany, in the Yeare of Our lord 1596*. London: Edward Blount, pp. 31–2.

14 Ibid., p. 34.

15 Gallo, A. (2003 [1569]), *Le vinti giornate dell'agricoltura e dei piaceri della villa*. L. Crosato (ed). Treviso: Canova, pp. 129–39.

16 Heresbach, *Foure Bookes of Husbandry*.

17 De Serres, O. (1600), *Le théâtre d'agriculture et mésnage des champs*. Paris: Jamet Métayer, pp. 508–70.

18 Du Chesne, *Le pourtraict de la santé, où est au vif representée la reigle universelle et particulière de bien sainement et longuement vivre*, pp. 369–410.

19 Coles, W. (1656), *The Art of Simpling: An Introduction to the Knowledge and Gathering of Plants*. London: Nathaniel Brook, p. 119.

20 Ibid., pp. 48, 49.

21 Ibid., p. 50.

22 Archivio di Stato, Mantua, *Archivio Gonzaga*, b. 2997, libro 36, fol. 32r, 27 February 1519, in Malacarne, G. (2001), *Sulla mensa del principe: alimentazione e banchetti alla corte dei Gonzaga*. Modena: il Bulino, pp. 108–9.

23 Archivio di Stato, Mantua, *Archivio Gonzaga*, b. 2997, libro 36, fols. 31v–32r, 26 February 1519, in Malacarne, *Sulla mensa*, p. 112.

24 Vigilio, G. B. (1992), *La Insalata: cronaca mantovana dal 1561 al 1602*. D. Ferrari and C. Mozzarelli (eds). Mantua: Arcari, pp. 34–5, 37.

25 Flecha, M. (1581), *Las Ensaladas de Flecha*. Prague: Iorge Negrino.

26 Bruyérin-Champier, *De re cibaria*, pp. 454–6.

27 Felici, C. (1987 [1572]), 'Del'insalata e piante che in qualunque modo vengono per cibo dell'homo', in Faccioli, E. (ed), *L'arte della cucina in Italia*. Turin: Einaudi, 469–90; Massonio, S. (1628), *Archidipno, ovvero dell'insalata e dell'uso di essa*. Venice: Marc'Antonio Brogiollo, pp. iv, 5.

28 Heresbach, *Husbandry*, p. 19r. He is favourably quoting the ancient Roman scholar Varro.

29 Jeanneret, M. (2007), 'Ma salade et ma muse', in T. Tomasik and J. Vitullo (eds), *At the Table: Metaphorical and Material Cultures of Food in Medieval and Early Modern Europe*. Turnhout: Brepols, p. 212; Flandrin, 'Dietary choices and culinary technique, 1500–1800', pp. 404–6.

30 Thirsk, J. (1997), *Alternative Agriculture: A History*. Oxford: Oxford University Press, pp. 23–42; Pinkard, S. (2009), *A Revolution of Taste: The Rise of French Cuisine, 1650–1800*. Cambridge: Cambridge University Press, pp. 35–43.

31 Nuñez de Oria, *Regimiento y aviso de sanidad*, p. 198v.

32 Bruyérin-Champier, *De re cibaria*, p. 453.

33 De Bonnefons, N. (1658 [1651]), *The French Gardiner: Instructing How to Cultivate All Sorts of Fruit-Trees and Herbs for the Garden*. Trans. Philocepos [John Evelyn]. London: John Crooke, p. 167.

34 De Bonnefons, *The French Gardiner*, pp. 166–82.

35 Sada, L. (1987), 'L'arte culinaria barese al celebre banchetto nuziale di Bona Sforza nel 1517', in B. Bilinski (ed), *La regina Bona Sforza tra Puglia e Polonia*. Warsaw: Ossolineum, p. 46 note 2.

36 Pospiech, A. (1997), 'Il ritmo annuale dell'alimentazione nella società tradizionale dell'Europa centrale: i piaceri della mensa', in S. Cavaciocchi (ed), *Alimentazione e nutrizione, secc. XIII–XVIII: atti della ventottesima settimana di studi*. Florence: Le Monnier, pp. 225–6.

37 Proceedings of the round-table discussion, in Cavaciocchi, *Alimentazione*, p. 494. I was unable to find the poem referred to, but Potocki's poem 'Italian banquet' ('Bankiet włoski'), gives an idea of the style. Online at: http://literat.ug.edu.pl/~literat/potocki/index.htm.

38 Court of Arches, Lambeth Palace Library, London, *Houston* no. 842, cit. in Pelling, M. (1982), 'Food, status and knowledge: attitudes to diet in early modern England', in idem, *The Common Lot: Sickness, Medical Occupations and the Urban Poor in Early Modern England*. London and New York: Longman, p. 47.

39 Le Roy Ladurie, E. (1966), *Les paysans de Languedoc*. Paris: SEVPEN, vol. 1, p. 62. The passage is absent from the later, abridged version.

40 Pisanelli, *Trattato*, p. 120.

41 De Serres, *Théatre*, pp. 516–17.

42 De Bonnefons, *The French Gardiner*, p. 157. Italics in the original.

43 De Bonnefons, *Les délices de la campagne*, pp. 133–7.

44 Heresbach, *Husbandry*, p. 63r.

45 Thirsk, *Alternative Agriculture*, p. 31.

46 Moffet, *Health's Improvement*, p. 215.

47 Castelvetro, *The Fruit, Herbs and Vegetables of Italy*, pp. 55–9.

48 Androutsos, G. (2006), 'Nicolas Venette (1633–1698): premier sexologue français et grand pionnier en matière de lithiase urinaire'. *Andrologie*, 16:2, 160–7.

49 Venette, *L'art de tailler des arbres fruitiers, avec … un traité de l'usage des fruits des arbres pour se conserver en santé ou pour se guérir lorsqu'on est malade*, pp. 8–14.

50 Quellier, F. (2007), 'Les fruits, le *Thrésor de santé* de la France classique (XVIIe–XVIIIe siècles)', in F. Audoin-Rouzeau and F. Sabban (eds), *Un aliment sain dans un corps sain: perspectives historiques*. Tours: Presses Universitaires François Rabelais, 185–98.

51 Calanius, P. (1533), *Traicté pour l'entretenement de santé*. Lyon: Temporal, p. 60; Goulin, *Le médecin des dames, ou l'art de les conserver en santé*, pp. 56–7.

52 Tissot, *Advice to the People in General, with Regard to Their Health*, pp. 68, 333, 342–3.

53 Gullino, G. (1983), 'Corner, Alvise', in *Dizionario biografico degli Italiani*. Rome: Treccani, vol. 29, online at: http://www.treccani.it/enciclopedia/alvise-corner_(Dizionario-Biografico)/; see also Milani, M. (2014), 'Introduction to Cornaro', in A. Cornaro, *Writings on the Sober Life: The Art and Grace of Living Long*. Trans. and ed. H. Fudemoto. Toronto, ON: University of Toronto Press, pp. 12, 13.

54 Cornaro, L. (1558), *Trattato de la vita sobria*. Venice: a San Luca al segno del Diamante.

55 Cardano, *Opus novum cunctis de sanitate tuenda*, p. 8.

56 Leys (1643 [1613]), *Hygiasticon: Or the Right Course of Preserving Life and Health unto Extream Old Age*, pp. 62–3.

57 Ibid., pp. 61, 66.

58 Ibid., pp. 98, 118.

59 Ibid., pp. 143, 145.

60 Ibid., pp. 151, 170–1.

61 Ibid., pp. 129–30, 181–4.

62 Spencer, C. (1993), *The Heretic's Feast: A History of Vegetarianism*. London: Fourth Estate, pp. 205–6.

63 Crab, R. (1655), *The English Hermite, or, Wonder of His Age. Being a Relation of the Life of Roger Crab*. London. Preface 'to the reader'.

64 Tryon, T. (1691), *Wisdom's Dictates: Or Aphorisms and Rules, Physical, Moral and Divine … to Which Is Added a Bille of Fare of Seventy-Five Noble Dishes of Excellent Food*. London: Thomas Salisbury, p. 139.

65 Ibid., p. 153.

66 Discussed in Houston, A. (2008), *Benjamin Franklin and the Politics of Improvement*. New Haven, CT: Yale University Press, pp. 211–12.

67 This is evident in Tryon's letter 'Of flesh-broths', which uses the vocabulary of chemical medicine: Tryon, T. (1700), *Tryon's Letters, Domestic and Foreign, to Several Persons of Quality*. London: Geo. Conyers, pp. 87–92.

68 Andry, N. (1713), *Traité des aliments de Caresme*. Paris: Jean-Baptiste Coignard, p. 7, cit. in Albala, K. (2002/3), 'Insensible perspiration and oily vegetable humor: an eighteenth-century controversy over vegetarianism'. *Gastronomica: The Journal of Food and Culture*, 3:1, p. 5.

69 *King James Bible*, first letter of St Paul to Timothy, 4:4.

70 Renan, Les bienfaits controversés du régime maigre, p. 426.

71 Evelyn, J. (1699), *Acetaria, a Discourse on Sallets*. London: B. Tooke, pp. 138–9.

72 Ibid., pp. 127–8.

73 Ibid., p. 77.

74 Lémery, *A Treatise of All Sorts of Foods, Both Animal and Vegetable*, p. 25.

75 Brockliss, The medico-religious universe of an early eighteenth-century Parisian doctor, pp. 191–221.

76 Baldini, U. (1982), 'Cocchi, Antonio', in *Dizionario biografico degli Italiani*. Rome: Treccani, vol. 26, online at: http://www.treccani.it/enciclopedia/antonio-cocchi_%28Dizionario -Biografico%29/.

77 Cocchi, A. (1743), *Del vitto pitagorico per uso della medicina*. Florence: Francesco Moücke; (1745), *The Pythagorean Diet of Vegetables Only Conducive to the Preparation of Health and the Cure of Diseases*. London: R. Dodsley; (1750), *Du régime de vivre Pythagoricien à l'usage de la médecine*. Geneva: Cramer.

78 Cocchi, A. (1791), *Consulti medici*. Bergamo: Vincenzo Antoine, p. 2.

79 Cocchi, *Pythagorean Diet*, pp. 34, 64–5. The book's English title is a bit misleading here.

80 Cocchi, A. (1769 [1762]), *The Grand Question: Is Marriage Fit for Literary Men?* Trans. P. Hiffernan. London: S. Bladon.

81 Manetti, S. (1759), *Lettera … sopra la malattia, morte e dissezione anatomica del corpo del cadavere di Antonio Cocchi*. Florence: Pietro Gaetano Viviani, pp. 5–6.

82 Ibid., p. 32.

83 Albala, 'Insensible perspiration', pp. 33–4.

84 Pujati, G. A. (1751), *Riflessioni sul vitto pitagorico*. Feltre: Odoardo Foglietta, pp. 36–7.

85 Ibid., pp. 33, 69–70.

86 Ibid., pp. 40–1, 65–6, 77–8.

87 Ibid., p. 77.

88 Pujati, *Della preservazione della salute de' letterati e della gente applicata e sedentaria*, pp. 334–54.

89 Corrado, V. (1773), *Il cuoco galante*. Naples: Stamperia Raimondiana.

90 Corrado, V. (2001 [1781]), *Del cibo pitagorico ovvero erbaceo per uso de' nobile e de' letterati*. Rome: Donzelli, pp. 11–12.

91 Buc'hoz, *L'art alimentaire ou methode pour préparer les aliments les plus sains pour l'homme*, pp. 18–19.

92 Harper, *The Oeconomy of Health: Or, a Medical Essay Containing New and Familiar Instructions for the Attainment of Health, Happiness and Longevity*, p. 42.

93 Sinclair, *The Code of Health and Longevity: Or a Concise View of the Principles Calculated for the Preservation of Health and the Attainment of Long Life*, vol. 1, pp. 421–30.

Chapter 7

1 Bruyérin-Champier, J. (1560), *De re cibaria libri XXII, omnium ciborum genera, omnium gentium moribus et usu probata complectentes*. Lyon: Sebast. Honoratum, pp. 122–36.

2 Ibid., pp. 831–2.

3 Ibid., p. 70.

4 Crosby, A. (1972), *The Columbian Exchange: Biological and Cultural Consequences of 1492*. Westport, CT: Greenwood Press.

5 The South American staple cassava (manioc) could have grown in the warmer parts of southern Europe but Europeans were put off eating it by its toxicity when not correctly prepared. They did, however, take it along with them on their conquests to feed to their labourers and slaves in Africa and elsewhere (in Ferrières, *Sacred Cow, Mad Cow*, pp. 83–4). On more deliberate strategies of ignorance towards New World products, see Schiebinger, L. (2008), 'West Indian abortifacients and the making of ignorance', in R. Proctor and L. Schiebinger (eds), *Agnotology: The Making and Unmaking of Ignorance*. Stanford, CA: Stanford University Press, pp. 149–62.

6 Greenblatt, S. (1991), *Marvelous Posession: The Wonder of the New World*. Chicago: University of Chicago Press, p. 19.

7 Monardes, N. (1885 [1545]), *Sevillana medicina, que trata el modo conservativo y curativo de los que habitan en la muy insigne ciudad de Sevilla*. Seville: Enrico Rasco, pp. 62–156.

8 Monardes, *Ioyfull Newes Out of the Newe Founde Worlde*.

9 Solomon, *Fictions of Well-Being*, pp. 37–8, 84–5.

10 Schiebinger, L. (2004), *Plants and Empire: Colonial Bioprospecting in the Atlantic World*. Cambridge, MA: Harvard University Press, p. 5. See also, Cook, *Matters of Exchange*, pp. 304–38.

11   Baley, *A Short Discourse of the Three Kindes of Peppers in Common Use*.

12   Albala, *Eating Right in the Renaissance*, p. 233.

13   Estienne, C. (1580), *De nutrimentis ad Baillyum*. Paris: Robertus Stephanus, pp. 35–8, 76–7.

14   Bruyérin-Champier, *De re cibaria*, pp. 122–3.

15   Nuñez de Oria, *Regimiento y aviso de sanidad*, p. 36v.

16   Parkinson, J. (1629), *Paradisi in Paradisus Terrestris: A Garden of All Sorts of Pleasant Flowers Which Our English Ayre Will Permit to Be Noursed Up*. London: Humfrey Lownes and Robert Young.

17   Pisanelli, B. (1589), *Trattato de' cibi et del bere*. Carmagnola: Marc'Antonio Bellone, pp. 136–7.

18   Darrow, G. (1966), *The Strawberry: History, Breeding and Physiology*. New York: Holt, Rinehart and Winston, pp. 15–72.

19   Parkinson, *Paradisi*, p. 521, cit. in Dickenson, V. (2008), 'Cartier, Champlain and the fruits of the New World: botanical exchange in the 16th and 17th centuries'. *Scientia Canadensis: Canadian Journal of the History of Science, Technology and Medicine/Scientia Canadensis: revue canadienne d'histoire des sciences, des techniques et de la médecine*, 31:1–2, p. 41.

20   De los Rios, G. (1777 [1592]), *Agricultura general: que trata de la labranza del campo y sus particularidades, crianza de animales, propriedades de las plantas que en ella se contienen, y virtudes provechosas a la salud humana*. Madrid: Antonio de Sancha, p. 454.

21   Kaplan, Lawrence and Kaplan, Lucille (2007), 'Beans of the Americas', in N. Foster and L. Cordell (eds), *From Chilies to Chocolate: Food the Americas Gave the World*. Tucson, AR: University of Arizona Press, pp. 61–79; Albala, *Beans*, pp. 135–7.

22   Bock, H. (1546), *Kreuter Buch. Darin Vnderscheid/Wuerckung und Namen der Kreüter*. Strasbourg: W. Rinel, pp. 235–6, cit. in Johnson, *The German Discovery of the World*, pp. 151–2.

23   Lémery (1745 [1705]), *Treatise of All Sorts of Foods*, p. 84.

24   Lémery, L. (1755), *Traité des alimens … par M. Louis Lémery … revue, corrigée et augmentée … par M. Jacques-Jean Bruhier*. Paris: Durand, p. 322.

25   Andrews, J. (1992), 'The peripatetic chili pepper: diffusion of the domesticated capsicums since Columbus', in N. Foster and L. Cordell (eds), *From Chilies to Chocolate: Food the Americas Gave the World*. Tucson, AR: University of Arizona Press, pp. 81–93.

26   De Acosta, *The Naturall and Morall History of the East and West Indies*, pp. 269–70.

27   Collingham, L. (2006), *Curry: A Tale of Cooks and Conquerors*. London: Vintage, pp. 47–73.

28   Baley, *Short Discourse*.

29   Soderini, G. (1814), *Della coltura degli orti e dei giardini*. Florence: del Giglio, pp. 201–2.

30   Bertaldi, L. (1620), *Regole della sanità et natura de' cibi di Ugo Benzo senese … arricchite dal sig. Lodovico Bertaldi*. Turin: Gio. Domenico Tarino, p. 428.

31   Evelyn, J. (1699), *Acetaria: A Discourse of Sallets*. London: B. Tooke, pp. 52–3.

32   Fleuriot, J.-M.-J. (1784), *Voyage de Figaro en Espagne*. Paris, cit. Flandrin, 'Dietary choices and culinary technique, 1500–1800', p. 410. Flandrin's reference here is tongue-in-cheek, discussing him in the context of other travellers, even though the marquis Fleuriot never set foot in Spain.

33   Lang, G. (1990 [1971]), *The Cuisine of Hungary*. New York, NY: Bonanza Books, p. 46.

34   Keating, J. and Markey, L. (2011), ' "Indian" objects in Medici and Austrian-Hapsburg inventories: a case study of the sixteenth-century term'. *Journal of the History of Collections*, 23:2, esp. pp. 286–8.

35   Schorger, A. W. (1966), *The Wild Turkey: Its History and Domestication*. Norman, OK: University of Oklahoma Press, pp. 3–4.

36   Pisanelli, *Trattato*, pp. 26–7; Heresbach, C. (1577), *Four Books of Husbandry*. Trans. B. Googe. London: Richard Watkins, pp. 166–8; Du Chesne, J. (1620), *Le pourtraict de la santé*. Paris: Claude Morel, p. 423; Muffet, *Healths Improvement*, p. 84.

37   Lémery, *Treatise of All Sorts of Foods*, p. 84. *Coq d'Inde* in the original French: Lémery, *Traités des aliments*, p. 295.

38   Schorger, *Wild Turkey*, pp. 472, 475, 485–6.

39   Schorger, *Wild Turkey*, pp. 9, 464.

40   On representations of the turkey in Renaissance Italy, see Eiche, S. (2004), *Presenting the Turkey: The Fabulous Story of a Flamboyant and Flavourful Bird*. Florence: Centro Di, pp. 16, 22–4.

41   Schorger, *Wild Turkey*, pp. 465, 468.

42   De Ruble, A. (1877), *Le mariage de Jeanne d'Albret*. Paris: Labitte, p. 7. Available online at: http://www.mediterranee-antique.info/Fichiers_PdF/PQRS/Ruble/Mariage_J_Albret.pdf.

43   Sabban, F. and Serventi, S. (1996), *A tavola nel Rinascimento: con 90 ricette della cucina italiana*. Rome: Laterza, pp. 112–13.

44   Stefani, B. (2002 [1662]), *L'arte di ben cucinare et instruire i men periti in questa lodevole professione*. Mantua: Osanna, in L. Turrini (ed), *La cucina ai tempi dei Gonzaga*. Milan: Rizzoli, pp. 33–4.

45   De Bonnefons, *Les délices de la campagne*, pp. 230–4; Rodrigues, D. (1821 [1680]), *Arte de cozinha dividida em quatro partes*. Lisbon: Viuva de Lino da Silva Godinho.

46   Schorger, *Wild Turkey*, pp. 479–80.

47   Loring Bailey, S. (1880), *Historical Sketches of Andover*. Boston: Houghton, Mifflin and Co., pp. 44–5.

48   Estienne, C and Liebault, J. (1600), *Maison rustique or the Countrie Farme*. Trans. R. Surflet. London: Edmond Bollifant, pp. 116–17.

49   Sebisch, *De Alimentorum Facultatibus*, frontespiece and pp. 814–16.

50   De Thou, J.-A. (1691), *Perroniana et Thuana*. Cologne: G. Scagen, p. 71, cit. in Schorger, *Wild Turkey*, p. 466.

51   Anon., *Le thrésor de santé*, pp. 203–4.

52   Cheyne, *Essay of Health*, p. 12.

53   Pinkard, S. (2009), *A Revolution of Taste: The Rise of French Cuisine*. Cambridge: Cambridge University Press, p. 175.

54   Schorger, *Wild Turkey*, pp. 468–9.

55   Corrado (1786 [1773]), *Il cuoco galante*, pp. 54–6.

56   Janick, J. and Caneva, G. (2005), 'The first images of maize in Europe'. *Maydica*, 50, 71–80.

57   Nuñez de Oria, *Regimiento*, p. 41r.

58   Fuchs, L. (1542), *De historia stirpium commentarii insignes*. Basilea, p. 824, cit. in Finan, J. (1950), *Maize in the Great Herbals*. Waltham, MA: Chronica Botanica, p. 159.

59   Mattioli, P. A. (1570), *Commentarii in sex libros Pedacio Dioscoridis Anazarbei de medica materia*. Venice: Valgrisio, p. 305.

60   Gerard, J. (1597), *The Herball or Generall Historie of Plantes*. London: John Norton, pp. 75–7.

61   Soderini, *Coltura degli orti*, p. 302.

62   Tanara, V. (1674 [1644]), *L'economia del cittadino in villa*. Venice: Stefano Curti, p. 454.

63   Earle, *Body of the Conquistador*, p. 145.

64   López Lázaro, F. (2007), 'Sweet food of knowledge: botany, food and empire in the early modern Spanish kingdoms', in J. Vitullo and T. Tomasik (eds), *At the Table: Metaphorical and Material Cultures in Medieval and Early Modern Europe*. Turnhout: Brepols, p. 11.

65   Norton, M. (2008), *Sacred Gifts, Profane Pleasures: A History of Tobacco and Chocolate in the Atlantic World*. Ithaca, NY: Cornell University Press, p. 87; Earle, *Body of the Conquistador*, p. 136.

66   De Cárdenas, *Problemas y secretos*. Discussed in Pardo-Tomás, J. (2011), 'Natural knowledge and medical remedies in the book of secrets: uses and appropriations in Juan de Cárdenas' *Problemas y secretos maravillosos de las Indias* (Mexico, 1591), in S. Anagnostou, F. Egmond and C. Friedrich (eds), *Passion for Plants: Materia Medica and Botany in Scientific Networks from the 16th to 18th Centuries*. Stuttgart: Wissenschafliche Verlagsgesellschaft, pp. 93–108.

67   Cárdenas, *Problemas y secretos*, p. 147r.

68   Mood, F. (1937), 'John Winthrop, Jr., on Indian corn'. *The New England Quarterly*, 10:1, p. 125.

69   Ibid., p. 130.

70   Eden, *The American Table*, pp. 140–1.

71   Thwaites, *The Jesuit Relations and Allied Documents*, vol. 20, p. 53, cit. in Millones Figueroa, Staff of life, p. 309.

72   Lafitau, J.-F. (1974 [1714]), *Customs of the American Indians Compared with the Customs of Primitive Times*. Trans. W. Fenton and E. Moore. Toronto: The Champlain Society, vol. 2, pp. 59, 61.

73   Ibid., vol. 2, p. 63.

74   Warman, A. (2003), *Corn and Capitalism: How a Botanical Bastard Grew to Global Dominance*. Trans. N. Westrate. Chapel Hill, NC: University of North Carolina Press; Finzi, R. (2009), '*Sazia assai ma dà poco fiato*': il mais nell'economia e nella vita rurale italiane, secoli XVI–XIX. Bologna: CLUEB.

75   Bertaldi, *Regole della sanità*, p. 579.

76   Lafitau, *Customs of the American Indians*, vol. 2, p. 63.

77   D'Aulnoy, *Rélation du voyage d'Espagne*, pp. 113–14.

78   Lémery, *Treatise of All Sorts of Foods*, pp. 97–8.

79   Tanara, *Cittadino in villa*, p. 39.

80   Gallo, A. (1775), *Le venti giornate dell'agricoltura e de' piaceri della villa*. Brescia: Giambattista Bossini [photostatic reprint Brescia: Scaglia, 2003], 'Aggiunta sopra il formentone', pp. 533–58.

81   Ibid., pp. 553–4.

82   García Guerra, D. and Álvarez Antuña, V. (1993), *Lepra Asturiensis: la contribución asturiana en la historia de la pelagra (siglos XVIII y XIX)*. Madrid: CSIC, pp. 4–16.

83   Gentilcore, D. (2013), ' "Italic scurvy", "pellarina", "pellagra": medical reactions to a new disease in Italy, 1770–1830', in J. Reinarz and K. Siena (eds), *A Medical History of Skin: Scratching the Surface*. London: Pickering and Chatto, pp. 57–69.

84   Parkinson, *Paradisi*, p. 518, cit. in Dickenson, 'Fruits of the New World', pp. 39, 46.

85   De Champlain, S. (1922), *The Works of Samuel de Champlain*. H. P. Biggar (ed). Toronto, NO: The Champlain Society, vol. 1, 351, cit. in Dickenson, 'Fruits of the New World', p. 38.

86 Gerard, J. (1633), *The Herball or Generall Historie of Plantes… Very Much Enlarged and Emended by Thomas Johnson*. London: Adam Norton and Richard Whitakers, p. 752.

87 Lémery, *Treatise of All Sorts of Foods*, pp. 128–9.

88 Dickenson, 'Fruits of the New World', p. 46.

89 Gerard, *Herball* (1633 edn.), p. 753.

90 Ferrières, *Sacred Cow, Mad Cow*, pp. 82–110.

91 Ibid., p. 92.

92 Sebisch, *Alimentorum Facultatibus*, p. 410.

93 Gerard, *Herball* (1597 edn.), pp. 781–2.

94 Moffett, *Health's Improvement*, pp. 33, 226.

95 Venner, *Via Recta ad Vitam Longam*, pp. 141–2.

96 Bidloo, L. (1683), *Dissertatio de re herbaria*. Amsterdam: H. & viduam T. Boom, p. 73, cit. in Cooper, *Inventing the Indigenous*, p. 48.

97 Forster, J. (1664), *Englands Happiness Increased, or a Sure and Easie Remedy against All Succeeding Dear Years, by a Plantation of the Roots Called Potatoes*. London: A. Seile.

98 Salaman, R. (2000), *The Social History of the Potato*. Cambridge: Cambridge University Press, pp. 142–58; O'Riordan, T. (2001), 'The introduction of the potato into Ireland'. *History Ireland*, 9:1, online at: http://www.historyireland.com/early-modern-history-1500-1700/the-introduction-of-the-potato-into-ireland/; McNeill, W. (1999), 'How the potato changed the world's history'. *Social Research*, 66:1, p. 71.

99 Moryson, F. (1908), *The Itinerary of Fynes Moryson*. Glasgow: Robert Maclehose, vol. 4, pp. 200–1.

100 Connell, K. H. (1962), 'The potato in Ireland'. *Past and Present*, no. 23, 57–71, at pp. 58–9.

101 Buchan, W. (1797), 'Observations concerning the diet of the common people, recommending a method of living less expensive, and more conducive to health, than the present', added to the 1797 edition of his *Domestic Medicine: Or, a Treatise on the Prevention and Cure of Diseases by Regimen and Simple Medicines*. London: A. Strahan, pp. 666–9.

102 Morineau, M. (1979), 'The potato in the eighteenth century', in R. Forster and O. Ranum (eds), *Food and Drink in History: Selections from the Annales. Economies, Sociétés, Civilisations*. Baltimore and London: Johns Hopkins University Press, p. 24.

103 McNeill, W. (2007), 'Frederick the Great and the propagation of potatoes', in B. Hollinshead and T. Rabb (eds), *I Wish I'd Been There: Twenty Historians Revisit Key Moments in History*. London: PanMacmillan, pp. 176–89, and, McNeill, 'How the potato changed the world's history', 67–83.

104 Zuckerman, L. (1998), *The Potato: How the Humble Spud Rescued the Western World*. New York, NY: North Point Press; Reader, J. (2008), *Propitious Esculent: The Potato in World History*. London: Heinemann; Mann, C. (2011), *1493: How Europe's Discovery of the Americas Revolutionized Trade, Ecology and Life on Earth*. London: Granta, pp. 197–237.

105 Cheyne, *Essay of Health*, pp. 33–4.

106 Pressavin, *L'art de prolonger la vie et de conserver la santé, ou traité d'hygiene*, pp. 111–12.

107 Ferrières, *Sacred Cow*, p. 103.

108 Quellier, F. (2013), *La table des Français: une histoire culturelle (XVe–XIXe siècle)*. Rennes and Tours: Presses Universitaires de Rennes and Presses Universitaires de Tours, pp. 202–7;

Gentilcore, D. (2012), *Italy and the Potato: A History, 1550–2000*. London: Continuum, pp. 65–91.

109 Michiel, P. A. (1940), *I cinque libri di piante*. E. De Toni (ed). Venice: Carlo Ferrari, pp. 175–6 and 227, discussed in Gentilcore, *Pomodoro! A History of the Tomato in Italy*, pp. 11–12.

110 Sebisch, *Alimentorum facultatibus*, pp. 348–9.

111 Ferrières, *Sacred Cow*, p. 93.

112 Gentilcore, *Pomodoro*, pp. 45–68.

113 López Lázaro, 'Sweet food of knowledge', p. 26.

114 Gentilcore, *Pomodoro*, p. 100.

115 Schorger, *Wild Turkey*, pp. 478–9; Lima-Reis, J. P. (2008), 'Da viagem transatlântica do peru e cenas do seu destino'. *Alimentação Humana*, 14:2, 74–6.

116 López Lázaro, 'Sweet food of knowledge', p. 17.

Chapter 8

1   Pisanelli, *Trattato de' cibi et del bere*, p. 216.

2   Josselin, R. (1976), *The Diary of Ralph Josselin, 1616–1683*. A. Macfarlane (ed). Oxford: Oxford University Press, p. 584.

3   Locatelli, *Voyage de France*, p. 167.

4   Lecoutre, M. (2012), 'L'ivresse, un bien traître remède', *Le Point-l'Histoire: Histoire insolite du vin de Bacchus à Pétrus*, September–October, pp. 40–1; Lecoutre, M. (2011), *Ivresse et ivrognerie dans la France moderne*. Tours and Rennes: Presses Universitaires.

5   Martin, A. L. (2003), 'Alcohol and the clergy in traditional Europe', in L. P. Wandel (ed), *History Has Many Voices*. Kirksville MS: Truman State University Press, p. 23.

6   Unger, R. (2004), *Beer in the Middle Ages and the Renaissance*. Philadelphia, PA: University of Pennsylvania Press, pp. 128–32; Meyzie, *L'Alimentation en Europe à l'époque moderne*, pp. 110–11.

7   Moryson, F. (1617), *An Itinerary*. London: John Beale.

8   Cornaro, A. (2014), 'Draft of the letter written to Messer Zan Paolo da Ponte', 1 December 1559, in idem, *Writings on the Sober Life: The Art and Grace of Living Long*. Trans. and ed. H. Fudemoto. Toronto, ON: University of Toronto Press, p. 173.

9   Simon-Muscheid, K. (2007), 'Des vertus de l'eau-de-vie à l'excess de l'alcool (Allemagne/ Alsace, XIIIe–XVIe siècles)', in F. Audoin-Rouzeau and F. Sabban (eds), *Un aliment sain dans un corps sain: perspectives historiques*. Tours: Presses Universitaires François Rabelais, p. 176.

10 Holt, M. (2006), 'Europe divided: wine, beer and the Reformation in sixteenth-century Europe', in idem (ed), *Alcohol: A Social and Cultural History*. Oxford and New York: Berg, p. 33.

11 Camporesi, P. (1998), *Exotic Brew: The Art of Living in the Age of Enlightenment*. Trans. C. Woodall. Cambridge: Polity Press, p. 88.

12 Meyzie, *Alimentation*, p. 98.

13 Le Bègue de Presle, *Conservateur de la santé*, p. 97.

14 Joubert, *The Second Part of the Popular Errors*, p. 27.

15 Redi, F. (1825), *Bacchus in Tuscany (Bacco in Toscana)*. Trans. L. Hunt. London: John Hunt; Redi, F. (1831), *Consulti medici*. L. Martini (ed). Capolago: Tipografia Elvetica.

16 Cheyne, *Essay of Health*, p. 22.

17 Tissot, S. A. (1771 [1770]), *An Essay on the Disorders of People of Fashion*. Trans. F. B. Lee. London: Richardson and Urquhart, p. 90.

18 Redi, *Consulti medici*.

19 Meyzie, *Alimentation*, p. 99.

20 De Ségur, P. (1897), *Le Royaume de la rue Saint-Honoré: Madame Geoffrin et sa fille*. Paris: Calmann Lévy, p. 356.

21 Calaresu, M. (2013), 'Making and eating ice cream in Naples: rethinking consumption and sociability in the eighteenth century'. *Past and Present*, 220, pp. 43–4.

22 Meyzie, *Alimentation*, p. 99.

23 Calaresu, 'Ice cream', pp. 59–60.

24 Baldini, F. (1775), *De' sorbetti: saggio medico-fisico*. Naples: Stamperia Raimondiana.

25 Albala, *Eating Right in the Renaissance*, p. 74.

26 Bacci, A. (1596), *De naturali vinorum historia de vinis Italiae et de conviviis Antiquorum*. Rome: Nicholai Mutii.

27 Martin, A. L. (2001), 'Old people, alcohol and identity in Europe, 1300–1700', in P. Scholliers (ed), *Food, Drink and Identity: Cooking, Eating and Drinking in Europe since the Middle Ages*. Oxford and New York: Berg, 119–37.

28 Elyot, T. (1539 [1534]), *The Castel of Helth*. London: Thomas Berthlet, p. 34.

29 Cornaro, *Writings on the Sober Life*, pp. 22–3, 86.

30 But this only applied to those who had been abstemious until forty, killjoy Trotter added in a footnote, and six daily glasses remained the upper limit however old one got. Trotter, T. (1804), *An Essay, Medical, Philosophical and Chemical, on Drunkenness and Its Effects on the Human Body*. London: Longman, Hurst, Rees and Orme, pp. 156–7.

31 Locatelli, *Voyage de France*, p. 53.

32 Evans, K. (2012), *Colonial Virtue: The Mobility of Temperance in Renaissance England*. Toronto: University of Toronto Press, pp. 39–41.

33 Pardo, G. (1661), *Trattado del vino aguado y agua envinada*. Valladolid: Valdilmelso, p. 2.

34 Archivio di Stato, Rome, *Fondo Spada Veralli*, B.410, 22/7/1657, cit. in Cavallo and Storey, *Healthy Living in Late Renaissance Italy*, p. 212.

35 Fridaevallis, H. (1568), *De tuenda sanitatis*. Antwerp: Christopher Plantin, cit. in Albala, *Eating Right*, p. 121.

36 Quellier, *La table des Français*, pp. 63–4.

37 Ludington, C. (2013), *The Politics of Wine in Britain: A New Cultural History*. New York: Palgrave Macmillan, pp. 46–59.

38 Porter, R. (1985), 'The drinking man's disease: the "pre-history" of alcoholism in Georgian Britain'. *British Journal of Addiction*, 80:4, p. 386.

39 Cheyne, *Essay of Health*, p. 44.

40 Weston, *Medical Consulting by Letter in France, 1665–1789*, p. 180.

41 Fox, L. (ed) (1965), *The Correspondence of the Reverend Joseph Greene: Parson, Schoolmaster and Antiquary*. London: HMSO, p. 136, cit. in Lane, 'The doctor scolds me', p. 218.

42 Sinclair, *Code of Health*, vol. 1, pp. 309–10.

43 Le Paulmier, J. [Palmarius] (1589 [1588]), *Traité du vin et du sidre*. Trans. J. de Cahaignes. Caen: Pierre Le Chandelier.

44 Le Paulmier, *Traité*, p. 40r.

45 Cogan, T. (1584), *The Haven of Health*. London: Henrie Midleton, pp. 224–5.

46 Harrison, W. (1890 [1577]), *Elizabethan England: 'A Description of England'*. London: Walter Scott, p. 35.

47 Schorger, *The Wild Turkey*, pp. 467.

48 Harrison, *Description of England*, p. 102.

49 Cardano, G. (1663), *De usu ciborum liber, Oper omina*. Lyon. vol. 7, p. 53, cit. in Siraisi, *The Clock and the Mirror*, p. 88.

50 Grataroli, G. [Gratarolus] (1565), *De vini natura, artificio et usu deque omni re potabili*. Stasbourg: Theodosius Ribelius, pp. 31–2.

51 Cheyne, *Essay of Health*, p. 31.

52 Brettschneider, J. [Placotomus] (1550), *De tuenda bona valetudine*. Frankfurt: Christ. Egenolph, 'De Cerevisia', pp. 70v.–102r.

53 Unger, *Beer*, p. 151.

54 Hans Folz, *Wem der gebrennt wein schad oder nutz sei und wie er gerecht oder felschlich gemacht sei* (1493), in Arntz, H. (1974), *Weinbrenner: die Geschichte vom Geist der Weines*. Stuttgart: Seewald, pp. 139–41.

55 Simon-Muscheid, 'Vertus', pp. 180–1.

56 Conroy, D. (2006), 'In the public sphere: efforts to curb the consumption of rum in Connecticut, 1760–1820' in M. Holt (ed), *Alcohol: A Social and Cultural History*. Oxford and New York: Berg, p. 45.

57 Buc'hoz, *L'art alimentaire ou methode pour préparer les aliments les plus sains pour l'homme*, pp. 69–71.

58 Le Bègue, *Conservateur de la santé*, p. 118.

59 Sinclair, *Code of Health*, vol. 1, p. 346.

60 Spary, *Eating the Enlightenment*, p. 151.

61 Dubuisson, F.-R.-A. (1779), *L'art du distillateur et marchand de liqueurs considérées comme aliments médicamenteux*. Paris: Dubuisson, vol. 1, p. 24, cit. in Spary, *Eating the Enlightenment*, p. 186.

62 Moore, J. (1781), *A View of Society and Manners in Italy with Anecdotes Relating to Some Eminent Characters*. London: W. Strahan and T. Cadell, vol. 2, p. 129, cit. in Calaresu, 'Ice cream', p. 50.

63 Cheyne, *Essay of Health*, p. 22.

64 Cowan, B. (2005), *The Social Life of Coffee: The Emergence of the British Coffeehouse*. New Haven, CT: Yale University Press, p. 44.

65 Dufour, P. S. (1671), *De l'usage de caphe du thé et du chocolate*. Lyon: Jean Girin and Barthélémy Rivière.

66 De Acosta, *The Naturall and Morall History of the East and West Indies*, p. 271.

67 Norton, *Sacred Gifts*, p. 87.

68 Colmenero de Ledesma, A. (1640 [1631]), *A Curious Treatise of the Nature and Quality of Chocolate*. London: I. Okes, p. 12.

69 De Cárdenas, *Problemas y secretos maravillosos de las Indias*, pp. 140, 143.

70 Forrest, B. and Najjaj, A. (2007), 'Is sipping sin breaking fast? The Catholic controversy and the changing world of early modern Spain'. *Food and Foodways*, 15:1, 37.

71   Norton, *Sacred Gifts*, p. 166.

72   Hernández, F. (1959), *Historia natural, de Nueva España*. Mexico City: Universidad Nacional de México, vol. 1, p. 305, cit. in Norton, *Sacred Gifts*, p. 126.

73   Albala, K. (2007), 'The use and abuse of chocolate in 17th-century medical theory'. *Food and Foodways*, 15:1, p. 54.

74   Norton, *Sacred Gifts*, pp. 234–5; Forrest and Najjaj, 'Sipping sin'.

75   Archivio di Stato, Rome, *Fondo Spada Veralli*, B.618, 9/3/1679, 5/10/1678 and 26/3/1678, cit. in Cavallo and Storey, *Healthy living*, p. 230.

76   Camporesi, *Exotic Brew*, pp. 109–11. The recipe did eventually leak out, but the instructions to add 'a sufficient quantity of fresh jasmine' to ten pounds of chocolate is less than helpful.

77   Dufour, P. S. (1684), *Traitez nouveaux et curieux du café du té et du chocolat*. Lyon: Girin and Rivière, p. 100.

78   Rosee, P. (1652), *The Vertue of the Coffee Drink*. London; and Ellis, M. (2004), 'Pasqua Rosee's coffee-house, 1652–1666'. *London Journal*, 29:1, 1–24.

79   Tryon, *Wisdom's Dictates*, p. 128.

80   Spary, *Eating the Enlightenment*, p. 93.

81   Aignan, *Le prestre medecin*, p. 147.

82   Cowan, *Social Life*, pp. 94, 154.

83   Galanti, G. M. (1792), *Breve descrizione della città di Napoli e del suo contorno*. Naples: Gabinetto Letterario, p. 271, cit. in Calaresu, M. (2005), 'Coffee, culture and consumption: reconstructing the public sphere in late eighteenth-century Naples', in A. Gatti and P. Zanardi (eds), *Filosofia, scienza, storia: il dialogo fra Italia e Gran Bretagna*. Padua: il Poligrafo, p. 163.

84   Horowitz, E. (1989), 'Coffee, coffeehouses, and the nocturnal rituals of early modern Jewry'. *Association for Jewish Studies Review*, 14:1, p. 28.

85   Liberles, R. (2012), *Jews Welcome Coffee: Tradition and Innovation in Early Modern Germany*. Waltham, MA: University Press of New England.

86   Goulin, *Le médecin des dames*, pp. 74–6.

87   Mai, F. A. (1793), *Medicinische Fastenpredigten*. Mannheim, cit. in Bergdolt, *Wellbeing*, pp. 245–6.

88   Schlözer, A. L. (1780), 'Revolutionen in der Diät von Europa seit 300 Jaren', in idem, *Briefweschel meist historischen und politischen Inhalts*. Gottinghen. vol. 7, pp. 93–120, cit. in Liberles, *Jews Welcome Coffee*, pp. 33–4.

89   Delattre, A. (ed) (1950), *Correspondence avec les Tronchin*. Paris: Mercure de France, p. 196, cit. in Spary, *Eating the Enlightenment*, p. 212.

90   Bibliotèque Centrale et Universitaire, Lausanne, *Fonds S-A Tissot*, IS 3784/II/144.03.05.05 and 144.02.03.24, cit. in Spary, *Eating the Enlightenment*, p. 285.

91   Biancolelli, P.-F. and Romagnesi, J.-A. (1730), *La Foire des poètes*. Paris: Briasson, scene II, pp. 13–14.

92   Cowan, *Social Life*, p. 32.

93   Francioni, G. and Romagnoli, S. (eds) (1998), *Il Caffè (1764–1766)*. Turin: Bollati Boringheri, vol. 1, p. 12.

94   Liberles, *Jews Welcome Coffee*, p. 15.

95   Sinclair, *Code of Health*, vol. 1, p. 287.

96   Cheyne, *Essay of Health*, p. 32.

97 Harper, *The Oeconomy of Health: Or, a Medical Essay Containing New and Familiar Instructions for the Attainment of Health, Happiness and Longevity,* pp. 38–9.

98 Camporesi, *Exotic Brew,* p. 83.

99 Spary, *Eating the Enlightenment,* p. 109.

100 Brennan, T. (1984–85), 'Beyond the barriers: popular culture and Parisian *guinguettes'. Eighteenth-Century Studies,* 18: 2, 153–69.

Conclusion

1 Audoin-Rouzeau, F. and Sabban, F. (eds) (2007), *Un aliment sain dans un corps sain: perspectives historiques.* Tours: Presses Universitaires François Rabelais, editors' preface, p. 9.

BIBLIOGRAPHY

Primary Sources

Abraham, N. (1600), *Gouvernement nécessaire à chacun pour vivre longuement en santé*. Paris: Michel Sonnius.

Aignan, F. M. (1696), *Le prestre medecin, ou discours physique sur l'établissement de la medecine. Avec un traité du caffé e du thé de France*. Paris: Laurent D'Houry.

Álvarez de Miraval, B. (1601), *De la conservación de la salud del cuerpo y del alma*. Salamanca: Andres Renaut.

Andry, N. (1713), *Traité des aliments de Caresme*. Paris: Jean-Baptiste Coignard.

Anon. (1561), *Régime de vivre et conservation du corps humain*. Paris: Vincent Sertenas.

Anon. (1607), *Le thresor de santé, ou mesnage de la vie humaine*. Lyon: Jean Ant. Huguetan.

Anon. (1608), *The Englishmans Doctor: Or the Schoole of Salerne, or Physicall Observations for the Perfect Preserving of the Body of Man in Continuall Health*. Trans. J. Harington. London: J. Helme. Available online at: http://user.icx.net/~richmond/rsr/ajax/harington.html.

Anon. (1702), *L'anti-Cornaro ou remarques critiques sur le traité de la vie sobre de Louis Cornaro venitien*. Paris: Claude Barré.

Archer, J. (1673 [1671]), *Every Man His Own Doctor... Shewing How Every One May Know His Own Constitution, the Nature of All Food, What Is Good or Hurtful to Any*. London: Peter Lillicrap for the author.

Audiger. (1692), *La maison reglée et l'art de deriger une maison d'un grand seigneur*. Paris: Nicolas Le Gras.

Bacci, A. (1596), *De naturali vinorum historia de vinis Italiae et de conviviis Antiquorum*. Rome: Nicholai Mutii.

Bacon, F. (1831 [1638]), 'History of life and death', in B. Montagu (ed), *The Works of Francis Bacon*. London: William Pickering, vol. xiv.

Baker, G. (1772), 'The case of Mr Thomas wood, a miller, of Billericay, in the county of Essex... read at the College on September 9, 1767'. *Medical Transactions*, vol. 2, 259–74.

Baldini, F. (1775), *De' sorbetti: saggio medico-fisico*. Naples: Stamperia Raimondiana.

Baley, W. (1588), *A Short Discourse of the Three Kindes of Peppers in Common Use*. London: Eliot's Court Press.

Benedict of Norcia, *The Rule of St Benedict* (1989 [c.530]). Trans. J. McCann. London: Sheed and Ward.

Bernini, D. (1786), *Vita di S. Giuseppe da Copertino sacerdote professo dell'Ordine de' Minori Conventuali di S. Francesco*. Florence: stamperia Bonducciana.

Bertaldi, L. (1620), *Regole della sanità et natura de' cibi di Ugo Benzo senese... arricchite dal sig. Lodovico Bertaldi*. Turin: Gio. Domenico Tarino.

Biancolelli, P.-F. and Romagnesi, J.-A. (1730), *La Foire des poètes*. Paris: Briasson.

Black, W. (1782), *An Historical Sketch of Medicine and Surgery*. London: J. Johnson.

Boorde, A. (1547 [1542]), *Compendyous Regyment of a Dyetary of Helth*. London: Wyllyam Powell.

Boorde, A. (1555), *The Fyrst Boke of the Introduction of Knowledge. The whych Dothe Teache a Man to Speake Parte of all Maner of Languages, and to Knowe the Usage and Fashion of al Maner of Countreys*. London: William Copland.

Brettschneider, J. [Placotomus] (1550), *De tuenda bona valetudine*. Frankfurt: Christian Egenolph.

Bright, T. (1580), *Treatise: Wherein Is Declared the Sufficiencie of English Medicines, for Cure of All Diseases*. London: Henry Midleton.

Bruyérin-Champier, J. (1560), *De re cibaria, libri xxii. Omnium ciborum genera, omium gentium moribus et usu probata complectentes*. Lyon: Sebast. Honoratum. Available online at: http://reader.digitale-sammlungen.de/resolve/display/bsb10191089.html, and in French translation by S. Amundsen (1998), *L'Alimentation de tous les peuples et de tous les temps jusqu'au XVIe siècle*. Paris: Dumas.

Buc'hoz, P. (1783), *L'art alimentaire ou methode pour préparer les aliments les plus sains pour l'homme*. Paris: chez l'auteur.

Buchan, W. (1774 [1769]), *Domestic Medicine: Or, a Treatise on the Prevention and Cure of Diseases by Regimen and Simple Medicines*. London: W. Strahan.

Buchan, W. (1797), 'Observations concerning the diet of the common people, recommending a method of living less expensive, and more conducive to health, than the present', in idem, *Domestic Medicine*. London: A. Strahan, ch. 56, 647–79.

Calanius, P. (1533), *Traicté pour l'entretenement de santé*. Lyon: Temporal

Calderón de la Barca, P. (1983), *Los Guisados (mojiganga)*, in E. Rodríguez and A. Tordera (eds), *Entremeses, jácaras y mojigangas*. Madrid: Castalia, 404–14. Available online at: http://www.cervantesvirtual.com/obra/los-guisados-mojiganga.

Cardano, G. (1580), *Opus novum cunctis de sanitate tuenda*. Rome: Francesco Zanetti.

Cardano, G. (1654 [1576]), *De vita propria liber*. Amsterdam: Johannem Ravesteinium, 1654.

Cardano, G. (1663), *Opera omnia*. Lyon: Huguetan and Ravaut.

Castelvetro, G. (1989 [1614]), *The Fruit, Herbs and Vegetables of Italy*. Trans. and ed. G. Riley. London: Viking/Penguin. Italian original available online at: http://www.liberliber.it/mediateca/libri/c/castelvetro/brieve_racconto_di_tutte_le_radici_etc/pdf/brieve_p.pdf.

Cepari, V. (1762), *Vita di S. Luigi Gonzaga della Compagnia di Gesu*. Roma: Gioacchino Puccinelli.

Cheyne, G. (1725 [1724]), *An Essay of Health and Long Life*. Dublin: George Ewing.

Cocchi, A. (1745 [1743]), *The Pythagorean diet of Vegetables Only Conducive to the Preparation of Health and the Cure of Diseases*. London: R. Dodsley.

Cocchi, A. (1769 [1762]), *The Grand Question: Is Marriage Fit for Literary Men?* Trans. P. Hiffernan. London: S. Bladon.

Cocchi, A. (1791), *Consulti medici*. Bergamo: Vincenzo Antoine.

Cogan, T. (1584), *The Haven of Health Chiefely Gathered for the Comfort of Students, and Consequently of All Those That Have a Care of Their Health*. London: Henrie Midleton.

Coles, W. (1656), *The Art of Simpling: An Introduction to the Knowledge and Gathering of Plants*. London: Nathaniel Brook.

Colmenero de Ledesma, A. (1640), *A Curious Treatise of the Nature and Quality of Chocolate*. London: I. Okes.

Columbus, C. (1971), *Los cuatro viajes del almirante y su testamento*. I. Anzoátegui (ed). Madrid: Espasa.

Cornaro, A. (1634), 'A treatise of temperance and sobrietie', in L. Lessius (ed), *Hygiasticon: Or, the Right Course of Preserving Life and Health unto Extream Old Age*. Cambridge: R. Daniel and T. Buck.

Cornaro, L. [A.] (1558), *Trattato de la vita sobria*. Venice: a San Luca al segno del Diamante.

Cornaro, A. (2014), *Writings on the Sober Life: The Art and Grace of Living Long*. Trans. and ed. H. Fudemoto. Toronto, ON: University of Toronto Press.

Corrado, V. (1786 [1773]), *Il cuoco galante: opera meccanica*. Naples: Stamperia Raimondiana.

Corrado, V. (2001 [1781]), *Del cibo pitagorico ovvero erbaceo per uso de' nobile e de' letterati*. Rome: Donzelli.

Crab, R. (1655), *The English Hermite, or, Wonder of His Age. Being a Relation of the Life of Roger Crab*. London.

Croce, G. C. (1617), *Contrasto del pane di formento e quello di fava per la precedenza*. Bologna: Bartolomeo Cochi. Available online at: http://www.giuliocesarecroce.it/trascrizioni.html.

D'Aulnoy, M.-C. (1705), *Rélation du voyage d'Espagne*. La Haye: Henri van Bulderen.

Da Fonseca Henriques, F. (1731 [1721]), *Âncora medicinal para conservar a vida com saúde*. Lisbon: Miguel Rodrigues.

Da Fonseca, F. (1626), *Regimento pera conservar a saude e vida ... de qualidades do ar, de sitios e mantimentos do termo da cidade de Lisboa*. Lisbon: Geraldo da Vinha.

Dallington, R. (1605), *A Survey of the Great Dukes State of Tuscany, in the Yeare of Our lord 1596*. London: Edward Blount.

De Acosta, J. (1604), *The Naturall and Morall History of the East and West Indies*. Trans. E[dward] G[rimstone]. London: Val. Sims.

De Azara, F. (1846), *Viajes por la América del Sur desde 1789 hasta 1801*. Montevideo: Comercio del Plata.

De Bonnefons, N. (1655), *Les Délices de la campagne suitte du Jardinier françois*. Amsterdam: Raphael Smith.

De Bonnefons, N. (1658 [1651]), *The French Gardiner: Instructing How to Cultivate All Sorts of Fruit-Trees and Herbs for the Garden*. Trans. Philocepos [J. Evelyn]. London: John Crooke.

De Cárdenas, J. (1591), *Problemas y secretos maravillosos de las Indias*. Mexico: Pedro Ocharte.

De Cervantes, M. (1885 [1615]), *Don Quixote of La Mancha*. Trans. J. Ormsby. London: Smith, Elder and Co. Available online at: http://ebooks.adelaide.edu.au/c/cervantes/c41d/index.html.

De Champlain, S. (1922), *The Works of Samuel de Champlain*. H. P. Biggar (ed), Toronto: The Champlain Society.

De los Rios, G. (1777 [1592]), *Agricultura general: que trata de la labranza del campo y sus particularidades, crianza de animales, propriedades de las plantas que en ella se contienen, y virtudes provechosas a la salud humana*. Madrid: Antonio de Sancha.

De Montaigne, M. (1811 [1580]), *The Essays of Michel de Montaigne*. Trans. P. Coste. London: W. Miller, 3 vols.

De Sales, F. (1770 [1619]), *Philothea, or an Introduction to a Devout Life*. London: J. P. Coghlan.

De Serres, O. (1600), *Le théâtre d'agriculture et mésnage des champs*. Paris: Jamet Métayer.

De Thou, J.-A. (1691), *Perroniana et Thuana*. Cologne: G. Scagen.

Delattre, A. (ed) (1950), *Correspondence avec les Tronchin*. Paris: Mercure de France.

Della Porta, G. B. (1658 [1558]), *Natural Magick*. London: Young and Speed.

Du Chesne, J. (1620 [1606]), *Le pourtraict de la santé, où est au vif representée la reigle universelle et particulière de bien sainement et longuement vivre*. Paris: Claude Morel.

Dubois, J. [Sylvius] (1544), *Régime de santé pour les povres, facile à tenir*. Paris: Jacques Gazeau.

Dubois, J. [Sylvius] (1574), *De studiosorum et eorum qui corporis exercitationibus addicti non sunt*. Douai: Joannes Bogardi.

Dubuisson, F.-R.-A. (1779), *L'art du distillateur et marchand de liqueurs considérées comme aliments médicamenteux*. Paris: Dubuisson.

Dufour, P. S. (1671), *De l'usage de caphe du thé et du chocolate*. Lyon: Jean Girin et Barthélémy Rivière

Dufour, S. (1684), *Traitez nouveaux et curieux du café du té et du chocolat*. Lyon: Girin et Rivière.

Durante, C. (1586), *Tesoro della sanità, nel quale si dà il modo di conservar la sanità et prolungar la vita*. Rome: F. Zanetti.

Durante, C. (1686), *A Family-Herbal or the Treasure of Health*. Trans. J. Chamberlayne. London: W. Crooke.

Elyot, T. (1539), *The Castel of Helthe ... Whereby Every Man May Knowe the State of His Owne Body, the Preservation of Helthe, and How to Instruct Well His Phisition in Sicknes, That He Be Not Deceyved*. London: Thomae Bertheleti.

Erasmus, D. (1522), *De interdicto esu carnium ad Christophorum episcopum Basilien. epistola apologetica*.

Bibliography

Erasmus, D. (1964 [1526]), *Concerning the Eating of Fish*, in J. Dolan (ed), *The Essential Erasmus*. New York and London: Mentor, 276–326.

Estienne, C. (1580), *De nutrimentis ad Baillyum*. Paris: Robertus Stephanus.

Estienne, C. and Liébault, J. (1600 [1572]), *Maison rustique, or the countrie farme*. Trans. R. Surflet. London: E. Bollifant.

Evelyn, J. (1699), *Acetaria, a Discourse on Sallets*. London: B. Tooke.

Falconer, W. (1778), *Observations on Some of the Articles of Diet and Regimen Usually Recommended to Valetudinarians*. London: Edward and Charles Dilly.

Fanzago, F. (1815), 'Paralleli tra le pellagra ed alcune malattie che più le rassomigliano (1792)', in idem, *Sulla pellagra: memorie*. Padua: Tipografia del Seminario, 93–202.

Fanzago, F. (1816), *Istruzione catechistica sulla pellagra, divisa in tre dialoghi*. Venice: Francesco Andreola.

Farington, J. (1978–98), *The Diary of Joseph Farington*, K. Garlick and A. Macintyre (eds). New Haven and London: Yale University Press.

Felici, C. (1987 [1572]), 'Del'insalata e piante che in qualunque modo vengono per cibo dell'homo', in Faccioli, E. (ed), *L'arte della cucina in Italia*. Turin: Einaudi, 469–90.

Fioravanti, L. (1570), *Il tesoro della vita humana*. Venice: Eredi di Melchior Sessa.

Flecha, M. (1581), *Las Ensaladas de Flecha*. Prague: Iorge Negrino.

Forster, J. (1664), *Englands Happiness Increased, or a Sure and Easie Remedy against All Succeeding Dear Years, by a Plantation of the Roots Called Potatoes*. London: A. Seile.

Forster, W. (1746), *A Treatise on the Causes of Most Diseases*. London: J. Clarke, G. Hawkins and W. Reeve.

Fox, L. (ed) (1965), *The Correspondence of the Reverend Joseph Greene: Parson, Schoolmaster and Antiquary*. London: HMSO.

Francioni, G. and Romagnoli, S. (eds) (1998), *Il Caffè (1764–1766)*. Turin: Bollati Boringheri.

Fridaevallis, H. (1568), *De tuenda sanitatis*. Antwerp: Christopher Plantin.

Gage, T. (1648), *The English-American, His Travail by Sea and Land: Or, A New Survey of the West-India's*. London: R. Cotes.

Galanti, G. M. (1792), *Breve descrizione della città di Napoli e del suo contorno*. Naples: Gabinetto Letterario.

Galen. (2003), *On the Properties of Foodstuffs*. Trans. and ed. O. Powell. Cambridge: Cambridge University Press.

Gallo, A. (2003 [1569]), *Le vinti giornate dell'agricoltura e dei piaceri della villa*. L. Crosato (ed). Treviso: Canova.

Gallo, A. (2003) [1775]), *Le venti giornate dell'agricoltura e de' piaceri della villa*. Brescia: Giambattista Bossini; photostatic reprint Brescia: Scaglia, 2003.

Gerard, J. (1597), *The Herball, or Generall Historie of Plantes*. London: John Norton.

Gerard, J. (1633), *The Herball or Generall Historie of Plantes... Very Much Enlarged and Emended by Thomas Johnson*. London: Adam Norton and Richard Whitakers.

Gioia, M. (ed) (1977), *Gli scritti di Ignazio di Loyola*. Turin: UTET.

Goulin, J. (1771), *Le médecin des dames, ou l'art de les conserver en santé*. Paris: Vincent.

Goulin, J. (1772), *Le médecin des hommes, depuis la puberté jusqu'à l'extrême vieillesse*. Paris: Vincent.

Graham, J. (1790), *The Guardian of Health, Long-Life and Happiness*. Newcastle upon Tyne: S. Hodgson.

Grataroli, G. [Gratarolus] (1565), *De vini natura, artificio et usu deque omni re potabili*. Strasbourg: Theodosius Ribelius, 1565.

Grataroli, G. [Gratarolus] (1574), *A Direction for the Health of Magistrates and Studentes*. Trans. T. Newton. London: William How.

Green, R. (1951), *A Translation of Galen's 'Hygiene' (De sanitate tuenda)*. Springfield, IL: C. Thomas.

Hammond, J. (1656), *Leah and Rachel: Or, the Two Fruitfull sisters Virginia and Maryland: their Present Condition, Impartially Stated and Related*. London: T. Mabb. Available online at: http://etext.lib.virginia.edu/etcbin/jamestown-browse?id=J1026.

Harper, A. (1785), *The Oeconomy of Health: Or, a Medical Essay Containing New and Familiar Instructions for the Attainment of Health, Happiness and Longevity*. London: C. Stalker.

Harrington, J. (1607), *The Englishmans Doctor: Or the Schoole of Salerne*. London: John Busby.

Harrison, W. (1890 [1577]), *Elizabethan England: 'A Description of England'*. London: Walter Scott.

Hecquet, P. (1710 [1709]), *Traité des dispenses du Carême*. Paris: Francois Fournier.

Heresbach, K. (1578 [1568]), *Foure Bookes of Husbandry*. Trans. B. George. London: John Wight.

Hernández, F. (1658), *Rerum medicarum Novae Hispaniae thesaurus seu plantarum, animalium, mineralium mexicanorum historia*. Rome: Vitale Mascardi. Spanish translation: Hernández, F. (1959), *Historia natural, de Nueva España*. Mexico City: Universidad Nacional de México

Hoffmann, F. (1761), *A Treatise on the Nature of Aliments, or Foods in General*. London: L. Davis and C. Reymer.

Hoffmann, F. (1971 [1695]), *Fundamenta Medicinae*. Trans. L. King. London: Macdonald.

Howell, J. (1642), *Instructions for Forreine Travel*. London: Humphrey Mosley.

Huarte, J. (1594), *Examen de Ingenios, or The Examination of Mens Wits*. Trans. R[ichard] C[arew]. London: Adam Islip.

Hunter, A. (1810 [1804]), *Culina Famulatrix Medicinæ: Or, Receipts in Modern Cookery, with a Medical Commentary*. York: Wilson and Son.

István, M. (1762–64), *Diaetetica, az az, a' jó egészség' meg tartásának modját fundamentomoson elö-ado könyv*. Kolozsvár: István Páldi. Available online at: http://mek.oszk.hu/08500/08581/.

Jefferson, T. (1787), *Notes on the State of Virginia*. London: John Stockdale.

John of Gaddesden. (1314), *Rosa Anglica*. Available online at: http://www.ucc.ie/celt/.

Johnson, S. (1755), *Dictionary of the English language*. London: W. Strahan.

Josselin, R. (1976), *The Diary of Ralph Josselin, 1616–1683*. A. Macfarlane (ed). Oxford: Oxford University Press.

Joubert, L. (1989 [1578]), *Popular Errors*. Trans. G. D. De Rocher. Tuscaloosa, AL: University of Alabama Press.

Joubert, L. (1995 [1578]), *The Second Part of the Popular Errors*. Trans. G. D. De Rocher. Tuscaloosa, AL: University of Alabama Press.

Langton, C. (1547), *A Very Brefe Treatise, Ordrely Declaring the Pri[n]cipal Partes of Phisick*. London: Edward Whitchurch.

Le Bègue de Presle, A. (1763), *Le conservateur de la santé, ou avis sur les dangers qu'il importe à chacun d'éviter, pour se conserver en bonne santé et prolonger sa vie*. Paris: P. Didot.

Lémery, L. (1705), *Traité des aliments*. Paris: Pierre Witte.

Lémery, L. (1706), *A Treatise of Foods in General*. London: Andrew Bell.

Lémery, L. (1745), *A Treatise of All Sorts of Foods, Both Animal and Vegetable: Also of Drinkables*. Trans. D. Hay. London: T. Osborne.

Lémery, L. (1755), *Traité des alimens … augmenté … par Jacques Jean Bruhier*. Paris: Durand.

Le Paulmier, J. [Palmarius] (1589 [1588]), *Traité du vin et du sidre*. Trans. J. de Cahaignes. Caen: Pierre Le Chandelier.

Leys, L. [Lessius] (1634 [1613]), *Hygiasticon: Or the Right Course of Preserving Life and Health unto Extream Old Age*. Trans. G. Herbert. Cambridge: Roger Daniel.

Locatelli, S. (1905), *Voyage de France: moeurs et coutumes françaises (1664–1665)*. Trans. and ed. A. Vautier. Paris: Alphonse Picard.

Lotichius, J. P. (1643), *De casei nequitia, tractatus medico-philologicus novus*. Frankfurt am Main: Johannis Friderici Weissii.

Bibliography

Luther, M. (1961 [1520]), *Address to the nobility of the German nation*, in J. Dillenberger (ed), *Martin Luther: Selections from His Writings*. Garden City, NY: Anchor.

Malvasia, C. C. (1678), *Felsina pittrice. Vite de pittori bolognesi*. Bologna: Barbieri.

Manetti, S. (1759), *Lettera... sopra la malattia, morte e dissezione anatomica del corpo del cadavere di Antonio Cocchi*. Florence: Pietro Gaetano Viviani.

Marmontel, J.-F. (1804), *Œuvres posthumes... Mémoires*. Paris: Xhrouet.

Mason, H. (1627), *Christian Humiliation, or, the Christian's Fast*. London: John Clarke.

Massonio, S. (1628), *Archidipno, overo dell'insalata e dell'uso di essa*. Venice: Marc'Antonio Brogiollo.

Mattioli, P. A. (1544), *Di Pedacio Dioscoride anazarbeo libri cinque. Della historia et materia medicinale tradotti in lingua volgare...* Venice: N. De Bascarini.

Mattioli, P. A. (1570), *Commentarii in sex libros Pedacio Dioscoridis Anazarbei de medica materia*. Venice: ex Officina Valgrisiana.

Mattioli, P. A. (1595), *I discorsi... di Pedacio Dioscoride anazarbeo della materia medicinale*. Venice: Felice Valgrisio.

May, R. (1660), *The Accomplish't Cook, or the Art and Mystery of Cookery*. London: Nathaniel Brooke.

Méndez, G. (1562), *Regimiento de salud*. Salamanca: Pedro de Castro.

Mercier, L.-S. (1994 [1781–88]), *Tableau de Paris*. Paris: Jean-Claude Bonnet.

Mercurio, S. (1645 [1603]), *De gli errori popolari d'Italia*. Verona: Francesco Rossi.

Michiel, P. A. (1940), *I cinque libri di piante*. E. De Toni (ed). Venice: Carlo Ferrari.

Moffett, T. [also Muffett] (1655), *Health's Improvement: Or, Rules Comprizing and Discovering the Nature, Method, and Manner of Preparing All Sorts of Food Used in This Nation*. London: Thomas Newcomb.

Monardes, N. (1577), *Joyfull Newes out of the Newe Founde Worlde: Wherein is Declared the Rare and Singuler Vertues of Diverse and Sundrie Hearbes, Trees, Oyles, Plantes, and Stones, with their Aplications, as well for Phisicke as Chirurgerie*. Trans. J. Frampton. London: William Norton.

Monardes, N. (1885 [1545]), *Sevillana medicina, que trata el modo conservativo y curativo de los que habitan en la muy insigne ciudad de Sevilla*. Seville: Enrico Rasco.

Moore, J. (1781), *A View of Society and Manners in Italy with Anecdotes Relating to Some Eminent Characters*. London: W. Strahan and T. Cadell, 2 vols.

Moryson, F. (1908 [1617]), *The Itinerary of Fynes Moryson*. Glasgow: Robert Maclehose, 4 vols.

Nonnius, L. (1645 [1627]), *Diaeteticon, sive re cibaria*. Antwerp: Petri Belleri.

Nuñez de Oria, F. (1586), *Regimiento y aviso de sanidad*. Medina del Campo: Francisco del Canto.

Paracelsus, T. (1993 [c.1520]), *The Herbarius of Theophrastus [Paracelsus], Concerning the Powers of the Herbs, Roots, Seeds, etc. of the Native Land and Realm of Germany*. Trans. B. Moran, in 'The *Herbarius* of Paracelsus'. *Pharmacy in History*, 35:3, 99–127.

Pardo, G. (1661), *Trattado del vino aguado y agua envinada*. Valladolid: Valdilmelso.

Parkinson, J. (1629), *Paradisi in Paradisus Terrestris: A Garden of All Sorts of Pleasant Flowers Which Our English Ayre Will Permit to Be Noursed Up*. London: Humfrey Lownes and Robert Young.

Paschetti, B. (1602), *Del conservare la sanità et del vivere de' Genovesi*. Genoa: Giuseppe Pavoni.

Paulet, J.-J. (1793), *Traité des champignons*. Paris: Imprimerie nationale exécutive du Louvre, p. 21. Available online at: http://www.biodiversitylibrary.org/bibliography/5417#/summary.

Petronio, A. (1592), *Del vivere delli Romani et del conservare la sanità*. Rome: Domenico Basa.

Pinsonnat, F. [Sieur de la Cour] (1690 [1686]), *Régime de santé pour se procurer une longue vie et une vieillesse heureuse*. Paris: Maurice Villery.

Pisanelli, B. (1589), *Trattato de' cibi et del bere, con molte dotte et belle annotazioni di Francesco Gallina*. Carmagnola: Marc'Antonio Bellone.

Potocki, W. (c.1675–90), *Ogród nie Plewiony i inne wiesze* (c.1675–90). Available online at: http://literat.ug.edu.pl/~literat/potocki/index.htm.

Pressavin, J. B. (1786), *L'art de prolonger la vie et de conserver la santé, ou traité d'hygiene*. Lyon: J. S. Grabit.

Henry VIII. (1518), *Provysion Made by the Kynges Hyghness and His Counsayll for the Puttynge a Parte the Excessive Fare and Redusynge the Same*. London: Richard Pynson.

Pujati, G. A. (1751), *Riflessioni sul vitto pitagorico*. Feltre: Odoardo Foglietta.

Pujati, G. A. (1768), *Della preservazione della salute de' letterati e della gente applicata e sedentaria*. Venice: Antonio Zatta.

Rangoni, T. (1577 [1558]), *Come il serenissimo doge di Vinegia … e li Venetiani possano vivere sempre sani*. Venice: Marco Bindoni.

Rangoni, T. [Philologus] (1533), *De vita hominis ultra cxx annos potrahenda*. Venice: Nicolinus Sabiensis. Available online at: http://reader.digitale-sammlungen.de/resolve/display/bsb10166407.html.

Redi, F. (1825 [1685], *Bacchus in Tuscany (Bacco in Toscana)*. Trans. by Leigh Hunt. London: C. Hunt.

Redi, F. (1831), *Consulti medici*, L. Martini (ed). Capolago: Tipografia Elvetica.

Redman, B. (ed) (1977), *The Portable Voltaire*. Harmondsworth: Penguin.

Relations des Jésuites, 1611–1636. Contenant ce qui s'est passé de plus remarquable dans les missions des Pères de la Compagnie de Jésus dans la Nouvelle-France. (1972 [1858]). Montreal: Éditions du jour, 6 vols.

Rodrigues, D. (1821 [1680]), *Arte de cozinha dividida em quatro partes*. Lisbon: Viuva de Lino da Silva Godinho.

Rodriguez Cardoso, F. (1620), *Tractatus absolutissimus … de sex rebus non naturalibus*. Frankfurt: Paul Jacobi.

Rosee, P. (1652), *The Vertue of the Coffee Drink. First Publiquely Made and Sold in England, by Pasqua Rosee*. London.

Santorio, S. (1676 [1614]), *Medicina Statica, or Rules of Health, in Eight Sections of Aphorisms*. Trans. J. D. London: John Starkey.

Savonarola, M. (1991 [1515]), *Libreto di tutte le cose che se manzano*. Padua: Programma, 2 vols.

Schoock, M. [Schoockius] (1664), *Tractatus de butyro. Accessit ejusdem diatriba de adversatione casei*. Groningen: Johannis Cöllen.

Sebisch, M. [Sebizius] (1650), *De alimentorum facultatibis*. Strasbourg: Joannis Philippi Mülbii et Josiae Stedelii.

Sinclair, J. (1807–08), *The Code of Health and Longevity: Or, a Concise View of the Principles Calculated for the Preservation of Health and the Attainment of Long Life*. Edinburgh: Arch. Constable, 4 vols.

Smith, J. (1986), *The Complete Works of Captain John Smith*, P. Barbour (ed). Chapel Hill, NC: University of North Carolina Press.

Smith, W. (1776), *A Sure Guide in Sickness and Health, in the Choice of Food, and Use of Medicine*. London: J. Bew and J. Walter.

Soderini, G. (1814), *Della coltura degli orti e dei giardini*. Florence: del Giglio.

Sorapán de Rieros, J. (1616), *Medicina española contenida en proverbios vulgares de nuestra lingua*. Madrid: Martin Fernandez Zambrano.

Stefani, B. (2002 [1662]), *L'arte di ben cucinare et instruire i men periti in questa lodevole professione*, in L. Turrini (ed), *La cucina ai tempi dei Gonzaga*. Milan: Rizzoli.

Tanara, V. (1651 [1644]), *L'economia del cittadino in villa*. Rome: Gio. Battista e Giuseppe Corvo.

Thomas, W. (1549), *The Historie of Italy*. London: Thomas Berthelet.

Thomas, W. (1861 [1546]), *The Pilgrim*. J. A. Froude (ed). London: Parker, Son, and Bourne.

Thomson, G. (1675), *Orthomethodos Iatro Chimiche, or the Direct Method of Curing Chymically*. London: B. Billingsley.

Thwaites, R. (ed) (1896–1901), *The Jesuit Relations and Allied Documents*. Cleveland, OH: Burrows Brothers, 73 vols.

Bibliography

Tissot, S. A. (1765 [1761]), *Advice to the People in General, with Regard to Their Health*. Trans. J. Kirkpatrick. London: T. Becket.

Tissot, S. A. (1772 [1768]), *A Treatise on the Diseases Incident to Literary and Sedentary Persons*. Edinburgh: Donaldson. [*Essai sur les maladies des gens du monde*].

Trotter, T. (1804), *An Essay, Medical, Philosophical and Chemical, on Drunkenness and Its Effects on the Human Body*. London: Longman, Hurst, Rees and Orme.

Tryon, T. (1691), *Wisdom's Dictates: Or Aphorisms and Rules, Physical, Moral and Divine ... to Which Is Added a Bille of Fare of Seventy-Five Noble Dishes of Excellent Food*. London: Thomas Salisbury.

Tryon, T. (1700), *Tryon's Letters, Domestic and Foreign, to Several Persons of Quality*. London: Geo. Conyers.

Turler, J. (1575), *The Traveiler*. London: William How.

Valverda, J. (1552), *De animi et corporis sanitate tuenda libellus*. Paris: Carolus Stephanus.

Van den Berghe, A. [Montanus] (1662), *Diatriba de esu carnium et quadragesima pontificiorum*. Amsterdam: Aegidius Valkenier.

Van Helmont, J. B. (1662), *Oriatrike, or, Physick Refined*. Trans. J. Chandler. London: Lodowick Loyd.

Venette, N. (1683), *L'art de tailler des arbres fruitiers, avec ... un traité de l'usage des fruits des arbres pour se conserver en santé ou pour se guérir lorsqu'on est malade*. Paris: Charles de Sercy.

Venner, T. (1620), *Via Recta ad Vitam Longam, or A Plaine Philosophical Discourse of the Nature, Faculties, and Effects, of All Such Things, as by Way of Nourishments, and Dieteticall Obseruations, Make for the Preservation of Health*. London: Edward Griffin.

Verri, P. (1947), 'Articoli tratti dal "Caffè"', in idem, N. Valeri (eds), *Opere varie*. Florence: Le Monnier, vol. 1.

Vigilio, G. B. (1992), *La Insalata: cronaca mantovana dal 1561 al 1602*. D. Ferrari and C. Mozzarelli (eds). Mantua: Arcari.

Wesley, J. (1880 [1747]), *Primitive Physic*. Chicago, IL: O.W. Gordon.

Wesley, J. (1975–), *The Works of John Wesley*. Oxford: Clarendon Press.

Young, A. (1792), *Travels, During the Years 1787, 1788, and 1789, Undertaken More Particularly with a View of Ascertaining the Cultivation, Wealth, Resources, and National Prosperity, of the Kingdom of France*. London: W. Richardson.

Zacchia, P. (1636), *Il vitto quaresimale ... ove insegnasi come senza offender la sanità si possa viver nella Quaresima*. Rome: Pietro Antonio Facciotti.

Secondary Sources

Abad, R. (1999), 'Un indice de déchristianisation? L'évolution de la consommation de viande à Paris en carême sous l'Ancien Régime'. *Revue historique*, CCCI:2, 237–75.

Ackerknecht, E. (1973), *Therapeutics: From the Primitives to the Twentieth Century, with an Appendix History of Dietetics*. London: Collier-Macmillan.

Albala, K. (2002), *Eating Right in the Renaissance*. Berkeley, CA: University of California Press.

Albala, K. (2002/3), 'Insensible perspiration and oily vegetable humor: an eighteenth-century controversy over vegetarianism'. *Gastronomica: The Journal of Food and Culture*, 2:3, 29–36 and 3:1, 2–5.

Albala, K. (2003), *Food in Early Modern Europe*. Westport, CT: Greenwood Press.

Albala, K. (2006), 'To your health: wine as food and medicine in mid-sixteenth-century Italy', in M. Holt (ed), *Alcohol: A Social and Cultural History*. Oxford and New York: Berg, 11–23.

Albala, K. (2007), 'The use and abuse of chocolate in 17th-century medical theory'. *Food and Foodways*, 15:1, 53–74.

Albala, K. (2007), *Beans: A History*. Oxford: Berg.

Albala, K. (2007), *The Banquet: Dining in the Great Courts of Late Renaissance Europe*. Urbana, IL: University of Illinois Press.

Andrews, J. (1992), 'The peripatetic chili pepper: diffusion of the domesticated capsicums since Columbus', in N. Foster and L. Cordell (eds), *From Chilies to Chocolate: Food the Americas Gave the World*. Tucson, AR: University of Arizona Press, 81–93.

Androutsos, G. (2006), 'Nicolas Venette (1633–1698): premier sexologue français et grand pionnier en matière de lithiase urinaire'. *Andrologie*, 16:2, 160–7.

Apperson, G. (2006), *The Wordsworth Dictionary of Proverbs*. Ware: Wordsworth.

Arntz, H. (1974), *Weinbrenner: die Geschichte vom Geist der Weines*. Stuttgart: Seewald.

Audoin-Rouzeau, F. and Sabban, F. (eds) (2007), *Un aliment sain dans un corps sain: perspectives historiques*. Tours: Presses Universitaires François Rabelais.

Baldini, U. (1982), 'Cocchi, Antonio', in *Dizionario biografico degli Italiani*. Rome: Treccani, vol. 26. Available online at: http://www.treccani.it/enciclopedia/antonio-cocchi_%28Dizionario -Biografico%29/.

Bell, R. (1987), *Holy Anorexia*. Chicago, IL: University of Chicago Press.

Bergdolt, K. (2008), *Wellbeing: A Cultural History of Healthy Living*. Trans. J. Dewhurst. Cambridge: Polity Press.

Blake, J. (ed) (1942), *Europeans in West Africa, 1450–1560*. London: The Hakluyt Society.

Braudel, F. (1972), *The Mediterranean and the Mediterranean World in the Age of Philip II*. Trans. S. Reynolds. London: William Collins, 2 vols.

Braudel, F. (1981), *The Structures of Everyday Life: The Limits of the Possible*. Trans. S. Reynolds. London: William Collins.

Brennan, T. (1984–85), 'Beyond the barriers: popular culture and Parisian *guinguettes*'. *Eighteenth-Century Studies*, 18:2, 153–69.

Bruegel, M., J.-M. Chevet and S. Lecocq (2014), 'Animal protein and rational choice: diet in the eighteenth century', *Journal of Interdisciplinary History*, 44:4, 427–52.

Brockliss, L. (1989), 'The medico-religious universe of an early eighteenth-century Parisian doctor: the case of Philippe Hacquet', in R. French and A. Wear (eds), *The Medical Revolution of the Seventeenth Century*. Cambridge: Cambridge University Press, 191–221.

Brown, A. (1890), *The Genesis of the United States: A Narrative of the Movement in England, 1605–1616, Which Resulted in the Plantation of North America by Englishmen*. Boston: Houghton, Mifflin and Co.

Burke, P. (2012), 'Cultural history and its neighbours'. *Culture & History: Digital Journal*, 1:1. Available online at: http://dx.doi.org/10.3989/chdj.2012.006.

Calaresu, M. (2005), 'Coffee, culture and consumption: reconstructing the public sphere in late eighteenth-century Naples', in A. Gatti and P. Zanardi (eds), *Filosofia, scienza, storia: il dialogo fra Italia e Gran Bretagna*. Padua: il Poligrafo, 135–73.

Calaresu, M. (2013), 'Making and eating ice cream in Naples: rethinking consumption and sociability in the eighteenth century'. *Past and Present*, 220, 35–78.

Camporesi, P. (1989), *Bread of Dreams: Food and Fantasy in Early Modern Europe*. Trans. D. Gentilcore. Cambridge: Polity Press.

Camporesi, P. (1995), *La terra e la luna: alimentazione, folclore, società*. Milan: Garzanti.

Camporesi, P. (1998), *Exotic Brew: The Art of Living in the Age of Enlightenment*. Trans C. Woodall. Cambridge: Polity Press.

Capone, P. (2005), *L'arte del vivere sano. Il 'Regimen Sanitatis Salernitanum' e l'età moderna*. Milan: Guerini e Associati.

Carbonelli, G. (ed) (1906), *Il 'De sanitatis custodia' di maestro Giacomo Albini di Moncalieri: con altri documenti sulla storia della medicina negli stati sabaudi nei secoli XIV e XV*. Pinerolo: Tip. Sociale.

Bibliography

Carrington, J. (2000), 'Rangoni, Tommaso, Italian physician, philologist and patron', in J. Turner (ed), *Encyclopedia of Italian Renaissance and Mannerist Art*. London and New York: Macmillan, Grove's Dictionaries, vol. 2, 1315–16.

Cavallo, S. and Storey, T. (2013), *Healthy Living in Late Renaissance Italy*. Oxford: Oxford University Press.

Céard, J. (1982), 'La diététique dans la médecine de la Renaissance', in J.-C. Margolin and R. Sauzet (eds), *Pratiques et discours alimentaires à la Renaissance: actes du colloque de Tours 1979*. Paris: Maisonneuve et Larose, 21–36.

Chambers, D., Fletcher, J. and Pullan, B. (eds) (1992), *Venice: A Documentary History, 1450–1630*. Oxford: Blackwell.

Chen, N. (2009), *Food, Medicine, and the Quest for Good Health: Nutrition, Medicine, and Culture*. New York, NY: Columbia University Press.

Claflin, K. (2012), 'Food among the historians: early modern Europe', in K. Claflin and P. Scholliers (eds), *Writing Food History: A Global Perspective*. London and New York: Berg, 38–58.

Coe, S. (1994), *America's First Cuisines*. Austin, TX: University of Texas Press.

Coleman, W. (1974), 'Health and hygiene in the *Encyclopédie*: a medical doctrine for the bourgeosie'. *Journal of the History of Medicine and Allied Sciences*, 29, 399–421.

Collingham, L. (2006), *Curry: A Tale of Cooks and Conquerors*. London: Vintage.

Conlin, J. (1977), 'Another side to William Byrd of Westover: an explanation of the food in his secret diaries'. *Virginia Cavalcade*, 26:3, 124–33.

Connell, K. H. (1962), 'The potato in Ireland'. *Past and Present*, 23, 57–71.

Conroy, D. (2006), 'In the public sphere: efforts to curb the consumption of rum in Connecticut, 1760–1820', in M. Holt (ed), *Alcohol: A Social and Cultural History*. Oxford and New York: Berg, 41–60.

Cook, H. (2007), *Matters of Exchange: Commerce, Medicine and Science in the Dutch Golden Age*. New Haven, CT: Yale University Press.

Cooper, A. (2007), *Inventing the Indigenous: Local Knowledge and Natural History in Early Modern Europe*. Cambridge: Cambridge University Press.

Cowan, B. (2005), *The Social Life of Coffee: The Emergence of the British Coffeehouse*. New Haven, CT: Yale University Press.

Crignon-De Oliveira, C. (2011), 'Peut-on vieillir sans médecins? La réponse des auteurs de régimes de santé ou «conseils pour vivre longtemps» aux xviie et xviiie siècles'. *Astérion*. Available online at: http://asterion.revues.org/2018.

Crosby, A. (1972), *The Columbian Exchange: Biological and Cultural Consequences of 1492*. Westport, CT: Greenwood Press.

Dacome, L. (2005), 'Useless and pernicious matter: corpulence in eighteenth-century England', in C. Forth and A. Carden-Coyne (eds), *Cultures of the Abdomen: Diet, Digestion and Fat in the Modern World*. Houndmills: Palgrave Macmillan, 185–204.

Darrow, G. (1966), *The Strawberry: History, Breeding and Physiology*. New York: Holt, Rinehart and Winston.

De Castro, T. (2002), 'L'émergence d'une identité alimentaire. Musulmans et chrétiens dans le royaume de Granade', in M. Bruegel and B. Laurioux (eds), *Histoire et identités alimentaires en Europe*. Paris: Hachette, 199–215.

De Ruble, A. (1877), *Le mariage de Jeanne d'Albret*. Paris: Labitte, p. 7. Available online at: http://www.mediterranee-antique.info/Fichiers_PdF/PQRS/Ruble/Mariage_J_Albret.pdf.

De Ségur, P. (1897), *Le Royaume de la rue Saint-Honoré: Madame Geoffrin et sa fille*. Paris: Calmann Lévy.

Dickenson, V. (2008), 'Cartier, Champlain and the fruits of the New World: botanical exchange in the 16th and 17th centuries'. *Scientia Canadensis: Canadian Journal of the History of*

Science, Technology and Medicine/Scientia Canadensis: revue canadienne d'histoire des sciences, des techniques et de la médecine, 31:1–2, 27–47.

Dupèbe, J. (1982), 'La diététique et l'alimentation des pauvres selon Sylvius', in J.-C. Margolin and R. Sauzet (eds), *Pratiques et discours alimentaires à la Renaissance: actes du colloque de Tours 1979*. Paris: Maisonneuve et Larose, 41–56.

Earle, R. (2012), *The Body of the Conquistador: Food, Race and the Colonial Experience in Spanish America, 1492–1700*. Cambridge: Cambridge University Press.

Eden, T. (2008), *The Early American Table: Food and Society in the New World*. DeKalb, IL: Northern Illinois University Press.

Eiche, S. (2004), *Presenting the Turkey: The Fabulous Story of a Flamboyant and Flavourful Bird*. Florence: Centro Di.

Ellis, M. (2004), 'Pasqua Rosee's Coffee-House, 1652-1666'. *London Journal*, 29:1, 1–24.

Emch-Dériaz, A. (1992), 'The non-naturals made easy', in R. Porter (ed), *The Popularization of Medicine, 1650–1850*. London: Routledge, 134–59.

Ercolani, G. L. (2001), *Il pane dei santi. Storia e curiosità sull'alimentazione dei santi*. Lugano: Todaro.

Estes, J. W. (1996), 'The medical properties of food in the eighteenth century'. *Journal of the History of Medicine and Allied Sciences*, 51, 127–54.

Evans, K. (2012), *Colonial Virtue: The Mobility of Temperance in Renaissance England*. Toronto: University of Toronto Press.

Fara, P. (2004), *Pandora's Breeches: Women, Science and Power in the Enlightenment*. London: Pimlico.

Ferrières, M. (2006), *Sacred Cow, Mad Cow: A History of Food Fears*. Trans. J. Gladding. New York, NY: Columbia Univesity Press

Ferrières, M. (2007), *Nourritures canailles*. Paris: Seuil.

Finan, J. (1950), *Maize in the Great Herbals*. Waltham, MA: Chronica Botanica.

Findlen, P. (1995), 'Translating the New Science: women and the circulation of knowledge in Enlightenment Italy'. *Configurations*, 3:2, 167–206.

Finzi, R. (2009), '*Sazia assai ma dà poco fiato': il mais nell'economia e nella vita rurale italiane, secoli XVI–XIX*. Bologna: CLUEB.

Fissell, M. (2007), 'The marketplace of print', in M. Jenner and P. Wallis (eds), *Medicine and the Market in England and its Colonies, c. 1450–c. 1850*. Houndmills: Palgrave Macmillan, 108–32.

Flandrin, J.-L. (1999), 'Dietary choices and culinary technique, 1500–1800', in J.-L. Flandrin and M. Montanari (eds), *Food: A Culinary History*. New York, NY: Columbia University Press, 403–17.

Flandrin, J.-L. (1999), 'From dietetics to gastronomy, the liberation of the gourmet', in J.-L. Flandrin and M. Montanari (eds), *Food: A Culinary History*. New York, NY: Columbia University Press, 418–33.

Flandrin, J.-L. (2007), *Arranging the Meal: A History of Table Service in France*. Trans. J. Jonshon. Berkeley, CA: University of California Press.

Fleischer, M. (1981), 'The first German agricultural manuals'. *Agricultural History*, 55:1, 1–15.

Food & History, 10:2 (2012), Special issue: 'Studia alimentorum 2003–2013. Une décennie de recherche/A Decade of Research'.

Forrest. B. and Najjaj, A. (2007), 'Is sipping sin breaking fast? The Catholic controversy and the changing world of early modern Spain'. *Food and Foodways*, 15:1, 31–52.

Galinier-Pallerola, J.-F. (2005), 'La gourmandise: péché capitale ou vertu mondaine? Le discours sur le goût en France au XVIIIe siècle', in A.-M. Cocula and J. Pontet (eds), *Au contact des Lumières. Mélanges offerts à Philippe Loupès*. Bordeaux: Presses Universitaires de Bordeaux, 129–38.

García Guerra, D. and Álvarez Antuña, V. (1993), *Lepra Asturiensis: la contribución asturiana en la historia de la pelagra (siglos XVIII y XIX)*. Madrid: CSIC.

Bibliography

García-Ballester, L. (1993), 'On the origin of the six non-natural things in Galen', in J. Kollesch and D. Nickel (eds), *Galen und das hellenistische Erbe*. Stuttgart: Steiner, 105–15.

Gasparini, D. (2002), *Polenta e formenton: il mais nelle campagne venete tra XVI e XX secolo*. Verona: Cierre.

Gentilcore, D. (2010), 'The *Levitico*, or how to feed a hundred Jesuits'. *Food & History*, 8, 87–120.

Gentilcore, D. (2010), *Pomodoro! A History of the Tomato in Italy*. New York, NY: Columbia University Press.

Gentilcore, D. (2011), 'Body and soul, or "living physically" in the kitchen', in B. Kumin (ed), *A Cultural History of Food*, vol. 4, *The Early Modern Age*. Oxford: Berg, 143–64.

Gentilcore, D. (2012), *Italy and the Potato: A History, 1550–2000*. London: Continuum.

Gentilcore, D. (2013), ' "Italic scurvy", "pellarina", "pellagra": medical reactions to a new disease in Italy, 1770–1830', in J. Reinarz and K. Siena (eds), *A Medical History of Skin: Scratching the Surface*. London: Pickering and Chatto, 57–69.

Giacomotto-Charra, V. (2012), 'Un médecin géographe: voyages, chorographie et médecine pratique dans *Le pourtraict de la santé* de Joseph Du Chesne'. *Camenæ*, 14. Available online at: http://www.paris-sorbonne.fr/article/camenae-14.

Giannetti, L. (2010), 'Italian food-fashioning, or the triumph of greens'. *California Italian Studies Journal*, 1:2, 1–16. Available online at: http://escholarship.org/uc/item/1n97s00d.

Gil, J. (2009), 'Berenjeneros: the aubergine-eaters', in K. Ingram (ed), *The Conversos and Moriscos in Late Medieval Spain and Beyond*, vol. 1, *Departures and Change*. Leiden: Brill, 125–42.

Grafe, R. (2012), *Distant Tyranny: Markets, Power and Backwardness in Spain, 1650–1800*. Princeton, NJ: Princeton University Press.

Green, M. (2009), 'The sources of Eucharius Rösslin's "Rosegarden for Pregnant Women and Midwives" (1513)', *Medical History*, 53:2, 167–92.

Greenblatt, S. (1991), *Marvelous Posession: The Wonder of the New World*. Chicago, IL: University of Chicago Press.

Grieco, A. (1991), 'The social politics of pre-Linnaean botanical classification', *I Tatti Studies*, 4, 131–49.

Grumett, D. and Muers, R. (2010), *Theology on the Menu: Asceticism, Meat and Christian Diet*. London: Routledge.

Guerrini, A. (2000), *Obesity and Depression in the Enlightenment: The Life and Times of George Cheyne*. Norman, OK: University of Oklahoma Press.

Gullino, G. (1983), 'Corner, Alvise', in *Dizionario biografico degli Italiani*. Rome: Treccani, vol. 29. Available online at: http://www.treccani.it/enciclopedia/alvise-corner_(Dizionario -Biografico)/.

Guptill, A., Copelton, D. and Lucal, B. (2013), *Food and Society: Principles and Paradoxes*. Cambridge: Polity Press, 2013.

Hand-Meacham, S. (2003), 'They will be adjudged by their drink, what kinde of housewives they are: gender, technology and household cidering in England and the Chesapeake, 1690–1760'. *The Virginia Magazine of History and Biography*, 111:2, 117–50.

Holt, M. (2006), 'Europe divided: wine, beer and the Reformation in sixteenth-century Europe', in M. Holt (ed), *Alcohol: A Social and Cultural History*. Oxford and New York: Berg, 25–40.

Horowitz, E. (1989), 'Coffee, coffeehouses, and the nocturnal rituals of early modern Jewry'. *Association for Jewish Studies Review*, 14:1, 17–46.

Houston, A. (2008), *Benjamin Franklin and the Politics of Improvement*. New Haven, CT: Yale University Press.

Hurren, E. (2013), 'Cultures of the body, medical regimen, and physic at the Tudor court', in T. Betteridge and S. Lipscomb (eds), *Henry VIII and the Court: Art, Politics and Performance*. Farnham: Ashgate, 65–89.

Jamieson, R. (2001), 'The essence of commodification: caffeine dependencies in the early modern world'. *Journal of Social History*, 35:2, 269–94.

Janick, J. and Caneva, G. (2005), 'The first images of maize in Europe'. *Maydica*, 50, 71–80.

Jarcho, S. (1970), 'Galen's six non-naturals'. *Bulletin of the History of Medicine*, 44, 372–7.

Jeanneret, M. (2007), 'Ma salade et ma muse', in T. Tomasik and J. Vitullo (eds), *At the Table: Metaphorical and Material Cultures of Food in Medieval and Early Modern Europe*. Turnhout: Brepols, 211–20.

Johnson, C. (2008), *The German Discovery of the World: Renaissance Encounters with the Strange and Marvelous*. Charlottesville VA: University of Virginia Press.

Jordanova, L. (1993), 'Has the social history of medicine come of age?'. *The Historical Journal*, 36, 437–49.

Jordanova, L. (1995), 'The social construction of medical knowledge'. *Social History of Medicine*, 8, 361–81.

Kaplan, L. and Kaplan, L. (2007), 'Beans of the Americas', in N. Foster and L. Cordell (eds), *From Chilies to Chocolate: Food the Americas Gave the World*. Tucson, AR: University of Arizona Press, 61–79.

Keating, J. and Markey, L. (2011), ' "Indian" objects in Medici and Austrian-Hapsburg inventories: a case study of the sixteenth-century term'. *Journal of the History of Collections*, 23:2, 283–300.

Killerby, C. (2002), *Sumptuary Law in Italy, 1200–1500*. Oxford: Oxford University Press.

Knoeff, R. (1997), 'Practicing chemistry "after the Hippocratical manner": Hippocrates and the importance of chemistry in Boerhaave's medicine', in L. Principe (ed), *New Narratives in Eighteenth-Century Chemistry*. Dordrecht: Springer, 63–76.

La France, R. (2013), 'Bronzino and his friends: the Medici-Toledo tapestries', in Gáldy, A. (ed), *Agnolo Bronzino: Medici Court Artist in Context*. Newcastle upon Tyne: Cambridge Scholars, 2013), 67–80.

LaCombe, M. (2012), *Political Gastronomy: Food and Authority in the English Atlantic world*. Philadelphia, PE: University of Pennsylvania Press.

Lane, J. (1985), ' "The doctor scolds me": the diaries and correspondence of patients in eighteenth century England', in R. Porter (ed), *Patients and Practitioners: Lay Perceptions of Medicine in Pre-Industrial Society*. Cambridge: Cambridge University Press, 205–48.

Lang, G. (1990 [1971]), *The Cuisine of Hungary*. NewYork, NY: Bonanza Books, 1990.

Laudan, R. and Pilcher, J. (1999), 'Chilies, chocolate and race in New Spain: glancing backward to Spain or looking forward to Mexico'. *Eighteenth-Century Life*, 24, 59–70.

Le Roy Ladurie, E. (1966), *Les paysans de Languedoc*. Paris: SEVPEN, two vols. English translation (abridged): Le Roy Ladurie, E. (1976), *The Peasants of Languedoc*. Trans. J. Day. Urbana, IL: University of Illinois Press.

Le Roy Ladurie, E. (1987), *The French Peasantry, 1450–1660*. Trans. A. Sheridan. Aldershot: Scolar.

Lecoutre, M. (2011), *Ivresse et ivrognerie dans la France moderne*. Tours and Rennes: Presses Universitaires.

Lecoutre, M. (2012), 'L'ivresse, un bien traître remède', *Le Point-l'Histoire: Histoire insolite du vin de Bacchus à Pétrus*, September–October, p. 40–1.

Lemasson, J.-P. (2011), *L'incroyable odyssée de la tourtière*. Montréal: Del Busso.

Liberles, R. (2012), *Jews Welcome Coffee: Tradition and Innovation in Early Modern Germany*. Waltham, MA: University Press of New England.

Lima-Reis, J. P. (2008), 'Da viagem transatlântica do peru e cenas do seu destino'. *Alimentação Humana*, 14:2, 74–6.

Livi-Bacci, M. (1991), *Population and Nutrition: An Essay on European Demographic History*. Trans. T. Croft-Murray. Cambridge: Cambridge University Press.

Lloyd, P. (2012), 'Dietary advice and fruit-eating in late Tudor and early Stuart England'. *Journal of the History of Medicine and Allied Sciences*, 67:4, 553–86.

Bibliography

López Lázaro, F. (2007), 'Sweet food of knowledge: botany, food and empire in the early modern Spanish kingdoms', in J. Vitullo and T. Tomasik (eds), *At the Table: Metaphorical and Material Cultures in Medieval and Early Modern Europe*. Turnhout: Brepols, 3–28.

Loring Bailey, S. (1880), *Historical Sketches of Andover*. Boston: Houghton, Mifflin and Co.

Ludington, C. (2013), *The Politics of Wine in Britain: A New Cultural History*. New York, NY: Palgrave Macmillan.

Malacarne, G. (2001), *Sulla mensa del principe: alimentazione e banchetti alla corte dei Gonzaga*. Modena: il Bulino.

Mann, C. (2011), *1493: How Europe's Discovery of the Americas Revolutionized Trade, Ecology and Life on Earth*. London: Granta.

Martin, A. L. (2001), *Alcohol, Sex, and Gender in Late Medieval and Early Modern Europe*. New York, NY: Palgrave Macmillan.

Martin, A. L. (2001), 'Old people, alcohol and identity in Europe, 1300–1700', in P. Scholliers (ed), *Food, Drink and Identity: Cooking, Eating and Drinking in Europe since the Middle Ages*. Oxford and New York: Berg, 119–37.

Martin, M. (2005), 'Doctoring beauty: the control of women's *toilettes* in France, 1750–1820'. *Medical History*, 49, 353–68.

McNeill, W. (2007), 'Frederick the Great and the propagation of potatoes', in B. Hollinshead and T. Rabb (eds), *I Wish I'd Been There: Twenty Historians Revisit Key Moments in History*. London: PanMacmillan, 176–89.

McNeill, W. (1999), 'How the potato changed the world's history', *Social Research*, 66, 67–83.

Meyzie, P. (2010), *L'alimentation en Europe à l'époque moderne: manger et boire, XIVe siècle–XIXe siècle*. Paris: Armand Colin.

Mikkeli, H. (1999), *Hygiene in the Early Modern Medical Tradition*. Helsinki: Academia Scientiarum Fennica.

Milani, M. (2014), 'Introduction to Cornaro', in Cornaro, A. (ed), *Writings on the Sober Life: The Art and Grace of Living Long*. Trans. and ed. H. Fudemoto. Toronto, ON: University of Toronto Press, 3–69.

Millones Figueroa, L. (2010), 'The staff of life: wheat and "Indian bread" in the New World'. *Colonial Latin American Review*, 19:2, 301–22.

Montanari, M. (2008), *L'Europa a tavola. Storia dell'alimentazione dal Medioevo a oggi*. Rome: Laterza.

Montanari, M. (2012), 'Civiltà del vino', in idem, *Gusti del Medioevo: i prodotti, la cucina, la tavola*. Rome-Bari: Laterza, 155–82.

Montenach, A. (2001), 'Esquisse d'une économie de l'illicite. Le marché parallèle de la viande à Lyon pendant le Carême (1658–1714)'. *Crime, histoire et société/Crime, History and Societies*, 5:1, 7–25.

Montenach, A. (2011), 'Formal and informal economy in an urban context: the case of food trade in seventeenth-century Lyon', in T. Buchner and P. R. Hoffmann-Rehnitz (eds), *Shadow Economies and Irregular Work in Urban Europe, 16th to Early 20th Centuries*. Vienna: Verlag, 91–106.

Mood, F. (1937), 'John Winthrop, Jr., on Indian corn'. *The New England Quarterly*, 10:1, 123–33.

Moran, B. (1993), 'The *Herbarius* of Paracelsus'. *Pharmacy in History*, 35:3, 99–127.

Morineau, M. (1979), 'The potato in the eighteenth century', in R. Forster and O. Ranum (eds), *Food and Drink in History: Selections from the Annales. Economies, Sociétés, Civilisations*. Baltimore and London: Johns Hopkins University Press, 17–36.

Moyer, J. (2013), '"The food police": sumptuary prohibitions on food in the Reformation', in K. Albala and T. Eden (eds), *Food and Faith in Christian Culture*. New York, NY: Columbia University Press, 59–81.

Nadeau, C. (2005), 'Spanish culinary history in Cervantes' "Bodas de Camacho"'. *Revista Canadiense de Estudios Hispánicos*, 29:2, 347–61.

Natale, A. (2011), 'Formaggi', in G. M. Anselmi and G. Ruozzi (eds), *Banchetti letterari: cibi, pietanze e ricette nella letteratura italiana da Dante a Camilleri*. Rome: Carocci, 181–9.

Nestle, M. (2007), *Food Politics: How the Food Industry Influences Nutrition and Health*. Berkeley, CA: University of California Press.

Neves Abreu, J. L. (2010), 'Higiene e conservação da saúde no pensamento médico luso-brasileiro do século XVIII'. *Asclepio: Revista de Historia de la Medicina y de la Ciencia*, 62, 225–50.

Newton, H. (2012), *The Sick Child in Early Modern England, 1580–1720*. Oxford: Oxford University Press.

Nicoud, M. (2007), *Les régimes de santé au moyen âge*. Rome: École Française de Rome, two vols.

Nicoud, M. (2013), 'I *regimina sanitatis*: un genere medico tra salute, prevenzione e terapia', in M. Conforti, A. Carlino and A. Clericuzio (eds), *Interpretare e curare. Medicine e salute nel Rinascimento*. Rome: Carocci, 43–54.

Niebyl, P. H. (1971), 'The non-naturals'. *Bulletin of the History of Medicine*, 45, 486–92.

Norton, M. (2006), 'Tasting empire: chocolate and the European internalization of Mesoamerican aesthetics'. *The American Historical Review*, 111:3, 660–91.

Norton, M. (2008), *Sacred Gifts, Profane Pleasures: A History of Tobacco and Chocolate in the Atlantic World*. Ithaca, NY: Cornell University Press.

O'Reilly, W. (2009), 'Last chances of the House of Hapsburg'. *Austrian History Yearbook*, 40, 53–70.

O'Riordan, T. (2001), 'The introduction of the potato into Ireland'. *History Ireland*, 9:1. Available online at: http://www.historyireland.com/early-modern-history-1500-1700/the-introduction-of-the-potato-into-ireland/.

Olsen, T. (2003), 'Poisoned figs and Italian sallets: nation, diet and the early modern English traveler'. *Annali d'Italianistica*, 21, 233–53.

Pahta, P. and Ratia, M. (2010), 'Treatises on specific topics', in I. Taavitsainen and P. Pahta (eds), *Early Modern English Medical Texts: Corpus Description and Studies*. Amsterdam and Philadelphia: John Benjamins, 73–99.

Palmer, R. (1991), 'Health, hygiene and longevity in Medieval and Renaissance Europe', in Y. Kawakita, S. Sakai and Y. Otsuka (eds), *History of Hygiene*. Tokyo: Ishiyaku EuroAmerica, 75–98.

Pardo-Tomás, J. (2011), 'Natural knowledge and medical remedies in the book of secrets: uses and appropriations in Juan de Cárdenas' *Problemas y secretos maravillosos de las Indias* (Mexico, 1591)', in S. Anagnostou, F. Egmond and C. Friedrich (eds), *Passion for Plants: Materia Medica and Botany in Scientific Networks from the 16th to 18th Centuries*. Stuttgart: Wissenschafliche Verlagsgesellschaft, 93–108.

Pardo-Tomás, J. and Martínez-Vidal, A. (2008), 'Stories of disease written by patients and lay mediators in the Spanish republic of letters (1680–1720)'. *Journal of Medieval and Early Modern Studies*, 38:3, 467–92.

Past, E. (2011),'Una ricetta per *longo* e *iocundo* vivere: il *Libreto di tutte le cosse che se magnano*', in C. Crisciani and G. Zuccolin (eds), *Michele Savonarola. Medicina e cultura di corte*. Florence: SISMEL-Galluzzo, 113–25.

Pelling, M. (1982), 'Food, status and knowledge: attitudes to diet in early modern England', in idem, *The Common Lot: Sickness, Medical Occupations and the Urban Poor in Early Modern England*. London and New York: Longman, 38–62.

Pennell, S. (1998), 'Pots and pans history: the material culture of the kitchen in early modern England'. *Journal of Design History*, 11:3, 201–16.

Pilloud, S. (2013), *Les mots du corps. Expérience de la maladie dans les lettres de patients à un médecin du 18e siècle: Samuel Auguste Tissot*. Lausanne: BHMS.

Bibliography

Pinkard, S. (2009), *A Revolution in Taste: The Rise of French Cuisine*. Cambridge: Cambridge University Press.

Pleij, H. (2001), *Dreaming of Cockaigne: Medieval Fantasies of the Perfect Life*, Trans. D. Webb. New York, NY: Columbia University Press.

Plunian, G. (forthcoming), 'L'alimentation du "Sauvage" dans les récits de voyage français. Perceptions et évolutions du regard sur la Nouvelle-France (1603–1704)', *Food & History*.

Ponsonby, A. (1923), *English Diaries: A Review of English Diaries from the Sixteenth to the Twentieth Century*. London: Methuen.

Porter, R. (1985), 'The drinking man's disease: the "pre-history" of alcoholism in Georgian Britain'. *British Journal of Addiction*, 80:4, 385–96.

Porter, R. (1985), 'Laymen, doctors and medical knowledge in the eighteenth century: the evidence of the *Gentlemen's Magazine*', in R. Porter (ed), *Patients and Practitioners: Lay Perceptions of Medicine in Pre-Industrial Society*. Cambridge: Cambridge University Press, 283–314.

Pospiech, A. (1997), 'Il ritmo annuale dell'alimentazione nella società tradizionale dell'Europa centrale: i piaceri della mensa', in S. Cavaciocchi (ed), *Alimentazione e nutrizione, secc. XIII–XVIII: atti della ventottesima settimana di studi*. Florence: Le Monnier, 217–30.

Proctor, R. (2008), 'Agnotology: a missing term to describe the cultural production of ignorance (and its study)', in R. Proctor and L. Schiebinger (eds), *Agnotology: The Making and Unmaking of Ignorance*. Stanford, CA: Stanford University Press, 1–33.

Prosperi, L. (2007), 'Le pouvoir de la nourriture sur la reproduction humaine: discours diététique et différences de genre d'après l'ouvrage de Giovanni Marinello (Italie-France, XVIe et XVIIe siècles)', in F. Audoin-Rouzeau and F. Sabban (eds), *Un aliment sain dans un corps sain: perspectives historiques*. Tours: Presses Universitaires François Rabelais, 291–307.

Quellier, F. (2007), 'Les fruits, le *Thrésor de santé* de la France classique (XVIIe–XVIIIe siècles)', in F. Audoin-Rouzeau and F. Sabban (eds), *Un aliment sain dans un corps sain: perspectives historiques*. Tours: Presses Universitaires François Rabelais, 185–98.

Quellier, F. (2008), 'Le repas de funéilles de Bonhomme Jacques. Faut-il reconsidér le dossier de l'alimentation paysanne des temps modernes?', *Food & History*, 6:1, 9–30.

Quellier, F. (2013), *La table des Français: une histoire culturelle (XVe–XIXe siècle)*. Rennes and Tours: Presses Universitaires de Rennes and Presses Universitaires François Rabelais.

Radeff, A. (1996), *Du café dans le chaudron. Économie globale d'ancien régime: Suisse Occidentale, Franche-Compté et Savoie*. Lausanne: Société d'Histoire de la Suisse Romande.

Rankin, A. (2013), *Panaceia's Daughter: Noblewomen as Healers in Early Modern Germany*. Chicago, IL: University of Chicago Press.

Reader, J. (2008), *Propitious Esculent: the Potato in World History*. London: Heinemann.

Renan, L. (2009), 'Les bienfaits controversés du régime maigre: le *Traité des dispenses du carême* de Philippe Hecquet et sa réception (1709–1714)'. *Dix-huitième siècle*, 41:1, 409–30.

Revel, J. (1975), 'Les privilèges d'une capitale: l'approvisionnement de Rome à l'époque moderne'. *Mélanges de l'École française de Rome. Moyen-Age, Temps modernes*, 87:2, 461–93. A short version of the article, without the tables and most of the notes, can be found in: R. Forster and O. Ranum (eds), *Food and Drink in History: Selections from the Annales*. Baltimore, MD: Johns Hopkins University Press, 37–49.

Rhodes, D. (1968), *La vita e le opere di Castore Durante e della sua famiglia*. Viterbo: Agnesotti.

Sabban, F. and Serventi, S. (1996), *A tavola nel Rinascimento: con 90 ricette della cucina italiana*. Rome: Laterza.

Sada, L. (1987), 'L'arte culinaria barese al celebre banchetto nuziale di Bona Sforza nel 1517', in B. Bilinski (ed), *La regina Bona Sforza tra Puglia e Polonia*. Warsaw: Ossolineum, 1987), 41–61.

Salaman, R. (2000), *The Social History of the Potato*. Cambridge: Cambridge University Press.

Saldarriaga, G. (2011), *Alimentación e identidades en el Nuevo Reino de Granada, siglos XVI y XVII*. Bogotá: Editorial Universidad del Rosario.

Sboarina, F. (2000), *Il lessico medico nel* Dioscoride *di Pietro Antionio Mattioli*. Frankfurt: Peter Lang.

Schaechter, E. (1997), *In the Company of Mushrooms: A Biologist's Tale*. Cambridge, MA: Harvard University Press.

Schäfer, D. (2011), *Old Age and Disease in Early Modern Medicine*. London: Pickering and Chatto.

Scheurer, R. (1985), 'Passage, accueil et intégration des réfugiés huguenots en Suisse', in M. Magdelaine and R. van Thadden (eds), *Le refuge huguenot*. Paris: Armand Colin, 45–62.

Schiebinger, L. (2004), *Plants and Empire: Colonial Bioprospecting in the Atlantic World*. Cambridge, MA: Harvard University Press.

Schiebinger, L. (2008), 'West Indian Abortifacients and the Making of Ignorance', in R. Proctor and L. Schiebinger (eds), *Agnotology: The Making and Unmaking of Ignorance*. Stanford, CA: Stanford University Press, 149–62.

Schorger, A. W. (1966), *The Wild Turkey: Its History and Domestication*. Norman, OK: University of Oklahoma Press.

Shapin, S. (2003), 'How to eat like a gentleman: dietetics and ethics in early modern England', in C. Rosenberg (ed), *Right Living: An Anglo-American Tradition of Self-Help Medicine and Hygiene*. Baltimore, MD: Johns Hopkins University Press, 21–58.

Shapin, S. (2003), 'Trusting George Cheyne: scientific expertise, common sense, and moral authority in early eighteenth-century dietetic medicine'. *Bulletin of the History of Medicine*, 77, 263–97.

Sigerist, H. (1956), *Landmarks in the History of Hygiene*. Oxford: Oxford University Press.

Siraisi, N. (1997), *The Clock and the Mirror: Girolamo Cardano and Renaissance Medicine*. Princeton, NJ: Princeton University Press.

Simon-Muscheid, K. (2007), 'Des vertus de l'eau-de-vie à l'excess de l'alcool (Allemagne/Alsace, XIIIe–XVIe siècles)', in F. Audoin-Rouzeau and F. Sabban (eds), *Un aliment sain dans un corps sain: Perspectives historiques*. Tours: Presses Universitaires François Rabelais, 175–84.

Slack, P. (1979), 'Mirrors of health and treasures of poor men: the uses of the vernacular medical literature of Tudor England', in C. Webster (ed), *Health, Medicine and Mortality in the Sixteenth Century*. Cambridge: Cambridge University Press, 237–73.

Smith, G. (1985), 'Prescribing the rules of health: self-help and advice in the late eighteenth century', in R. Porter (ed), *Patients and Practitioners: Lay Perceptions of Medicine in Pre-Industrial Society*. Cambridge: Cambridge University Press, 249–82.

Solomon, M. (2010), *Fictions of Well-Being: Sickly Readers and Vernacular Medical Writing in Late Medieval and Early Modern Spain*. Philadelphia, PA: University of Pennsylvania Press.

Sorcinelli, P. (1998), *Storia sociale dell'acqua: riti e culture*. Milan: Bruno Mondadori.

Spary, E. M. (2012), *Eating the Enlightenment: Food and the Sciences in Paris, 1670–1760*. Chicago, IL: University of Chicago Press.

Spencer, C. (1993), *The Heretic's Feast: A History of Vegetarianism*. London: Fourth Estate.

Stannard, J. (1969), 'P. A. Mattioli: sixteenth century commentator on Dioscorides'. *Bibliographical Contributions*, 1, 59–81.

Stolberg, M. (2011), *Experiencing Illness and the Sick Body in Early Modern Europe*. Trans. L. Unglaub and L. Kennedy. London: Palgrave Macmillan.

Suhr, C. (2010), 'Regimens and health guides', in I. Taavitsainen and P. Pahta (eds), *Early Modern English Medical Texts: Corpus Description and Studies*. Amsterdam and Philadelphia: John Benjamins, 111–18.

Szlatky, M. (1992), 'Tissot as part of the medical Enlightenment in Hungary', in R. Porter (ed), *Patients and Practitioners: Lay Perceptions of Medicine in Pre-Industrial Society*. Cambridge: Cambridge University Press, 194–214.

Bibliography

Thirsk, J. (1997), *Alternative Agriculture: A History*. Oxford: Oxford University Press.

Thomas, D. (1996), *Henri IV: images d'un roi entre réalité et mythe*. Pau: Heracles.

Thomas, K. (1983), *Man and the Natural World: Changing Attitudes in England, 1500–1800*. London: Allen Lane.

Toaff, A. (2000), *Mangiare alla giudia: la cucina ebraica in Italia dal Rinascimento all'età moderna*. Bologna: il Mulino.

Topolski, J. (1997), 'Religious fasting as a kind of the food taboo in Poland in the 16th–17th centuries', in S. Cavaciocchi (ed), *Alimentazione e nutrizione, secc. XIII–XVIII*. Prato: Istituto Datini, 555–68.

Toussaint-Samat, M. (1992), *A History of Food*. Trans. A. Bell. Oxford: Blackwell.

Turner, B. (1982), 'The discourse of diet'. *Theory, Culture and Society*, 1:1, 23–32.

Turner, B. (1982), 'The government of the body: medical regimens and the rationalization of diet'. *The British Journal of Sociology*, 33:2, 254–69.

Turrini, M. (2006), *Il 'giovin signore' in Collegio. I Gesuiti e l'educazione della nobiltà nelle consuetudini del Collegio ducale di Parma*. Bologna: CLUEB.

Tyrkkö, J. (2010), 'Sign terms in specific medical genres in early modern medical texts', in I. Taavitsainen and P. Pahta (eds), *Early Modern English Medical Texts: Corpus Description and Studies*. Amsterdam and Philadelphia: John Benjamins, 167–89.

Unger, R. (2004), *Beer in the Middle Ages and the Renaissance*. Philadelphia, PA: University of Pennsylvania Press.

Van Bavel, B. and Gelderblom, O. (2009), 'Land of milk and butter: the economic origins of cleanliness in the Dutch golden age'. *Past and Present*, 205, 41–69.

Vigarello, G. (1993), *Le sain et le malsain. Santé et mieux-être depuis le Moyen Age*. Paris: Seuil.

Von Hoffmann, V. (2013), *Goûter le monde. Une histoire culturelle du goût à l'époque moderne*. Bruxelles: Peter Lang.

Walker Bynum, C. (1987), *Holy Feast and Holy Fast: The Religious Significance of Food to Medieval Women*. Berkeley, CA: University of California Press.

Wallace, C. (2003), 'Eating and drinking with John Wesley: the logic of his practice'. *Bulletin of the John Rylands University Library of Manchester*, 85:2, 137–55.

Walsh, M. and S. Kuhn (2012), 'Developments in personalised nutrition', *Nutrition Bulletin*, 37:4, 380–3.

Warman, A. (2003), *Corn and Capitalism: How a Botanical Bastard Grew to Global Dominance*. Trans. N. Westrate. Chapel Hill, NC: University of North Carolina Press.

Watts, S. (2013), 'Enlightened fasting: religious conviction, scientific inquiry, and medical knowledge in early modern France', in K. Albala and T. Eden (eds), *Food and Faith in Christian Culture*. New York, NY: Columbia University Press, 105–23.

Wear, A. (1992), editor's introduction, in A. Wear (ed), *Medicine in Society: Historical Essays*. Cambridge: Cambridge University Press.

Wear, A. (2000), *Knowledge and Practice in English Medicine, 1550–1680*. Cambridge: Cambridge University Press.

Weston, R. (2013), *Medical Consulting by Letter in France, 1665–1789*. Farnham: Ashgate.

Willard, T. (2011), 'Living the long life: physical and spiritual health in two early Paracelsian tracts', in A. Classen (ed), *Religion und Gesundheit: der heilkundliche Diskurs im 16.Jahrhundert*. Berlin: de Gruyter, 347–80.

Zuccolin, G. (2011), 'Nascere in latino e in volgare. Tra la *Practica maior* e il *De regimine pregnantium*', in C. Crisciani and G. Zuccolin (eds), *Michele Savonarola. Medicina e cultura di corte*. Florence: SISMEL-Galluzzo, 137–209.

Zuckerman, L. (1998), *The Potato: How the Humble Spud Rescued the Western World*. New York, NY: North Point Press.

Unpublished PhD Theses

Moyer, J. (1997), *Sumptuary Law in Ancien Regime France, 1229–1806*, University of Syracuse, NY.

Williams, J. (2013), *Flesh and Faith: Meat-Eating and Religious Identities in Late Medieval and Early Modern Valencia*, Department of Historical Studies, University of Bristol.

Woodburn, R. (1975), *Proverbs in Health Books of the English Renaissance*, Texas Tech University, TX. Available online at: http://repositories.tdl.org.

INDEX

Note: Locators followed by the letter 'n' refer to notes

Index

Chen, Nancy 2
chestnuts 59, 60, 64, 65, 150, 153
Cheyne, George 3, 27, 29, 38, 40, 41, 47, 85, 90, 92,
    113, 129, 143–4, 153, 160, 168, 172, 179
chicken 7, 17, 20, 55, 57, 65
chick peas 61, 87
chicory 117, 121
Chigi, Agostino 144
chilli peppers 20, 68, 116, 134, 135, 138–40,
    155, 172
chocolate 110, 136, 147, 172–5, 179–80
    as food 157
Cholmley, Richard 52
Christian VII 72
Christmas 96
    Twelve Days of 49
chronicles, as source 133–4
cider 15, 83, 157, 166–7, 181
cinnamon 26, 69, 71, 89, 109, 162
circumcision 108
Cisneros, Diego 84
Claflin, Kyri 2
class 55, 76, 124, 148
climate 77, 85, 86, 89, 90, 91, 93, 177, 182
cloves 69, 71
clubs, private 180
Cocchi, Antonio 129–30
Cockaigne, Land of 66
cod 69, 97, 112, 127
coffee 45, 69, 162, 168, 175–80
    as antidote to drink 158, 172
coffee-houses 172, 175, 176, 178, 180
Cogan, Thomas 18, 63, 64, 86, 167
Coles, William 118
colewort 125
    see also cabbage
College of Physicians (London) 27
Collegio dei Nobili (Parma) 112
Collegio Romano (Rome) 103
Colmenero de Ledesma, Antonio 172–3
colour 68
Columbian exchange 64, 134, 155
Columbus, Christopher 75, 82, 133
Comédie Française 176
Comédie Italienne 177
complexion, bodily 5, 15–16, 17, 20, 51, 84, 107,
    116, 124, 163
concoction 19, 33, 39, 104, 119, 125, 139, 163
    see also digestion
condiments 19–20, 47, 136, 140, 154
Connecticut 146, 169
constipation 40, 89
constitution
    bodily 15, 24, 37, 44, 55, 59, 63, 82, 91, 103
    political 77

consumption
    compared to dietary advice 116–20
    meat 51–2, 57, 58
conversation 70
cookery 29, 73, 165, 181
    books 83, 100, 140, 142
    and medicine 18–22, 46–8
Cornaro, Alvise 6, 22, 27, 37, 42, 113, 124, 125, 126,
    159, 164
Corrado, Vincenzo 47, 131, 144
Cosimo III 174
courgettes (zucchini) 121
courts
    princely 9–10, 18, 21, 48, 87, 119, 131, 183
    royal 52, 53, 70, 103
Cowan, Brian 177
Crab, Roger 125–6
Crakow 122
cream 71, 72
Croce, Giulio Cesare 61
crocus 141
Cromwell, Thomas 80–1
Crosby, Allen 134
Cuba 88
cucumbers 15, 20, 35, 115, 128
cumin 109
curiosity 136
curriculum, medical 30
custom, role of 88
Cutò, Francesco Procopio 176

da Fonseca, Francisco 46
d'Albret, Jeanne 142
Dallington, Robert 117
Dapper, Olfert 89
darnel 61
da Udine, Giovanni 144
d'Aulnoy, Madame 72, 147
Dauphiné 62
Davis, William 6
Davy du Perron, Jacques 142
de Acosta, José 110, 139, 172
de Aviñon, Juan 135
de Azara, Félix 59
de Bonnefons, Nicolas 47, 70, 72, 107, 120, 122,
    128, 142
de Cárdenas, Juan 84, 145–6, 173
de Cervantes, Miguel 9, 87
de Champlain, Samuel 149
de Durfort, Aymeric Joseph 72
de Gouberville, Gilles 25, 57
de Langle, marquis 140
de la Roque, Pierre 175
de La Salle, Jean-Baptiste 103–4
de la Ville Gille, Madame 177

Index

Index

Index